Managing your patients' data in the neonatal and pediatric ICU

An introduction to databases and statistical analysis

Managing your patients' data in the neonatal and pediatric ICU

An introduction to databases and statistical analysis

**Includes eNICU software
for the neonatal intensive care unit,
which may be modified for
local use or other clinical settings**

Joseph Schulman M.D., M.S.
Division of Newborn Medicine
Weill Medical College of Cornell University
New York-Presbyterian Hospital
New York, New York 10021

BMJ
Books

Blackwell
Publishing

© 2006 J. Schulman
Published by Blackwell Publishing Ltd
BMJ Books is an imprint of the BMJ Publishing Group Limited, used under licence

Blackwell Publishing, Inc., 350 Main Street, Malden, Massachusetts 02148-5020, USA
Blackwell Publishing Ltd, 9600 Garsington Road, Oxford OX4 2DQ, UK
Blackwell Publishing Asia Pty Ltd, 550 Swanston Street, Carlton, Victoria 3053, Australia

First published 2006

1   2006

Library of Congress Cataloging-in-Publication Data

Schulman, Joseph, 1950–
    Managing your patients' data in the neonatal and pediatric ICU : an introduction to
databases and statistical analysis / Joseph Schulman.
        p. ; cm.
    "Includes eNICU software for the neonatal intensive care unit, which may be
modified for local use or other clinical settings."
    Includes bibliographical references.
    ISBN-13: 978-0-7279-1870-3 (pbk.)
    ISBN-10: 0-7279-1870-2 (pbk.)
    1. Neonatology—Databases.   2. Neonatology—Statistical methods.   3. Medical
records—Data processing.   I. Title.
    [DNLM: 1. Database Management Systems—Infant, Newborn.   2. Medical
Records—Infant, Newborn.   3. Models, Statistical.   4. Neonatology—methods.   WS
26.5 S386m 2006]
    BI253 S375 2006.

ISBN-13: 978-0-727918-70-3
ISBN-10: 0-727918-70-2

A catalogue record for this title is available from the British Library

Set in Meridien 9.5/12 by TechBooks, New Delhi, India
Printed and bound by Replika Press Pvt Ltd, Harayana, India

Commissioning Editor: Mary Banks
Development Editor: Veronica Pock
Production Controller: Debbie Wyer

For further information on Blackwell Publishing, visit our website:
http://www.blackwellpublishing.com

The publisher's policy is to use permanent paper from mills that operate a sustainable
forestry policy, and which has been manufactured from pulp processed using acid-free
and elementary chlorine-free practices. Furthermore, the publisher ensures that the text
paper and cover board used have met acceptable environmental accreditation standards.

Contents

"Microsoft, Access, SQL Server, and Windows are either registered trademarks or trademarks of Microsoft Corporation in the United States and/or other countries."

A man must carry knowledge with him,
if he would bring home knowledge.
Samuel Johnson

eNICU installation and administration instructions

This folder contains an assortment of documents about a wide variety of eNICU-related topics not essential to the central narrative of the book, but essential to using the eNICU software itself. Most file content will seem arcane until you install eNICU and begin to configure it to serve your particular needs. Therefore, begin by following the installation instructions provided in the file, "BEGIN HERE_automated installation." Braver souls who desire to understand more of what goes on "backstage" can tackle installation via the instructions in the file, "BEGIN HERE_do it yourself" (or at least read what's in the file). Many of the procedures specified in that file are described in detail in other eNICU Operational Details files bearing corresponding names. Defer this do-it-yourself experience until you feel rather knowledgeable about eNICU software overall. Only as a last resort in the event of difficulty installing eNICU by either of these two approaches, the file "If neither set of BEGIN HERE instructions work" provides a work-around. This is not to suggest that the automated installation will be problematic. In fact, the intent mainly is to provide further insight to the application's structure.

A few eNICU lookup lists contain choices suitable only to the setting in which the software was developed. Lookup lists of physician and hospital names are two examples. Although site-specific lookup lists could have been provided as empty files for users to populate, the provided choices may help guide the user in populating them with the locally relevant choices. Instructions for working with these lookup lists may be found within the book as well as in the Pendragon Forms manual.

Please explore all the files and do not worry if any seem irrelevant at first. As you make progress configuring the software to suit your needs, the role of each file in guiding you or expanding your understanding of the application will become increasingly clear.

Acknowledgments

To compile diverse, complicated information into a book that adds to readers' knowledge requires protracted time and lots of interacting with good people. I wish to express my gratitude publicly to several good people who helped me with this project.

Before EMR – electronic medical records – became a buzzword, Michael J. Horgan, M.D. and David A. Clark, M.D., of the Albany Medical College, understood that a prerequisite for implementing an EMR was to understand explicitly the fine structure of the daily clinical work and how to track its associated data. They provided the academic environment that enabled me to write this book and software.

Mary Banks, my publisher, championed this companion volume to my first project for BMJ Books: *Evaluating the Processes of Neonatal Intensive Care*. And with great insight, Mary appreciated the sense of combining in one place material traditionally considered to belong to at least two distinct disciplines.

I am indebted to Andrew G. James, M.B., of the University of Toronto and The Hospital for Sick Children, and Robert Reitter, M.A., President, Guideline Legal Division, Find Market Research. They carefully read the manuscript and provided much constructive advice that made the book clearer and more practical.

I am so fortunate to belong to a close and supportive family. Ahead of the refinement brought about by my colleagues and friends, my daughter, Sara Schulman Brass, and my son, Joshua Schulman, worked magic on the manuscript. Sara, a public health consultant, and Joshua, a student at Harvard Medical School, are both highly accomplished authors. Where you may find clarity, coherence, even grace, they have had a part. As I endeavored to make my story compelling for readers outside my own area of clinical practice and to guard against excessive abstraction, I kept in mind both Joshua and my new son, Steven Brass, a neurologist at the Massachusetts General Hospital. Their encouragement helped persuade me that this book would be welcomed by a wide range of readers. And of course, my deepest enablers are my parents, Ben and Rose, and my wife, Janis.

CHAPTER 1
Introduction

Good patient care, at all levels, depends upon competently managing and analyzing patient data. Good patient care also depends on understanding the determinants of desirable outcomes and on applying dependable criteria for evaluating care. To identify these determinants and criteria we must explicitly connect the data about our patients and what we do to them with the data about how things turn out. That is what this book is about.

We commonly believe that because we work hard and care deeply about what we do, we must be doing a good job.[1] Rarely do outcomes data support this relationship. Although one may have years of experience in these areas, experience does not reliably enhance competence.[2–5] For experience to inform future action, we must reflect on all that has happened, not just what was most memorable; we must give proper weight to each observation; and we must discern how some observations relate to others.

We may manage and analyze patient data at multiple levels. At the individual level, we work with the data to formulate a patient's problems and plan of care. At the group level, we work with the data to determine how well our system of care serves our patients. Together, the data from these two levels can largely describe our work. However, in actuality, we seldom achieve such comprehensive description of our work and we have few dependable criteria by which to evaluate it.

School-age children ask the riddle: "Why do you always find things in the last place you'd think to look for them?" The answer, of course, is "Because that's when you stop looking." Our daily work is too complicated and demanding to accept having to rummage through a patient chart, with little idea of exactly where to find the information we seek. A central aim of patient information management is to ensure that you get the information you need in the first place you look. But this may require profound advances in how an organization's members collect, manage, and interpret data; how they learn from their experience; and how they share the learning among all who can benefit.

Many of us work in organizations that continue in some degree to rely on handwritten records – a technology essentially unchanged for about 100 years. What has changed is the amount of information and processing activity such records reflect. It is now vast. Of course, we have tools to help, but commonly these are mismatched to the complexity of the problems we tackle.

This book aims at this mismatch of problems with tools. Part I introduces you to getting your arms around data: designing, implementing, and administering an electronic database of patient information. Part II introduces you to asking questions of data, obtaining well-founded answers, and making sense of those answers.

The subject matter is complex. I have strived to present it simply and clearly, mindful of Albert Einstein's observation: "You do not really understand something unless you can explain it to your grandmother." Even so, I encourage you to read this book unhurriedly and be sure every idea is clear before you move on. Ahead lays new competence to manage the ever-growing amount of information you must handle and new ways to interpret what you see.

When the only tool you have is a hammer, everything looks like a nail

ABRAHAM MASLOW

I think we clinicians often succumb to the vast amount of complex information in our daily work by changing our perception of reality or by not letting it all in. We formulate simplified versions of complicated situations, confident that we have included the essence of the problem (see Ch. 30 in Ref. 6; and Ch. 4, especially p. 87, in Ref. 7). In making a complex medical decision we may need to process in our heads more information than we can handle.[8] Perhaps for this reason, we apply to this vast amount of information decision-making methods that are often tacit (see p. 28 in Ref. 9). Of course, the resulting knowledge is tacit too.[9] Applying such imprecise methods as we do, is it any wonder that our care and documentation vary widely?[10,11] Some claim this variation is integral to the "art of medicine," a notion traditionally thought to embody the wisdom of experience. I think Eddy counters best: "When different physicians are recommending different things for essentially the same patients, it is impossible to claim that they are all doing the right thing."[8]

Here's the point. By our traditional information processing methods, we can't account for all important determinants of the outcomes we observe, nor do we have a sound basis to determine exactly which outcomes we ought to observe. We poorly understand the quantitative dimension of our work. We cannot accurately account for all the relevant evidence. The ever-growing demands of processing information in our heads are overwhelming. We are in trouble.

This information overload was recognized to some extent long ago when paper-based information systems were set up. But a paper-based system is inadequate.[12,13] To recall a lab value or remember to check on an X-ray, we may jot the information down on an index card or on the back of an envelope. Even better, so we don't lose it, we might write it on the leg of our scrub pants. A computer-based information system is potentially far better.

A computer is a wonderful tool to keep track of more things than we can in our heads. But most computers and the programs they run are not designed to handle tacit knowledge and implicit processes. If we are to benefit from the things computers can do enormously better than humans can, we must think *explicitly* about clinical data elements. This entails articulating precise methods for collecting, managing, and analyzing this data – methods quite different from traditional, paper-based, tacit approaches. Few clinicians are solidly trained in these skills.[14] It's understandable, therefore, that when many clinicians imagine a computer managing their patient information, they imagine the computer doing it the same way the clinicians have always done it, but just faster and with less direct clinician involvement. But to "computerize" patient information management, that is, to represent and conduct our daily work with the aid of a computer, *we must change the way we typically think and work*. To represent our work in a computer we must precisely specify as many essential details about our work as possible. And to conduct our work we must understand the structural relationships among the data elements.

Changing the way we think and work can be enormously disruptive, affecting workflow, and framing what we perceive. For the same reason, it can be positively transformative. Incorporating computer-aided information management processes in our daily work can enable us with capabilities we never before dreamed of. Computer-aided information management forces us to think about the fine structure of our work and our results, can help us make fewer errors (see Framework for Strategic Action, p. 2–3, in Ref. 15), and can help us understand quantitative dimensions of our work (see Ch. 30 in Ref. 6).

To understand quantitative dimensions of our work is to make sense of the enormous amounts of data generated by our work, both at the individual and the group level. It is to know explicitly why we collect each data element that we do, to know what might be different by knowing the value of each data element we collect. It is to progress from relying on what appears intuitively obvious to suspending judgment until results emerge from a carefully analyzed and interpreted body of data. And it is to connect that body of data to other established knowledge. The key tools for making sense of our data are database software and statistical software.

Database software facilitates collecting data, but it only provides data to admire. Statistical software facilitates interpreting aggregate data, but it does not do the interpreting, it only entails computing. Reasoning from the data is something we still must do in our heads. This book explains how to collect data worth admiring and explains powerful methods to analyze that data. The book also explains interpretive reasoning from the analytic results. Because I am a neonatologist, I shall illustrate concepts using data sets from neonatal situations. I assure you, the exposition is nonetheless ecumenical.

Part I of this book is about data management. Section I frames the problems of managing health care data. Section II describes how to plan solutions. Sections III and IV describe how to implement the plan, largely illustrated by the actual patient information management solution that I developed and use daily: eNICU. The eNICU software is on the CD accompanying this book.

What you learn here about database theory, software implementation, and administration should enable you to

- appreciate how these things contribute to managing patient information.
- recognize, understand, and interact productively with the database interfaces you increasingly encounter in your daily work.

- use and modify the accompanying eNICU software to support your daily clinical work and evaluation activities.
- recognize the boundaries of your new knowledge and select appropriate further reading material.

If you worry that the software platforms or the hardware that anchor the exposition will become outdated, then don't. They will – as will any other tool you use to manage data. My focus is on illustrating essential concepts that I expect will remain relevant to future software and hardware.

You may question why you need to know about database theory, software implementation, and administration at all, particularly if you plan to invest in a ready-to-use electronic medical record (EMR) product. Well, if that is your plan, then that is precisely why you should learn about these things. You must evaluate the EMR model and implementation – not just its bells and whistles. You must understand why a well-designed database product will nonetheless disappoint you if it is not properly administered. And because others use some of our data, you must understand how to share it.

Part II of this book is about why, and how, you must review collected data to learn accurately from clinical and investigational experience. The patterns in data and the connections among factors contributing to an outcome may be obscure and may surface only after carefully planned analysis. Intuitively "obvious" associations may fade in the light of careful analysis. Part II is also about how to formulate questions that pilot these activities. Some questions, better than others, point the way toward informative analysis and interpretation. Moreover, it is largely by explicitly formulating the questions you seek to answer that you determine the data you really need to collect. And that is the reason for combining in a single book the topics typically covered by two.

What you learn here about data analysis and interpretation should enable you to

- develop genuine analytical competence.
- clearly identify the boundaries of your new skills.
- add coherence and functionality to what you already know – though previous biostatistics coursework is not a prerequisite to master the material presented here.

To develop competence in managing and analyzing vast amounts of data, you must work with database and statistical software. Following are the software applications you'll need in conjunction with your reading:

- Microsoft® Access 2002 or 2003 (Part of Microsoft® Office XP or 2003 Professional).
- Pendragon Forms 4.0 or 5.0: by installing eNICU, provided on the CD at the back of this book, you activate a complementary 2-week trial version of Pendragon Forms. Version 5.0 operates on both Palm OS® and Microsoft® Windows Mobile 2003™ devices.
- Stata[16] (preferably Version 8 or 9; many graphics commands have changed from earlier versions and earlier versions cannot retrieve data directly from a database).

Before we move on to Part I, let's make sure we share a common understanding of key terms.

- *Database*: A collection of data. Surprisingly simple? The term does not necessarily imply computers or software program applications. The card catalog that is now disappearing from libraries is an example of a useful, low-tech database. Computerized, high-tech databases aren't just faster versions of low-tech databases; they usually reflect more sophisticated design principles than the traditional, low-tech databases. Computerized databases can also be connected to each other to achieve search results undreamed of with older technology.
- *Data management*: Meaning depends on context.
  - **(i)** As a clinical process, it refers to the overarching process that begins with planning which data to collect, collecting them, manipulating the data, interpreting them, and reporting both data and interpretation in a specified way.
  - **(ii)** As a database software process, it refers to the software features that control and manipulate the data that reside in the database.
- *Database management system (DBMS)*: A software application that manages data in a database. The DBMS is the means by which you can add, delete, and update data in a database. And it's the means by which you can configure the data in a myriad of ways for viewing or printing.
- *Table*: A container for holding data that share common attributes. Tables have rows (horizontal divisions) and columns (vertical divisions). Each column describes one attribute of whatever the table is intended to describe. Each row contains one instance of the table's attribute set, one observation of the thing the table describes. Each row is also called a record. Each column is also called a field. If you had a table for storing several attributes of your patients, each row would contain the information for one patient (one record), with each column recording the information for each attribute (field). In database jargon, a table is also called a relation.

  Even though you think of a table as a rectangular structure that's neatly subdivided and has data in each of those subdivisions, your computer doesn't. The table appears that way on the screen only because your computer is trying to relate to people. Your computer actually stores the data as magnetic charges distributed not so uniformly on the computer disk. This gives the computer and DBMS software lots of flexibility to manipulate and represent the data in tables.
- *Form*: A way to interface with the data in the database tables without direct risk to the base tables. If you have provided information to a page displayed by an Internet browser, then you have probably worked with a database form. The data you entered in the form went to one or more tables in the website's database.
- *Query*: A question you ask of a database. You ask the question operationally, providing a set of instructions for finding a subset of the data in the database.
- *Report*: Specifically designed printed output of a requested subset of data.

- *Relationship*: The logical connection between information in one table (relation) with the information in another table (relation). When one record in table A can relate to only one record in table B, that's a one-to-one relationship. Thus, each patient can have only one set of admission vital signs because a second set would no longer describe the condition at admission. When one record in table A can relate to many records in table B, that's a one-to-many relationship. One mother, for example, can have more than one infant.
- *Primary key*: One or more fields uniquely identifying each record in a table. That is, for each record, the value entered in the primary key field(s) is unique among all records in the table. Without a primary key, records in a database may become confused and the database content degraded.
- *Foreign key*: A good way to link a record in one table with a record in another table is for each record to share some common attribute value. Thus, if we wish to connect a particular record in a table of infant data with a particular record in another table of maternal data, we would ensure the infant data table includes a field containing the mother's unique identifier – primary key value. Such a linking field is called a foreign key. The linked records together describe one instance of a higher entity, the mother/infant dyad in our example, constituted by the various tables in aggregate.
- *Normalization*: A set of design rules specifying what each of the multiple tables in a database is about, and the attributes that belong with each table. These rules generally optimize data storage and retrieval by anticipating the things you'll want to do with the data, and ensuring you'll be able to carry them out. Normalization thus enables reliable queries.

If you want to work with the software straight away

Readers desiring to connect from the outset what they see on the pages of Part 1 with what they see on the PC or PDA screen may look ahead to Chapters 9, 11, 13, 17, and 14 – in that order – and then install eNICU from the accompanying CD. Be mindful, however: simply *owning* a specialized tool does not necessarily make you an expert *user*. To gain a coherent understanding of eNICU and database technology, return here to study the chapters in numerical (and logical) sequence – you will discover anew those to which you looked ahead.

Part I
Managing data
and routine reporting

A few observations and much reasoning lead to error;
many observations and a little reasoning to truth

Alexis Carrel

SECTION 1
The process of managing clinical data

CHAPTER 2
Paper-based patient records

Patient information systems have been mainly paper-based, but this is now changing. A paper-based system means we use paper media to store and manage data. Computer-based patient information systems may still produce paper chart notes, but the base data are stored and managed using electronic media, not paper.

I've heard the paper-based medical record being referred to as a WORN system: Write Once, Read Never. Specific limitations of paper-based records[16]:

- Paper charts facilitate data entry, but not retrieval.
- Paper charts are rarely indexed; it can take a long time to find what you're looking for.
- Often, the job to maintain the patient chart before it goes to the medical records department is specified, but the person to carry it out is not. The same may apply to checking to make sure the job is properly executed. As a result, the way work is represented in charts actually produced in such systems may be quite different from what we espouse is represented in a paper-based system.
- Criteria for completeness may be implicit or may not exist at all. The consequence is similar to the previous point.
- Handwriting is often illegible.
- Data you'd like to compare are often separated in the record. Consequently, intervals and patterns in data are obscure. Graphical displays are almost nonexistent.
- Context information that helps you interpret data may not be available when you need it. Data without interpretative context may be considered meaningless information, a notion we examine in Chapter 5.

How do we know our paper-based notes are good?

Two real examples from my own work setting are shown in Figs. 2.1 and 2.2. I have censored the patient identifiers. Do the tools in Figs. 2.1 and 2.2 succeed? This is an unanswerable question in many work settings because the

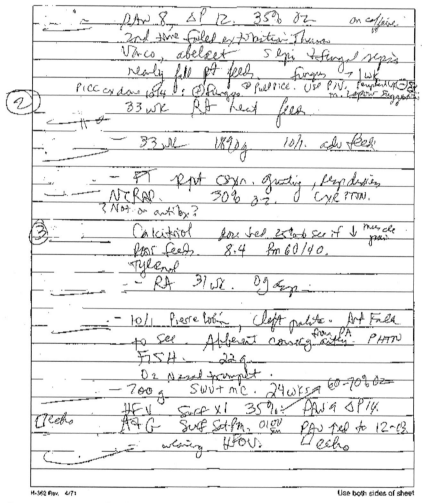

Figure 2.1 An example of a paper-based patient information product.

criteria of "success" are neither explicit nor shared. What *should* each tool achieve? Perhaps you think the answers are self-evident: in your experience, using similar methods, things have functioned quite well, thank you. To prepare for material presented in succeeding chapters, write down your current patient information system aims. Not the ones that sound admirable and lofty, but the ones that accurately describe reality; those that one might infer by

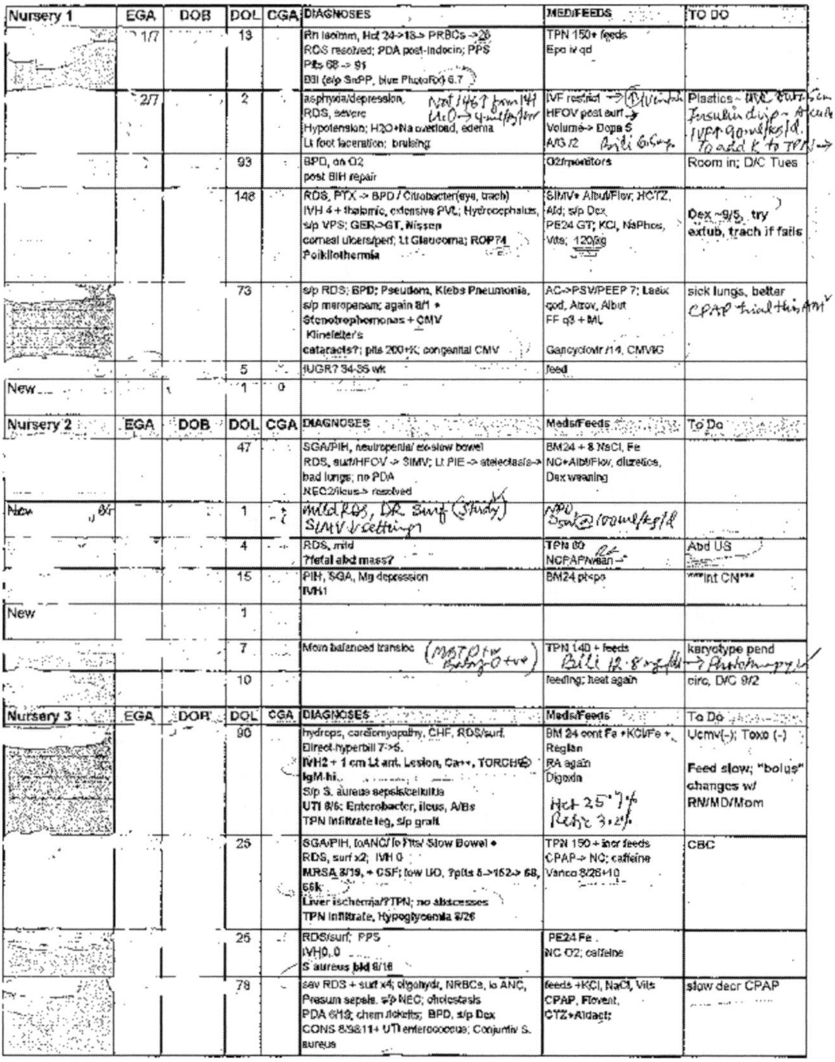

Nursery 1	EGA	DOB	DOL	CGA	DIAGNOSES	MED/FEEDS	TO DO
	1/7		13		Rh isoimm, Hct 24->18-> PRBCs ->26 ROS resolved; PDA post-Indocin; PPS Plts 68 -> 91 Bili (s/p SnPP, blue Photo) 6.7	TPN 150+ feeds Epo iv qd	
	2/7		2		asphyxia/depression, RDS, severe Hypotension; H2O+Na overload, edema Lt foot laceration; bruising	IVF restrict HFOV post surf Volume-> Dopa 5 A/B /2	Plastics
			93		BPD, on O2 post BIH repair	O2/monitors	Room in; D/C Tues
			148		RDS, PTX -> BPD / Citrobacter(eye, trach) IVH 4 + thalamic, extensive PVL; Hydrocephalus, s/p VPS; GER->GT, Nissen corneal ulcers/perf; Lt Glaucoma; ROP?4 Poikilothermia	SIMV+ Albut/Flov; HCTZ, Ald; s/p Dex PE24 GT; KCl, NaPhos, Vits; 120/kg	Dex ~9/5, try extub, trach if fails
			73		s/p RDS; BPD; Pseudom, Klebs Pneumonia, s/p meropenem; again 8/1 + Stenotrophomonas + CMV Klinefelter's cataracts?; plts 200+K; congenital CMV	AC->PSV/PEEP 7; Lasix qod, Atrov, Albut FF q3 + ML Gancyclovir /14, CMVIG	sick lungs, better
			5		IUGR? 34-35 wk	feed	
New			1	0			

Nursery 2	EGA	DOB	DOL	CGA	DIAGNOSES	Meds/Feeds	To Do
			47		SGA/PIH, neutropenia/ slow bowel RDS, surf/HFOV -> SIMV; Lt PIE -> atelectasis-> bad lungs; no PDA NEC2/ileus-> resolved	BM24 + 8 NaCl, Fe NC+Albt/Flov, diuretics, Dex weaning	
New			1				
			4		RDS, mild ?fetal abd mass?	TPN 80 NCPAP/wean	Abd US
			15		PIH, SGA, Mg depression IVH1	BM24 pt<po	***Int CN***
New			1				
			7		Mom balanced transloc	TPN 140 + feeds	karyotype pend
			10			feeding; heat again	circ, D/C 9/2

Nursery 3	EGA	DOB	DOL	CGA	DIAGNOSES	Meds/Feeds	To Do
			90		hydrops, cardiomyopathy, CHF, RDS/surf, Direct-hyperbili 7->5, IVH2 + 1 cm Lt ant. Lesion, Ca++, TORCH IgM-hi, S/p S. aureus sepsis/cellulitis UTI 8/6: Enterobacter, ileus, A/Bs TPN infiltrate leg, s/p graft	BM 24 cont Fe +KCl/Fe + Reglan RA again Digoxin	Ucmv(-); Toxo (-) Feed slow; "bolus" changes w/ RN/MD/Mom
			25		SGA/PIH, loANC/ lo Plts/ Slow Bowel + RDS, surf x2; IVH 0 MRSA 8/19, + CSF; low UO, ?plts 5->152-> 68, 66k Liver ischemia/?TPN; no abscesses TPN infiltrate, Hypoglycemia 8/26	TPN 150 + incr feeds CPAP-> NC; caffeine Vanco 8/26+10	CBC
			26		RDS/surf; PPS IVH0, 0 S aureus bld 8/16	PE24 Fe. NC O2; caffeine	
			78		sev RDS + surf x4; oligohydr, NRBCs, lo ANC, Presum sepsis. s/p NEC; cholestasis PDA 6/18; chem rickets; BPD, s/p Dex CONS 8/3&11+ UTI enterococcus; Conjunctiv S. aureus	feeds +KCl, NaCl, Vits CPAP, Flovent, CTZ+Aldact;	slow decr CPAP

Figure 2.1 (*Continued*).

MR	LastName	MotherID	Gender	IfMultGest	BirthDate	AdmitDate	ThisIsThe__AN	InfantID	FetalPresentation	DeliveryMode	AmnioticF	BirthWeight	AdmitWeight	HeadCirc	APGRA1
11121	Testpat1	02 12:26:31 PM	Male		9/4/2002	9/4/2002	1	111211	vertex	Spontaneous V	clear	2350	2350	32	6
112102	Testpat2	002 2:33:11 PM	Male		11/21/2002	11/21/2002	1	1121021		Spontaneous V	clear	3000	3000	35	9
123	Testpat3							1231							
123123	Testpat4	02 10:13:13 AM	Female		9/25/2002	9/25/2002	1	1231231	transverse	Caesarian	clear	1475	1475	30	6
1234567	Testpat5	002 9:51:10 AM	Male		11/19/2002	11/19/2002	1	12345671	transverse	Caesarian	clear	3456	3456	35	9

Figure 2.2 An example of a paper-based patient information product, produced using a computer.

observing your system operate. Have you ever given this careful thought? Might those aims be implicit, at best? You may believe you know what each component of your work should achieve, but try to explain these ideas to someone else and observe whether your explanation produces clear understanding, or confusion. The point is we need operational definitions of "good notes." We need to understand explicitly what our efforts are intended to achieve.

Patient information management that is not explicitly goal directed is problematic. Might paper be the root of the problem? I think it depends on how we *use* paper. What is problematic about paper is to use it to *base* an information management system that stores a large amount of data. As a *base* of a system, paper suffers from the limitations reviewed earlier. As a communication medium, paper continues to offer much usefulness. See Ref. 17 for a general discussion of this perspective.

At any time, work processes likely reflect adaptation to the current technology and objects. Therefore, a caveat: to introduce new technology and objects is to change work processes that evolved to use the displaced affordances (see Ch. 2 in Ref. 17). For many readers, we're about to enter new cognitive territory. If until now you've given little thought to the following considerations, by the end of the book expect to think differently about the information connected with your work, how you record it, and how you manage it. You shall gain appreciation of why managing patient information has engaged the serious attention of national governments[15–19]; why it matters *how* we think about representing, storing, and manipulating patient information – both to produce summary reports and to answer research and evaluative questions; why the design of our tools plays a crucial role in the results we can achieve; and why introducing new technology to a work process requires that each evolve interactively.[20–22]

CHAPTER 3
Computer-based patient records

Where are we going? How shall we get there?

The Institute of Medicine (IOM) articulated five objectives for future patient records and suggested how to achieve them[13]:

> First, future patient records should support patient care and improve its quality.
> Second, they should enhance the productivity of health care professionals and reduce the administrative costs associated with health care delivery and financing.
> Third, they should support clinical and health services research.
> Fourth, they should be able to accommodate future developments in health care technology, policy, management, and finance.
> Fifth, they must have mechanisms in place to ensure patient data confidentiality at all times.
> To achieve these objectives, future patient records must be computer based. However, merely automating the form, content, and procedures of current patient records will perpetuate their deficiencies and will be insufficient to meet emerging user needs. (Quoted from executive summary, p. 46)

In *Crossing the Quality Chasm*,[12] the Committee on Quality of Health Care in America found that

> health care delivery has been relatively untouched by the revolution in information technology . . . the growth in clinical knowledge and technology has been profound, [but] many health care settings lack basic computer systems to provide clinical information . . . The development and application of more sophisticated information systems is essential to enhance quality and improve efficiency. (p. 15)

The IOM believes that a "fully electronic medical record, including all types of patient information, is not needed to achieve many, if not most, of the benefits of automated clinical data" (see p. 16 in Ref. 12). It calls for "the elimination of most handwritten clinical data by the end of [this] decade" – a laudable goal and a daunting task.[23]

The term "electronic medical record" is not yet used uniformly. Stead *et al.* provide a helpful overview of key terms that describe subsets of the coming information infrastructure, terms that at present many use interchangeably.[24] They consider an electronic medical record (EMR) as a by-product of an electronic medical record *system* (EMRS). The latter automates order-entry, recording notes, scheduling, and billing. Thus framed, an EMR "lives within the specific EMRS that created it and is unique to that system."[24] Stead *et al.* consider an electronic health record (EHR) a broader concept: "any information in electronic form about a person that is needed to manage and improve their health"[24] Thus, an EHR might be constituted from electronic medical records originating in several different EMRS.

Whatever their hierarchical position, to ensure that computer-based patient records do not perpetuate deficiencies of traditional paper-based records and that they meet emerging user needs, we must think explicitly about those records.

Health care documentation

For our context, I consider a *record* as a saved description of a uniquely identifiable patient. The Consensus Workgroup on Health Information Capture and Report Generation considers *documentation* as those records that (a) conform to applicable regulations and standards and (b) describe health care process inputs, the interactions of health care processes with those inputs, and health care process outcomes. They reduce documentation to two component processes, with each process comprising a variety of methods.[25]

1 *Information capture*: the process by which we represent and record what we think, perceive, and do that relates to our patients and their care. This includes data generated by devices.
2 *Report generation*: the process by which we format and structure on any medium (electronic or paper), the captured information and its interpretation.

This decomposition distills from the complex and amorphous aggregate we call patient information, process elements amenable to reflection and analysis.

Information capture as a process

Consider these questions to help you think operationally about information capture:[26]

• How can collection of this data be incorporated into existing workflows?
• Is the data collection logically sequenced?
• Does a secondary process need to be put into place to ensure collection of the data at a later point?
• What is the best data-collecting tool?

Documentation guidelines

The Workgroup on Health Information Capture and Report Generation recommended a set of overarching principles to evaluate health care documentation and guide improvements:[25,27]

• Uniquely identify each patient and also the ways to correct errors.
• Promote accuracy by
  (a) requiring review of the data item before entering it in a patient record.
  (b) standardizing terminology.

- Allow users to append to a record, while preserving the original.
- Develop criteria for completeness while restraining nonessential or duplicated information; develop minimum data sets for particular documentation tasks.
- Ensure timely documentation to facilitate information sharing and minimize information loss or distortion related to human memory.
  (a) Provide a rapidly responsive system to enter and review data.
  (b) Ensure permanent time stamping of entries.
- Make systems able to interact with others outside the home organization "highest realistically achievable level of 'interoperability'."[27]
- Facilitate finding the desired information ("retrievability"[27]).
- Uniquely connect persons and devices with the data they create or generate ("authentication and accountability"[27]).
  (a) Discourage documents that are signed, but not reviewed.
  (b) Flag unsigned documents.
- Design information systems to
  (a) allow auditing of their design elements and access patterns.
  (b) inform appropriate individuals of errors, unauthorized changes or access, and system performance.
- Conform to relevant laws, policies, and guidelines protecting health information and signal when these are breached

This is a comprehensive framework for thinking about a health care information system. Reflect on your current system in the light of these criteria. Come back to this framework after you become familiar with the eNICU software provided with this book, and use it to evaluate other information systems.

Electronic Health Record

An IOM publication from 2003 provides further perspective on the changes brewing in the way we work with data. It summarizes recommendations to the Department of Health and Human Services of the United States for key care delivery-related capabilities of an EHR system.[28] The vision includes[28]

1 collecting individuals' health and health care information over time,
2 accessing individual- and population-level information whenever required, without delay, and only as appropriate for each authorized user,
3 supporting medical decision making, and
4 providing knowledge to improve quality, safety, and efficiency of patient care, and health care delivery for the population.

Exactly how do we implement these desiderata? The United Kingdom and the United States have 10-year plans to reach the goal.[15,19] If you already use a computer-based patient information system you may wonder why 10 years might be needed to reach the goal on a national level. On the other hand, some experts think the 10-year horizon is optimistic.[29] After surveying the current status of relevant technology, the IOM found that[13]

> no current system, however, is capable of supporting the complete CPR [computer-based patient record] . . . although no technological breakthroughs are needed to realize CPR systems, further maturation of a few emerging technologies, such as hand-held computers . . . may be necessary to develop state-of-the-art CPR systems . . . In some cases, promising technologies must be tested further in "real-life" situations. (Quoted from executive summary, p. 48[13])

A comprehensive discussion of the challenge is beyond our scope, involving organizational change at both the health care institution level and national level.[21,24] We touch on one tiny dimension of the problem here and another – the ontology problem – in Chapter 5.

The challenge of free-text data

Chances are that the computer-based system you may have experience with uses the so-called free-text fields. These are fields that allow you to write anything you'd like in them (within some size limit). People reluctant to abandon handwritten notes tend to like free-text fields. They make them feel good about "getting all the data into the computer." By using free-text fields, people can continue to think tacitly and implicitly. Never mind that the software can't reliably search this kind of data. What we typically get from such fields is exactly what we put in – clauses, rather than discrete ideas. This limits our ability to manipulate the information in these fields to support new learning. Understandably, Powsner et al. attribute most present benefits of computer-based records to data fields that contain structured, coded data.[30] Of course, searching of free-text fields is an active area of investigation.

Thoughts on building a complex system

A national-level health information system, such as the previously referenced visions of the UK and US governments, will be a huge construct. I wonder if the views of Zimmerman et al. about another huge information construct might apply to our subject too (p. 39 in Ref. 31). These authors describe the Internet as an example of a complex system that "no one" built. For the Internet, overall system growth and complexity occur after integrating *components* that were subject to testing and refinement.

> The only way to make a complex system that works is to begin with a simple system that works. Attempts to instantly install highly complex organization . . . without growing it inevitably lead to failure. . . . Time is needed to let each part test itself against all the others.(p. 40, Ref. 31).

My experience with eNICU, a comparatively simple, but nonetheless complex computer-based patient record system, seems to validate their advice.

CHAPTER 4
Aims of a patient data management process

Discriminating symptom from diagnosis in an information system

Did Chapter 3 leave you thinking that the solution to health care's problems with managing patient information is computer-based patient records? Let's not leap directly to a solution; let's reflect further on the problem.

As I am writing primarily for clinicians, I trust I need not elaborate much on the difference between a symptom and a diagnosis. A symptom is a manifestation of a problem. An ideal diagnosis identifies the root cause of the problem. In Chapter 2, we examined some symptoms stemming from the traditional way we have worked with patient information. Chapter 3 touched on symptomatic relief. However, I view computers less as a solution and more as a wonderful tool to facilitate implementing the real solution.

In my view, many concerns with our traditional approach to managing patient information cluster beneath one overarching problem: *We have tended to think about managing patient information in an ad hoc way.* Traditional, paper-based records seem to have developed in a makeshift fashion over a long time, to solve the apparent problems of the moment. Think of how cities – absent an overarching vision – tend to sprawl haphazardly into suburbs. Paper-based record systems often appear designed not to support the broader enterprise of health care but to accomplish ad hoc communication — whatever appears needed at the moment each record element is created according to that.

Exactly what should our information systems enable us regularly to accomplish? Most patient settings I've observed have few explicit aims that guide their information management processes – with the notable exception of those relating to regulatory compliance. Further, the processes themselves tend to vary among and within users. Laboratory and imaging systems, though explicitly implemented, often appear to have developed independently of a broader vision for the overarching task. That is, their aims commonly reflect local imperatives – the laboratory or imaging department – more than the needs of the wider system.

Toward explicit thinking about aims

Once again consider the IOM aims for patient records:[13]

> First ... support patient care and improve its quality.
> Second ... enhance the productivity of health care professionals and reduce the administrative costs associated with health care delivery and financing.
> Third ... support clinical and health services research.
> Fourth ... be able to accommodate future developments in health care technology, policy, management, and finance.
> Fifth ... have mechanisms in place to ensure patient data confidentiality at all times.

They are explicit, but articulated rather broadly. To achieve them, we require even more explicit aims for the individual components of patient records, described at a fine-grained level of detail. Many clinicians haven't thought pointedly about exactly what an admission note, or a "progress" note, or a "discharge" summary, should achieve. Our vague ideas about patient information stand in distinction to, at times, more precise ideas about what we want to achieve for our patient. This dichotomy should trouble you.

Our health care system hasn't forced us to tackle these problems. As Donald Berwick observes, "performance is embedded into the design of the system ... all systems are perfectly designed to achieve the results they get." (http://www.ihi.org/IHI/Topics/Improvement/ImprovementMethods/Literature/WantaNewLevelofPerformanceGetaNewSystem.htm; accessed 5 August 2004). In my experience, any document bearing the appropriate heading, the date and time, the physician's signature at the end, and some text in between – legibility optional – will do. If you don't know where you're going, it's easy to get there. What proportion of complaints about new information system technology might actually be about this technology's requirement for explicit thinking – about being forced to know exactly where we're going?

Not ready ... fire, but ready ... aim ... fire

This book is largely about implementing ideas. But it's crucial to appreciate that you can't rush headlong into implementation until you clearly understand the problem you intend to solve and exactly what you intend to achieve by your proposed solution. If you ignore these considerations you'll have trouble understanding your implementation as it unfolds and trouble understanding the results it produces.

To prime your thinking about your own patient information system, consider these additional aims:[32]

- To create an accurate data model: a formal data structure that faithfully represents the work and the results. It is a plan for what data you want and how you structure (link) the data so that you can answer the questions you want to and produce the documentation you need.

- Over time, to rapidly and inexpensively store and retrieve increasing amounts of patient data – to document what happened and whether it happened well.
- To foster decision support: systems to connect data elements in ways that produce new levels of meaning. For example, connecting data about a patient's renal function with data about drugs that are excreted through the kidneys and which you plan to give to a patient.
- To improve workflow.

See my previous book, *Evaluating the Processes of Neonatal Intensive Care,* for a practical guide to thinking about and evaluating the daily clinical work.[33]

Modeling data: Accurately representing our work and storing the data so we may reliably retrieve them

CHAPTER 5
Data, information, and knowledge

Overview

Does a database store information? Or, does it store data? Is there a difference? If there is, does it matter? What is the relationship between our information system and our knowledge of our daily work?

If we are to build a system that manages data and information, we ought to have a practical understanding of what those things are. To explore these ideas we shall brush against ideas from epistemology and communication theory – where, incidentally, information is a term associated with uncertainty and its resolution.

Data

Data, for our purpose, are mere symbols, representations. For example, the sequence of numbers "157" represents data. So does the sequence of letters "Smith." Floridi distinguishes four types of data:[34]
- Primary data, like "157" and "Smith."
- Metadata tells us about the nature of the primary data. For example, the data format (what *kind* of data), such as string (essentially letters and numeric symbols not subject to mathematical operations) or long (numeric symbols subject to mathematical operations).
- Operational data tells a data management system how to use the primary data.
- Derivative data derives from any of the preceding three categories.

Information

Think carefully: Is "Smith" something you recognize? Someone's last name, you say? If so, you're not thinking of "Smith" as data. You quickly performed two discrete operations: (a) you read some data and then (b) interpreted them. Devlin puts the concept this way:[35]

Information = Data + Meaning

Thus, a string of letters such as "Smith" within the closed quotes amounts to data. Once you attach meaning, you *may* conclude you're dealing with someone's last name. However, suppose the interpretive context is a map. Then "Smith" may be a town name. Note that by this formulation, data alone – just plain symbolic representation, are *meaningless information*!

Here's another way to think of the relationship between data and information:[34]

Information = Data + Queries

This is all the more intriguing because questions figure prominently in this book. You can think about this notion of information this way: information consists of a question *and* the binary (yes/no = 1/0) answer to some question(s) – not *just* the answer alone. For example, information emerges from combining the data, "yes (1)," with the query, "Did this mother receive prenatal care?." Notice, if you remove the answer to the query – the data – you're left with most of the semantic content but no information. If you remove the semantic content, the datum "1" *alone* doesn't do much for you. The datum "1," the value representing "yes," "works as a key to unlock the information contained in the query" (see p. 52 in Ref. 34).

It's important that the question be elementary, not one composed of multiple concepts; each demanding its respective binary choice before the overarching question is completely specified (see Ch. 27 in Ref. 36). The point is to focus on individual attributes of things that embody multiple attributes. The larger entity emerges by specifying the individual attributes. This focus is spot-on for data modeling, as you shall learn in further chapters. Information = Data + Queries is part of the communication theory view of data. Lucent Technologies provides a communication theory primer on the Internet, should you wish to explore these ideas further.[37]

Also, in contrast to the further chapters, my use of "query" here is not exactly synonymous with database query. A database query returns a data set, not *necessarily* a single datum – although it could. However, I suppose this query could be decomposed into a sequence of elementary questions.

You may find this next formulation more intuitive (see Bateson in Ref. 34).

Information = "A difference which makes a difference"

Philosophers insist it is more accurate to say "a *distinction* that makes a difference." Actually, to a philosopher, "a difference (or distinction) that makes a
difference" amounts to saying "data with meaning." Fascinating, we're back
to uninterpreted data as meaningless information.

Earlier I proposed that data are a representation. Perhaps you noticed that
I did not define representation. Or, that in speaking of information I used the
term meaning without defining what I mean. I shall tackle these problems via
yet another information formulation:[35]

Information = Representation + Constraint

Devlin suggests that representation can be constituted by anything we
want.[35] Essentially, if I say that *x represents y*, then in the context of the statement, I maintain that *x* is the *functional equivalent* of *y*. That is, *x stands* for *y* or *x*
symbolizes y.

Constraint is a more arcane notion. For our purpose, consider constraint to
refer to a data-encoding/decoding mechanism designed for a specific context.
From this perspective, the DNA contained in a complete set of human chromosomes does not contain the information to assemble a human being. The DNA
must be decoded in an appropriate environment (context). We overreach to
say that the DNA in a complete set of human chromosomes encodes the information to assemble a human. The DNA is a representation. In conjunction
with a suitable decoding device such as a fertilized human egg or appropriate
laboratory environment, we get information for assembling a human being.

Some people seem to think they sidestep the conundrum by considering
information as more than one idea: Information spelled with an upper case I
and referred to as big-I Information, and information spelled with a lower case
i and referred to as little-i information. In this framework, computers work
with little-i information: what I've been calling data. Computer *users* – people –
ultimately are after big-I Information. We, as computer users (and more
generally as communicators), must ensure that context-specific encoding/
decoding mechanisms accompany the representations, i.e. the data. Without
context-specific encoding/decoding mechanisms, we have only meaningless
information.

Knowledge

We may consider knowledge as information that a person can use (Ch. 16 in
Ref. 16). The obvious implication is that knowledge is something *in a person*,
not a machine. Perhaps this is why asking "Where is that information?" sounds
fine, but asking "Where is that knowledge?" sounds strange. Asking *"Who
knows that?"* seems more congruent with common experience (see Ch. 5 in
Ref. 38).

Shedroff relates knowledge to "the complexity of the experience used to
communicate it" (p. 28 in Ref. 39). To become knowledgeable about something

requires that the knower experience the data in varied ways. "This is . . . why education is so notoriously difficult . . . We all must build [knowledge] from scratch ourselves" (see Shedroff, p. 28, in Ref. 39). Thus, knowledge entails a person *assimilating information to achieve understanding*. Have you ever thought that you "knew" something only to become inarticulate when you tried to explain it to someone else? Perhaps this kind of "knowing" confuses information with knowledge: *assimilated* information that a person can use. (Read again the quotation by Albert Einstein, early in the Introduction.)

These views can explain why IBM® paid $3.5 billion for the Lotus software company when the company's book value was only $250 million (see Ch. 16 in Ref. 35). IBM appreciated that all the *information* stored in the Lotus company databases was insufficient to operate and grow the company. They also had to buy the *knowledge* in the Lotus employees, not accounted for in the book valuation. Another case in point: Microsoft® usually buys a company that has produced a successful software product rather than trying to reverse-engineer a similar product. The real source of value in many businesses is changing from hard assets to "employees – the so-called knowledge workers – [who] make the difference between success and failure."[40] In the past, workers tended to be interchangeable; increasingly, that is no longer the case.

The point is that introducing or augmenting (little-i) information technology in an organization provides no guarantee of establishing or augmenting knowledge.

Ontology

Even if we share a common idea of data, information, and knowledge, we may still have problems communicating. The term ontology describes a special kind of framework to represent our shared knowledge. Ontology in our context is how we *specify our idea* of our work. It includes precisely defining the vocabulary we use in our discourse. Workers in different settings come up with different terms and structures on their own for representing essentially similar information.

The lack of a common ontology has been called the Tower of Babel problem.[41] Within different databases, data with the same label may have different meaning. Other times, we may mean the same thing but use different labels. The potential for learning from our aggregate experience is awesome, but it requires that we resolve the inconsistencies among our data tools. This is an extremely important issue. Ultimately, we all can't create unique versions of our work. Uniform terminology, representation, and data structure are central to achieving the potential of the new information technology.[42] Calibrating all our data models and database applications to one common ontology could produce unimaginable opportunity to do our work better.

To learn more about uniform terminology for health care records, visit the websites of the standards-development organizations called Health Level 7 (HL7) at http://hl7.org/about/hl7about.htm (accessed 08 February 2005) and

Systematized Nomenclature of Medicine – Clinical Terms (SNOMED-CT) at http://www.snomed.org/snomedct/ (accessed 08 February 2005).

Conclusions

1 Ensure that your information technology, whether paper- or computer-based, incorporates context-specific encoding/decoding mechanisms: take care to attach appropriate meaning to your data. We return to this idea when we explore how to model data and how to implement a model in a software application.
2 To create and manage knowledge in your organization, use the information technology to facilitate consistent communication among people, the repositories of the knowledge.
3 As I opined earlier in this book, health care draws on a great deal of tacit knowledge. We're not yet skillful at either teasing out the underlying information or encoding it. To facilitate our learning on how to improve the way we work, knowers should try to communicate their insight to how they use big-I Information.

CHAPTER 6
Single tables and their limitations

Now that we share perspectives and vocabulary concerning data, we're ready to explore the typical way computers store data: in one or more tables.

Flat tables

A table is a container to store data that share common attributes. Each attribute, or column, is also called a field. A collection of attributes is called an attribute set. Each row of a table contains one occurrence of the thing the table describes – one instance of an attribute set, one observation. Each row is also called a record. In Fig. 6.1, each row describes one infant, each infant uniquely identified by the MR (medical record number) attribute. InfantID further discriminates a particular hospitalization for a particular infant.

The table shown in Fig. 6.1 is sometimes called a flat table, or a flat database. The modifier "flat" indicates the table has no other structural relationships, for example, to other tables. I created it using a database software application, but I could have used word processor or spreadsheet software. And I could maintain it using word processor or spreadsheet software – to a point. If the only attributes to keep track of are those in Fig. 6.1, then until the number of infants (records) became very large I wouldn't be bothered by declining computational efficiency. In real life, of course, we work with lots of data, much more complicated than this.

Flat tables tend to grow

In real life, we may add many more records to a table such as the one in Fig. 6.1. As the volume of our experience increases, we notice that the time required to obtain information about a particular record progressively increases. This must happen, since lots of records means lots of computation to filter and sort them. Thus, as our database grows in size we want to limit the amount of computation to what's essential.

However, in its current form, our table in Fig. 6.1 requires some nonessential computation. Specifically, the InfantID field uniquely identifies each record by

MR	LastName	MotherID	Gender	IfMultGest	BirthDate	AdmitDate	ThisIsThe____AN	InfantID	FetalPresentation	DeliveryMode	AmnioticF	BirthWeight	AdmitWeight	HeadCirc	APGRA1
11121	Testpat1	02 12:26:31 PM	Male		9/4/2002	9/4/2002	1	111211	vertex	Spontaneous V	clear	2350	2350	32	6
112102	Testpat2	002 2:33:11 PM	Male		11/21/2002	11/21/2002	1	1121021		Spontaneous V	clear	3000	3000	35	9
123	Testpat3							1231							
123123	Testpat4	02 10:13:13 AM	Female		9/25/2002	9/25/2002	1	1231231	transverse	Caesarian	clear	1475	1475	30	6
1234567	Testpat5	002 9:51:10 AM	Male		11/19/2002	11/19/2002	1	12345671	transverse	Caesarian	clear	3456	3456	35	9

Figure 6.1 A flat table.

25

MaternalLastName	MaternalFirstNa	LMP	GAByUS	OtherGAEst	DeliveryDate	MaternalZip	Race	Hispanic	MaternalAge	Gravida	Para	PrenatalCare	MaternalBloodT	RubellaImmunity	VDRLScreen
Testpat1	Jessica	10/11/2001			7/9/2002		Black	N	19	2	1001	Y	O+	immune	negative
Testpat2	Janet		40		7/10/2002	12186	White	N	40	3	0111	Y	O+	immune	negative
Testpat3	Julie	10/19/2001			7/10/2002	12137	White	N	24	4	0213	Y	O+	immune	negative
Testpat4	Amy		32.71		7/14/2002	12754	White	N	29	3	0111	Y	B+	immune	negative
Testpat5	Cynthia	10/11/2001			7/23/2002	12831	White	N	39	4	2012	Y	A+	immune	negative

Figure 6.2   Another flat table.

concatenating (combining) the MR number and the sequential hospitalization number (ThisIsThe__AM . . . ; denoting admission number) or a default value (=1) when the latter is missing (field value = null). The InfantID field represents derived data, containing all the primary data in the other two fields. Therefore, this table contains redundant data. To maximize efficiency we aim to minimize redundancy. Of the three fields, we need only InfantID.

Suppose we want to know more about each mother than merely some date/time information and last name. We might want to know about the attributes displayed in Fig. 6.2. We could just add these fields to the table in Fig. 6.1. While we're at it, why not also add: mother's medical complications during pregnancy; medications she took, and infant's problems and medications? Figure 6.3 expands on a portion of the table from Fig. 6.1, to show an example with four fields to describe some clinical problems.

Imagine Fig. 6.3 contains exactly four problem fields because I looked back at my experience – conducted a time-consuming, old-fashioned, "manual" chart review – and found that all my patients had four or fewer problems. Quite likely, eventually a patient will experience more than four problems. How shall we accommodate that additional data: add another column to the table when four problem fields will not do? Should we add, perhaps, another 10 columns, just to be on the "safe" side?

Suppose further, I wish to learn from my therapeutic interventions. I would like to keep track of medications in relation to an infant's problems. How can we represent these things? Well, we can always add *more* columns, can't we (see Fig. 6.4)?

As flat tables grow wider, so do their problems

To allow even the snippet of the complete table to fit on the page, Fig. 6.4 contains only three columns for problems, two for medications, and two for linking a particular problem with a particular medication. Do you think this configuration will work reliably over time?

Suppose that for a particular infant the Problem1 field contains the data value "sepsis," treated with ampicillin (the data value in the field Med1) and also treated with gentamicin (the data value in the field Med2). And the value

AdmitDate	ThisIsThe__A	InfantID	FetalPresentat	DeliveryMode	AmnioticFluid	BirthWeight	AdmitWeight	HeadCircumfere	APGAR1	APGAR5	Problem1	Problem2	Problem3	Problem4
9/4/2002	1	111211	vertex	Spontaneous V	clear	2350	2350	32	6	8				
11/21/2002	1	1121021		Spontaneous V	clear	3000	3000	35	9	9				
		1231												
9/25/2002	1	1231231	transverse	Caesarian	clear	1475	1410	30	6	7				
11/19/2002	1	12345671	transverse	Caesarian	clear	3456	3456	35	9	9				

Figure 6.3   An attempt to describe patient problems using a flat table.

BirthWeight	AdmitWeight	HeadCircumfere	APGAR1	APGAR5	Problem1	Problem2	Problem3	Med1	Med2	ProbAssocMed1	ProbAssocMed2
2350	2350	32	6	8							
3000	3000	35	9	9							

Figure 6.4 A flat table attempting to describe both patient problems and medications.

in the Problem2 field is "RDS," treated with surfactant: the data value in the field – oops, we've already run out of fields for meds. We need another Med field – Med3. Suppose Problem3 is another episode of sepsis, again treated with ampicillin and gentamicin. If the data value in the ProbAssocMed1 field is "sepsis," accurate accounting quickly becomes confused: which particular episode of sepsis does this refer to? Further, suppose 5 days go by and the cultures you obtained when you suspected sepsis remain sterile. Accordingly, you decide to change the working diagnosis. Despite your working with a computer, to update such data you must keep track of much information in your head. As the size of the database grows, the potential for errors in properly updating all the pertinent fields increases very rapidly.

Our problems in managing data in a flat table are just beginning. Suppose you record several attributes describing infants admitted to your NICU, along with data describing their mothers. Imagine you've just entered in this table data for one of triplets: infant "B." Remarkably, this set of triplets was born near term gestation. They all initially went to the well-baby nursery. Just as you finish entering the data for infant "B," you are informed that infant "C" has become cyanotic and tachypneic. Now you must enter a record in your flat table for infant "C." Two hours later, you establish a third record for this family, when infant "A" joins his siblings in the NICU.

Each of the fictional triplets described in the flat table displayed in Fig. 6.5 has the same mother, whose attributes are invariant. All these infants came to the NICU during the same neonatologist duty shift, so physician's name and number are also invariant: just a few of the unwanted, efficiency-degrading redundancies that can accumulate over time as a flat table grows.

If sometime in the future the hospital changed its system for identifying physicians by number, great potential for inaccuracy exists in updating existing records. Each physician number appears in the flat table many times. This data arrangement requires you go to each record and update the old physician number with the new.

Worse yet, our table currently requires that each physician be identified by name as well as by number. Suppose on one occasion you misspelled (as people are prone to do) the physician's name as Shulman, for example, instead of Schulman. Should you ever compute the number of patients Dr. Schulman has admitted, the result would underestimate the truth by the number of times

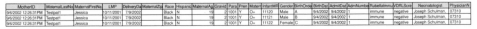

Figure 6.5 A flat table that describes several infants and their physician.

this name was misspelled. Also note, as far as your flat table is concerned, until a new neonatologist has admitted an infant to the NICU that neonatologist doesn't even exist.

Flat table limitations: summary

Let's now enumerate specific limitations of single table databases.

1 Redundancy: unnecessarily recording the same information more than once in different fields.
2 Typographical errors (e.g. Shulman vs. Schulman).
3 Inability to accommodate an unknown but multiple number of attributes (e.g. problems, meds).
4 Modification (insertion, deletion) and update anomalies: relying on human accuracy when you want to change some data.

Other sources expand on these concepts.[43–46]

Well, if a single table database often is inadequate to manage patient data, what's our recourse? Perhaps counter to your intuition, it is to use *more* tables. Multiple tables allow "lossless decomposition" of data, facilitating efficient data storage and retrieval.

CHAPTER 7

Multiple tables: Where to put the data, relationships among tables, and creating a database

Multiple tables store data efficiently and accurately

A multiple table database can entail as many tables as there are entities in our work. What is an "entity"? Consider the basic "things" that constitute your daily clinical work. When I thought about this, I decided – more about how, later – that some of the basic things include, for example, the following:

- mothers
- maternal complications
- maternal medications
- infants
- infant's admission examination
- infant's problems
- medications for each problem
- procedures performed for each problem
- neonatologists

Storing data in multiple tables tends to reduce redundant data and save computer storage space. Why care about saving computer storage space? Suppose you store 1 kilobyte (thousand bytes; kB) of data about each neonatologist, 5 kB of data about each infant, and you have data for about 1000 infants. In the flat table, each one of the 1000 infant records includes all the attributes describing the neonatologist who admitted that infant. With a two-table model, the information about the neonatologist is stored only once, as a unique record in a table about neonatologists. A link field, called a foreign key, in the infant table refers to a field in the neonatologist table, which uniquely identifies each neonatologist, called a primary key. As the amount of stored data increases, the savings in disk storage space and operating efficiency provided by multi-table solutions becomes enormous[46] – so much as to strongly influence user acceptance of the information system, because it runs quickly or wastes the user's time.

To update the neonatologist number attribute in the two-table model, one must change the data in one cell of that column on the neonatologist table. In the flat table model, one must change the same single datum, but must do so *in every row in which it occurs*. To use the more convenient update method requires that you work in a relational database management system.

Mother ID	MaternalLastNa	MaternalFirstN	LMP	DeliveryDate	MaternalZip	Race	Hispanic	MaternalAge	Gravida	Para	PrenatalCa	MaternalBl	Rubellalmm	VDRLScreen	HBsAgScreen	HIVScreen	GBSScreen	MaternalCigaret
9/6/2002 12:26:31 PM	Testpat1	Jessica	10/11/2001	9/4/2002		Black	N	19	2	1001	Y	O+	immune	negative	negative	negative	negative	0.5
7/14/2002 6:41:25 PM	Testpat2	Janet		7/10/2002	12186	White	N	40	3	0111	Y	O+	immune	negative	negative	negative	negative	0
7/14/2002 7:13:24 PM	Testpat3	Julie	10/19/2001	7/10/2002	12137	White	N	24	4	0213	Y	O+	immune	negative	negative	negative	negative	0
9/26/2002 12:26:31 PM	Testpat4	Amy		9/25/2002	12754	White	N	29	3	0111	Y	B+	immune	negative	negative	negative	unknown	0
7/23/2002 5:53:11 PM	Testpat5	Cynthia	10/11/2001	7/23/2002	12831	White	N	39	4	2012	Y	A+	immune	negative	negative	negative	negative	0

Figure 7.1 A flat table of maternal data.

There you specify how the tables relate to each other and to "cascade updates" (Chapter 10).

Multiple table data arrangements don't inherently prevent typographical errors but they make them more obvious. If I spelled my last name as "Shulman" when I set up the neonatologist table, then this misspelled entry will be what I see in every infant record that is linked to me and that displays my name. Also, it is simply less likely for me to misspell something if I enter it once rather than many times.

Lossless decomposition

At the end of the last chapter, I spoke of lossless decomposition of a flat table. Figures 7.1–7.3 partially illustrate the idea. Figure 7.1 contains maternal data from the larger flat table in Chapter 6, and Fig. 7.3 contains corresponding neonatologist data that might have populated that same larger table. Figure 7.2 shows what remains of this large flat table from Chapter 6, after removing the fields to constitute the tables in Figs. 7.1 and 7.3. What remains in Fig. 7.2 is now a table of mainly infant data. Each observation in each table is connected to the relevant observation in another table by a "pointer," a linking field. The database jargon for linking field is either "primary key" or "foreign key." MotherID is the linking field between the mothers (Fig. 7.1) and infants (Fig. 7.2) tables. AdmittingNeonatologist (see in Fig. 7.2) links an infant with a neonatologist, as displayed in Fig. 7.3. Linking is an essential aspect of a relational database (defined and discussed later).

Guiding questions for a multitable system

Exactly how shall we set up such a relational – for now, think multiple table – database system?
- How many tables do we need?
- What should each table describe?
- Exactly which attributes belong on each particular table?
- How shall the tables relate to each other?

Clearly, a multitable database does more than simply store data. In addition to data content, a multitable database also entails specific structure – relationships. Proper structure is what enables lossless decomposition of a flat

MR	LastName	MotherID	Gender	IsMultGestBirth	BirthDate	AdmitDate	NICU	InfantID	FetalPresentatio	DeliveryMode	AmnioticFluid	BirthWeight	AdmitWeight	HeadCirc	APGAR1	AdmittingNeonatolog
11120	Testpat1	9/6/2002 12:26:31 PM	Male	A	9/4/2002	9/4/2002	1	111201	vertex	Spontaneous V	clear	3500	3475	35		7310
11121	Testpat1	9/6/2002 12:26:31 PM	Male	b	9/4/2002	9/4/2002	1	111211	vertex	Spontaneous V	clear	2350	2350	32	6	7310
11122	Testpat1	9/6/2002 12:26:31 PM	Female	c	9/4/2002	9/4/2002	1	111221	vertex	Spontaneous V	clear	3000	3000	35	9	7310
123123	Testpat4	9/26/2002 10:13:13 AM	Female		9/25/2002	9/25/2002	1	1231231	transverse	Caesarian	clear	1475	1410	30	6	7310

Figure 7.2 Fields remaining after decomposing the larger table into multiple tables.

AttendingNeonatologist	AMCHNumber
M. J. Horgan, M.D.	226
J. M. B. Pinheiro, M.D., M.P.H.	570
M. A. Fisher, M.D.	5078
D. A. Clark, M. D.	7100
U. Munshi, M.D.	7249
A. Rios, M.D.	7294
J. Schulman, M.D., M.S.	7310

Figure 7.3 Table of physician names and identification numbers.

database, and is what enables flexible, accurate, and reliable recomposition of a desired subset of data.

Later in this chapter I provide a detailed framework of steps in designing a patient information database application that answers the preceding questions. But it draws upon additional concepts that I must now introduce.

Data modeling: overview

Formally, a data model is "an integrated collection of concepts for describing data, relationships between data, and constraints on the data in an organization" (see p. 49 in Ref. 43). A data model is an abstraction aimed at broadly representing the ideas and things that constitute an organization's work. It is the framework that specifies what kind of data to keep and how to store them.

A data modeler works with information system users much as an architect works with a building's future dwellers.[45] Both architects and data modelers are designers, people who work with problems that have more than one correct solution.[45] This aptly characterizes the problems that belong to patient information systems as well as the notion that designers often apply a relatively small number of key principles, design rules, to arrive at their solution.[47]

One models – maps – the important objects and events of the reality, so they may be "saved" and subsequently "manipulated." We shall concentrate on a particular type of data model called the relational data model. The relational model is so named because it is based on the notion of mathematical relations – for our purpose, tables. Although tables often are related to each other, this is not the reason why the model is called relational.

The relational model specifies a variety of table features. Each of the relations, or tables, must have a unique name, as must each of the columns, or attributes. The values each attribute may have are specified by a domain. This notion of domain introduces meaning to the data contained in an attribute (recall the discussion of data and information from Chapter 5) and helps to avoid incorrect relational operations. For example, a domain might dictate that telephone numbers contain only digits and may not be subjected to arithmetical operations. Each row (observation, record) in a table must be unique. Each cell, that is, each intersection of a row and column should contain only one value (jargon: field values should be atomic). In other words, *a single cell holds a single answer*. A form that allows you to tick off more than one answer to an elementary question does not work for a relational database. Uninformed users of a database application may consider a form permitting such multiple answers to be convenient. Informed users know such interfaces may be problematic.

Relational databases and languages

To work with data contained in relations (multiple tables) we use relational languages. I really don't mean to confuse you, but I must point out that a database composed of multiple relations in not necessarily a relational database. A relational database is "a collection of normalized relations" (see p. 77 in Ref. 43): a set of tables that are suitably structured. We consider what "suitably" means in the next chapter. I mention the concept here because I want you, as much as possible, to see where we're going with these initially confusing terms and ideas. They do come together to enable very powerful data manipulation.

The relational language we shall primarily focus upon is a type of relational algebra. It operates on one or more relations (tables) to yield a newly defined relation (table), while preserving the originals. Since tables go in and tables come out, we may nest operations, that is, sequentially use the output of one operation as the input of the next. Relational algebra specifies an operational order: exactly *how to go about obtaining the desired subset of data* – the answer to a specific query. Another language type, relational calculus, specifies *what you want to retrieve* by the query rather than how to obtain the answer. To delve further see Section 3.4 in Ref. 43.

Earlier, I said there may be more than one way to model your work. How do we decide among the possibilities? Any satisfactory solution must support the operations required to yield the desired subset of the data, the newly defined table. In other words, within any satisfactory solution we must be able to use relational algebra fluently. The main idea is that specific constraints apply to candidate models that purport to represent your work; these constraints anticipate the methods by which to extract subsets of data so they may be flexibly manipulated to meet users' information needs.

Database design approaches

Data modeling is not the same as database design. Database design involves more than modeling the data and has more practical aims: to support users' manipulating the data to meet their information needs. There are two basic approaches to database design: top–down and bottom–up.

Either approach is facilitated by working with a diagram of the design, called an *entity-relationship* (ER) diagram. This shows the *entities* – the essential, main things that constitute what you are modeling (relations, or tables), the attributes (columns, or fields) of each entity, and the *relationships,* how entities are linked. An ER diagram serves as the foundation, that is, the frame of reference for building the database application. The database application is the software for working with the stored data in the database. If the many application features that enable users to manipulate and present data are to work as desired, then these features must emerge from an exquisitely detailed understanding of the core data and their structure.

The *bottom–up* approach starts by the designer identifying all the attributes (fields) of whatever is being represented by the database. Next, the designer groups them into appropriate relations (tables) and establishes the relationships among them. Assuming that you know which attributes you need to adequately describe your work, the bottom–up approach can be a logical way to create a data model and database design. However, when the number of attributes is large relative to what you can keep track of in your head, this method can become enormously complicated at the point of establishing relationships among tables and tuning the design to perform effectively. I shall explain more about this in Chapter 8, when we consider normalization.

When the number of attributes is relatively large, the designer often takes a *top–down approach.* Instead of beginning with individual attributes and thinking about which belong together to form an entity (table), the designer begins by identifying a few of the highest level entities and their relationships, to work from the top (at the highest, most encompassing level of entities) down to identify lower level entities and their relationships.

A so-called mixed strategy[43] combines both approaches. This is the strategy I used to design eNICU (see Steps in Designing a Patient Database Application section later in this chapter).

Table relationship types

A relationship may be one-to-one. In eNICU, each infant has an admission physical exam recorded: one infant, one admission physical. *One* record in the Infants table maps to *one* and only one record in the AbnormalFindings table.

A relationship may be one-to-many. In eNICU, each mother has one record in the Mothers table. Although usually one mother will relate to only one infant admitted to the NICU, some mothers carry more than one fetus at a time. If more than one of her infants is admitted to the NICU, then that *one* mother will relate to *many* infants. Here's an example of how precisely you must think about your work when you model it. One mother may have more than one infant from more than one pregnancy admitted to the NICU. In the eNICU model a mother who has infants admitted to the NICU from more than one pregnancy is modeled as more than one mother. Yes, I should have called the Mothers table Pregnancies. I didn't, because that seemed to depersonalize each woman. However, I must always keep this point in mind when I design queries that draw upon maternal data.

Occasionally, a relationship may be many-to-many. In eNICU, each patient may have *many* problems, each of which may be treated with many medications. Similarly, *many* medications may be used to treat many different problems. More concretely, consider an infant who experiences multiple episodes of nosocomial infection, each instance treated with the same combination of antibiotics. In a relational database we cannot directly model the two tables in a many-to-many relationship. Each of the two tables must exist in a many-to-one relationship with a common linking table. In Fig. 7.5, tblInfants, tblMeds/Responses, and tblPatientProblems conform to this idea, but this not readily apparent. Figure 7.4 depicts the relationship without the distractions. A many-to-many relationship *exists* between tblMeds/Responses and tblPatientProblems. That relationship is *implemented* by using tblInfants as a linking table, in a one-to-many relationship with each of the other two

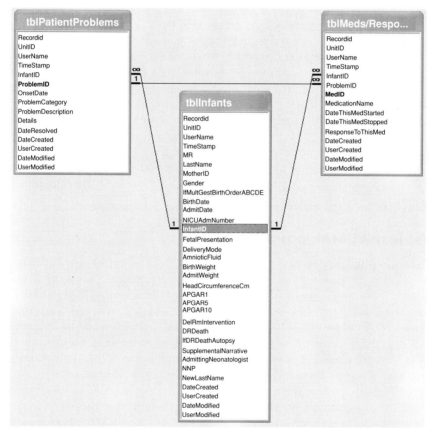

Figure 7.4 tblInfants is the common linking table for the many-to-many relationship between tblPatientProblems and tblMeds/Responses. Each listed attribute represents a table column. The "one" side of a relationship is denoted by the number 1 at the end of the connecting line. The many side of the relationship is denoted by the symbol ∞.

via the InfantID field. At another conceptual level, tblPatientProblems and tblMeds/Responses have a separate one-to-many relationship via the ProblemID field. This relationship models the idea that for each problem many medications may be used. To understand Fig. 7.4 completely, return to it after reading the next three sections.

Primary key

In a relational model each row in a table – each instance of the object, event, or classification – must be unique. The way to ensure row uniqueness is by designating one or more column (attribute) as a primary key. For each row, the value that appears in the primary key column must be unique. If the primary key is constituted from one column, it is called a simple key; if it is constituted from a combination of multiple columns, it is called a composite key. Whether simple or composite, only one primary key may be established per table.

Natural keys describe attributes that "naturally" describe an entity, in distinction to surrogate keys, wherein attributes are specifically created to uniquely identify an instance of an entity. For example, last name is a natural key, not necessarily a good primary key choice because different patients may have the same last name. Medical record number is a surrogate key, a better choice because it uniquely identifies a patient, although not a particular hospitalization. To uniquely identify a particular hospitalization for a particular patient we may use a composite key comprising each of these two attributes.

Sometimes a table contains more than one uniquely identifying column or combination of columns. If so, each is a candidate primary key. You must designate one as the primary key. The remaining candidates become alternate keys, and as such serve no structural role. Alternate keys are used neither to link nor to identify records.

How do we choose among the candidates? The best choice for primary key:[45]
- Must apply to all instances (rows) of the table.
- Must be unique; obvious, but can't be overemphasized.
- Is relatively minimal – fewer columns than other candidates.
- Represents an attribute that remains stable over time for each record.
- Prohibits null values (empty fields, distinguished from a value of zero).
- Is one with which users are familiar. [48]

Foreign key

To recap, the multitable solution to structuring data entails connecting rows in one table to another via linked fields. Located in different tables, and though they may be called by different names, these fields contain the same identifier value. In at least one of the related tables the linked field must be the primary key. In the other table, the field containing the common value is called the foreign key. The foreign key amounts to a reference to related data in another table. The foreign key points to a row containing a matching value in another table.

The eNICU relationship diagram

We're now ready to examine the eNICU data model. eNICU (provided on the CD accompanying this book) is a patient information software application that I developed for a neonatal intensive care unit (NICU).[32] It's not a "demo" or a "toy." I use it to perform the bulk of my patient information management in a very busy academic NICU. If used in conjunction with this book, eNICU can be much more than a clinical tool – it can be a learning laboratory. You also can modify it to reflect your own work needs and patient characteristics.

Refer to the relationship diagram in Fig. 7.5 for eNICU. I use the convention of naming a table with the prefix "tbl" and "camel caps" instead of a space between words that constitute a name. Relationships between tables are indicated by lines drawn from the primary key field, in bold font, of one table to the foreign key field of the other table. When the relationship is one-to-one, the number 1 appears at each end of the connecting line. When the relationship is one-to-many, the many side of the relationship is represented by the symbol ∞.

Figure 7.5 describes, but does not explain. Exactly how did I decide I needed a separate table for Infants, Patient Problems, Loose Ends, etc.? Truth be told, the scheme did not emerge from one exhilarating epiphany. It is the result of a reiterative process that reflected guidelines ranging from simple rules as "Provide a separate table for each class of 'real world' object about which you are trying to store information in the database," to complex ones as those that concern normalization (Chapter 8). The data model must also reflect the database aims: what you want to be able to do with the data. The following list outlines this reiterative process, framed for my NICU-specific implementation:[49]

Steps in designing a patient database application

1 Say what the database is to achieve. For example, this NICU database will maintain a core data set that attending neonatologists, neonatal nurse practitioners, and residents use in day-to-day patient record documentation and for NICU evaluation.

2 Specify exactly what you want to accomplish with the data.
  (a) List specific tasks the database will support, for example,
      (i) produce admission notes
      (ii) produce daily progress notes
      (iii) automatic attending sign-out summary
      (iv) report service charges
      (v) produce discharge summaries
      (vi) satisfy organizational chart audit requirements
      (vii) populate the fields required for other database projects
      (viii) support NICU-level evaluation

3 Describe the current reality.
   (a) At present, how do we collect data (forms, index cards, software application interfaces, etc.)?
      (i) Collect samples of each way you currently record data
         • for each, describe how it is used and for what purpose.
   (b) How do we currently present the information?
      (i) Collect sample chart notes, etc.
   (c) What information do users seem to need that they don't currently have?
      (i) Why do we need it?
      (ii) How do we know we need it?
      (iii) Exactly what will be different if we had it?
      (iv) What activities or documents rely on it?
4 Make a list of all fields and calculations gathered from steps 3a and 3b.
   (a) This is a preliminary field list; it contains current fundamental data requirements of the NICU and is the starting point for the design of the new database.
   (b) Identify apparent duplicate fields.
      (i) Do they represent the same attribute of the same entity?
         • If so, drop all but one.
         • If not, rename all but one so each uniquely describes a particular dimension of the entity.
   (c) Also look for fields with different names that actually describe the same attribute.
      (i) Drop all but one.
   (d) Place every calculated field (a field derived from other fields) on a separate calculated field list.
5 Ask for feedback on the list by all users. To encourage participation, schedule meetings by mutual assent and provide an appealing environment – refreshments.
6 Create the structures to contain the data.
   (a) Tables
      (i) Consider which fields appear to belong together.
         • Associate each field from the field list in step 4 with an appropriate table.
      (ii) Review each table to ensure that it
         • represents only one thing, or entity (object, event, or classification).
         • contains no duplicate fields.
      (iii) Describe in writing what each table represents and exactly how it contributes to what the database is to achieve. Return to this description days or weeks later and assure yourself what you wrote is clear and coherent. Next, get a co-worker's opinion of it.
      (iv) Edit the table names.
         • Use unique, descriptive, and plural names that make sense to all users.

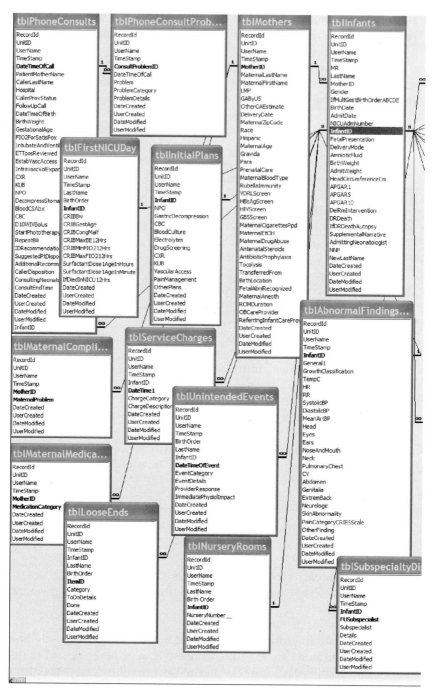

Figure 7.5 The eNICU data model.

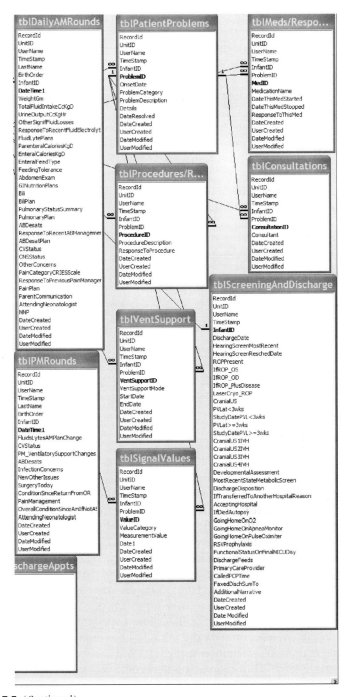

Figure 7.5 (*Continued*).

(b) Fields (attributes)

   (i) Assure yourself that each field is indeed an attribute of the object, event, or classification the table represents; relocate or delete fields as you think appropriate.

   (ii) Edit the fields.

   - Use unique, descriptive, and singular names that make sense to all users
   - Check that each field is designed to contain only a single (atomic) value.
     - Remodel a multivalued field as a discrete table.
       Designate the primary and foreign keys to link the original table to the new table.

   (iii) Identify each field that serves to link two tables; check that it appears in both tables, albeit under different respective field names

7 Create a table on paper using "dummy" (fabricated) data and look for anomalies: those you already know about and others to be described in Chapter 8.

8 Continue to refine the table structures.

   (a) Aim for redundant data only in linked fields.

   (b) Aim for duplicate fields only in linked fields.

9 Designate keys for each table

   (a) Start by identifying all candidate keys.

   (b) Next, select one primary key per table.

   (i) Designate the remaining candidate keys as alternate keys

Justifiable deviations

You should know that for practical reasons, the ER diagram in Fig. 7.5 deviates from the foregoing recommendations. To discuss now setting aside some rules I've just suggested to follow may confuse readers who have not yet tried modeling themselves. Therefore, readers with direct experience of the preceding content may please continue with this section; otherwise, may return here after you've tried some modeling yourself.

There are more fields than logically required, including RecordID, UnitID, UserName, TimeStamp, and LastName. Often, I departed from recommended practice to improve ease of use and data entry accuracy and to facilitate tracking users and input devices. Data entry forms on the handheld devices redundantly display patient identifier fields like LastName because users may be uncomfortable relying only on the primary key value. In general, the data model reflects an implementation using dual software platforms, one which is not truly relational. This statement will become more understandable over the next few chapters.

Some of the design compromises reflect my continuing efforts to learn about database theory and implementation as I progressed with building and modifying eNICU. This evolutionary approach encouraged refining existing solutions rather than scrapping the old and redesigning.

Here is one more point, especially for meticulous readers already familiar with Pendragon Forms and Microsoft® Access: Redundant fields in tbl DailyAMRounds, LooseEnds, NurseryRooms, PMRounds, and UnintendedEvents ensure that patient identifier data persists on the handheld after synchronization. If those fields on the handheld forms were not linked to tables in the eNICU Access application, subform records would seem to disappear from the handheld after a hot sync – but only when you look for those records from within the parent linking form. This problem stems from how Pendragon Forms maintains links between records in forms and subforms.

CHAPTER 8

Relational database management systems: normalization (Codd's rules)

Relations and relational

A database composed of multiple relations (tables) that have relationships with each other is not necessarily a *relational* database. To be considered part of a *relational* database, the tables must be "normalized," that is, they must conform to additional rules. These rules anticipate the ways you will want to be able to manipulate the data and are known as Codd's rules, after the man who formulated this way of thinking. Database management systems with tables that tend to conform to these rules are likely to remain robust over time. Those that flaunt Codd's rules are likely to encounter problems in keeping track of each data element and are likely to become degraded. With increasing data volume and frequency of use, it becomes increasingly likely that some data in those systems may not be reliably retrieved by a query that ought to work and that some data will not reflect the changes that an update ought to produce.

Let's look more closely at the notion of a relation. Earlier, I said that we may consider a relation to be a table. A relation is actually a mathematical concept: it is any subset of the Cartesian product of two or more sets (see Section 3.2.2 in Ref. 43). A Cartesian product is a relational algebra operation. If one set contains the elements $\{a, b\}$ and a second set the elements $\{x, y, z\}$, the Cartesian product is the set of all ordered pairs with the first element from the first set, the second element from the second set, or $\{(a, x), (a, y), (a, z), (b, x), (b, y), (b, z)\}$. Any subset of this set of six ordered pairs is a relation. Similarly, if we have a relation R, comprised of I rows and N columns, and a relation S, of J rows and M columns, the Cartesian product contains $I * J$ rows and $N + M$ columns: all possible pairs of rows from R and S. This material is not essential to what follows, but it may help you grasp the difference between the way a computer views a table and a non-mathematician views a table.

A relation always has a primary key – each row is unique. Operationally, neither the *order* of columns nor the *order* of rows matters (see Ch. 4 in Ref. 48).

Normalization: objectives and strategy

Normalization is a process applied to a set of relations so that
1 queries that logically may be asked of a set of relations indeed can be asked and will be answered correctly.
2 relations store a minimum of redundant data.

The point is that an informally determined set of relations that is not normalized may be incapable of handling all possible queries. Further, such a set of relations may take up more storage space than necessary and therefore perform more slowly. It may even provide *inaccurate* query results! Normalization assures the functionality of a database design and provides a nonarbitrary method for determining the appropriate tables. Without subjecting the tables of a database to this process, relational algebra operations performed upon the data may simply not work. Thus, understanding normalization is as important to developing a database application as it is to evaluating one you are considering for purchase.

Normalization entails applying a series of tests to a group of tables. You apply the tests at successively more detailed levels of scrutiny. Each level imposes greater restrictions on the tables, ensuring greater resistance to problems with data management. Normalizing to three levels usually provides satisfactory performance results. Four more levels may be applied, but these deal with situations that most people are exceedingly unlikely to create even accidentally, so I won't discuss them here (see Ch. 6 in Ref. 43 and Ch. 25 in Ref. 46).

First normal form

First normal form (1NF) is the only level that is absolutely critical (Ch 6 in Ref. 43). The process assumes a primary key is already established. To satisfy 1NF, all fields in a table must contain only *atomic* values – the data in each field must be indivisible; one field, one value. Secondly, data in all fields must be arranged in a two-dimensional matrix.[50] Look again at Fig. 6.5. Entering all three of the triplets' medical record numbers into the same cell of the InfantMR field would violate 1NF. As shown, the table in Fig. 6.5 conforms to 1NF. The table in Fig. 6.4 violates 1NF because of a third stipulation: no repeating of the same basic attribute as multiple columns. So it's incorrect to enter three different problems in one field describing patient problems and it's also incorrect to "solve" this difficulty by creating multiple columns that describe essentially the same attribute.

The correct solution to the problem of multiple instances of an attribute entails a distinct *row* for each unique instance of the attribute. Sometimes you can achieve this by modifying only the defective table. Often, normalization leads to generating a new table to contain each instance of the repeating group. This process is called decomposition. Normalization aims to produce "lossless decomposition," meaning no information from the source table is

LastName	InfantID	ProblemID	OnsetDate	ProblemCatego	ProblemDescription
Test6	111211	1112110	9/4/2002	CNS	brachial plexus paresis/palsy
Test6	111211	1112111	9/4/2002	PULMONARY	O2 requirement
Test6	111211	1112112	9/13/2002	PULMONARY	O2 requirement

Figure 8.1 A problematic compound primary key.

lost. Moreover, normalization, in conjunction with linkages via a common primary and foreign key, preserves the ability to recompose information (by running queries in a RDBMS).

Second normal form

To satisfy the test for second normal form (2NF), a table must be in 1NF and the value of one attribute must depend completely on the value of another. Every attribute that is not part of the primary key (remember, a primary key may be compound) is said to have full functional dependency on that key. For each row in a table, the value in every column that is not part of the primary key must depend completely on the value of the primary key for that row. In other words, the primary key value uniquely determines the attribute values of each observation. Restating the notion of alternate keys, we may say that all keys must qualify as defining attributes, but defining attributes need not be keys. Full functional dependency also means that if the table has a compound primary key, each part of the key is needed to determine the values in all the non-key attributes. Thus, 2NF problems occur in the context of compound keys. Avoid a compound key when a simple key will do.

To illustrate, imagine a table of patient problems with InfantID and Problem-ID as a two-part primary key, when ProblemID alone can uniquely identify a particular instance of a problem in a particular patient (Fig. 8.1). This table would not satisfy 2NF. In contrast, in Fig. 8.2 the InfantID and FUSubspecialist fields are both needed to determine uniquely the Subspecialist for a particular infant. Note, however, that MRNumber doesn't add useful information. In fact, MRNumber is only partially dependent on the primary key. You only need know InfantID (and not FUSubspecialist), to know MRNumber. This partial dependency can produce insertion, deletion, or update anomalies. For example, LastName, just as MRNumber, is only partially dependent on the primary key. Suppose a patient's last name changed after you already entered several such records. To update all relevant rows you need to know all relevant

LastName	InfantID	MRNumber	DischargeDate	FUSubspecialist	Subspecialist
Smith	111111	11111	1/8/2002	1	cardiology
Smith	111111	11111	1/8/2002	2	GI
Smith	111111	11111	1/8/2002	3	neurology

Figure 8.2 A sound compound key, but problems with partial dependency.

MotherID	MaternalLastName	MaternalFirstName	LMP	InfantID	ProblemID	ProblemDescription
9/6/2002 12:26:31 PM	Testpat1	· Jessica	10/11/2001	111201	1112010	meningitis
9/6/2002 12:26:31 PM	Testpat1	Jessica	10/11/2001	111211	1112110	RDS
9/6/2002 12:26:31 PM	Testpat1	Jessica	10/11/2001	111221	1112210	meningitis

Figure 8.3 An illustration of a transitively dependent field (ProblemID).

(compound) primary key values. If Fig. 8.2 satisfied 2NF, the LastName attribute would be contained in a separate base table, where each value would appear once in correspondence with its primary key value.

Third normal form

To satisfy the test for third normal form (3NF) a table must be in 2NF (therefore also in 1NF) and a non-key attribute value must depend only on the primary key and not on any other attribute. More formally, its non-primary-key attributes may not transitively depend on the primary key. Non-primary-key fields must be mutually independent. In discussing 2NF, I said that all keys must qualify as defining attributes, but defining attributes need not be keys. Thus, 3NF problems occur in the context of one or more attributes having a non-key attribute as its defining attribute. Formalism *may* help (see Ch. 6 in Ref. 43): if relation R contains attributes *a*, *b*, and *c*, and if *b* depends on *a* and *c* depends on *b* (and *a* is not functionally dependent on *b* or *c*), then *c* is transitively dependent on *a*, by means of *b*.

Suppose we have a table as the one shown in Fig. 8.3. MotherID is the primary key. To someone unfamiliar with database theory, all this apparently important information might suggest this is a good table. But InfantID is functionally dependent on MotherID and ProblemID is functionally dependent on InfantID. So the functional dependency of ProblemID on MotherID exists via InfantID. This table does not conform to 3NF. When an attribute is not a primary key and is transitively dependent on the primary key, we remove it and put it in a new table. Therefore, ProblemID requires its own table. In Fig. 7.5, patient problems appear on a separate table and ProblemID is the primary key.

3NF also prohibits calculated attributes. On the eNICU form for entering daily rounds data on the handheld device, there are fields for Parenteral Calories/kg/d, Enteral Calories/kg/d, and TotalCaloricIntakeKgD. The latter is a calculated field, representing the sum of the values in the other two. This field is useful on the handheld interface, because it provides some immediate decision support. To keep the calculated field in a database table would violate 3NF because the other two fields provide the information provided by TotalCaloricIntakeKgD.

Normalization summary

Must normalization seem arcane? Codd's rules would not occupy the pivotal position they do in database theory if people typically thought along these lines. Although I aimed for a conversational exposition, one thereby less rigorous than some would prefer, these ideas are nonetheless difficult to integrate after a single encounter. Here is the take-away message: In a normalized database, each table is a two-dimensional matrix describing only one of the essential entities that together constitute the work you wish to represent. For each table, attributes must either constitute the primary key or describe by a single value one nonrepeating characteristic fully dependent on the primary key in its entirety and otherwise independent of all other attributes in that table. So the answer appears to be yes, normalization is essentially an arcane notion.

Relational database management system

To manage the data in an electronic database we use a database management system (DBMS). This software is an integral part of a database development application. When the database is relational, we call its DBMS a relational database management system (RDBMS). I used two software development platforms to create the eNICU application: Pendragon Forms and Microsoft® Access. Pendragon Forms, running on a Palm OS® handheld device, is not relational. However, for eNICU it sometimes is procedurally relational. I tried to limit ways to use the application to those both correct and protective of data structures. The Access part of eNICU is where most data management occurs. Access is considered to have a RDBMS.

The person who developed the process for normalizing tables, E.F. Codd, also offered a set of rules to define a relational database management system. The essentials follow, in relatively plain English, based on Ch. 24 of Ref. 46:

- Store data only in tables.
- Every table must have a primary key.
  Any data item should be uniquely and clearly identified by its field name, associated primary key value, and the name of the table containing these two fields.
- Besides containing the data it was intended to store; a database must store data about its own structure – this is called a data dictionary. Data that describes the nature of data is called metadata. Since we store data only in tables, we store metadata in tables too.
- The data dictionary also stores the integrity rules (we discuss these in Chapter 10).
- You should be able to perform operations on the data (create the desired subset) by using a single language.
  You should be able both to retrieve and modify data with a single command.
  No language may allow you to compromise the integrity rules stored in the data dictionary (the importance of this will become clear in Chapter 10).

- As a user of the RDBMS, you should be unaware of changes the designer or administrator makes to logical design (the data model), data storage, or access methods.
- You should be able to modify the answers in a table resulting from a query, and those updates should propagate to the base tables – as long as this does not violate integrity and structural rules.
- A RDBMS must handle null values (*absent* information, meaning we *know* nothing, rather than some *representation* of "nothing" – a "0," e.g.) in a logical and consistent manner.

SECTION 3
Database software

CHAPTER 9
From data model to database software

Implementing a database application: technical and behavioral points

Now that you understand some core concepts in database theory, we may explore how to *implement* a relational data model. The elements include the following:

(a) Create the physical model – the actual tables to store the data and the relationships between the tables.

(b) Establish database integrity – the rules that protect data accuracy and the relational nature of the database.

(c) Enable queries to be run – ask questions of the data in the tables.

(d) Create forms – features for entering and reviewing data without risk of direct damage to the storage containers or their contents, and to navigate within the application.

(e) Create reports – features for sharing the results of information processing, by such documents as admission notes, daily progress notes, and discharge summaries.

In this chapter, we focus on creating the physical model (i.e. point a of the list; we discuss point b in Chapter 10 and points c to e in Chapter 11). Tables, queries, forms, and reports are the database objects we use to manage data. These are the means that support a wide variety of ends.

Carefully reflect on those ends, that is, exactly what the users want to achieve, at the earliest stages of developing a database software application. In my experience, users unfamiliar with database technology commonly ask for the same ends they believe the older technology has been achieving (notice the qualifier). This amounts to asking to impose the constraints of the old technology upon the capabilities of the new. To ask "Please make the computer help me write my notes more quickly, so I can devote a greater proportion of my time to patient care" is to miss a central point of improving the technology. Information management is at the core of what we do in health care, so think about how the new technology might *leverage* your information management efforts, not simply minimize them. Think about what our tools must do so that our professional activity accounts for all pertinent data.

Our work processes and expectations reflect the tools we use and vice versa. As we appreciate what new technology can do, we discover elements of our work that were rendered invisible by the old technology, for example, trends and patterns in data, made visible by graphical displays (Fig. 11.21d). These discoveries inspire us to imagine what new technology *might* help us do. Graphical data displays are just the beginning. New database technology can provide scheduled reminders (e.g. time to discontinue a drug), identify contraindications for an intervention, and illustrate text with images. Think about these things as you reflect on both the physical model and what activities you want it to be able to support.

Importantly, a new database application feature ought to represent the solution to an explicit problem, not merely programming prowess. Simply because a new feature *might* help us is not sufficient reason to add it to an information management system. Unless prompts, reminders, and the like, are calibrated to user needs and to facilitate workflow, a user may have no choice but to tune out items that appear on the screen. To force the user to interact with every prompt and alert when many are perceived to be excessive may doom the system.[23]

eNICU

To achieve point of care data entry and review capability, I developed eNICU upon two software development platforms. The workhorse of the application, where the data are stored (tables), the queries are run, and the reports are assembled, is a Microsoft® Access database application. You get the data into the tables primarily via a Palm® operating system (OS) or Microsoft® Windows Mobile 2003™ (formerly known as Pocket PC) handheld device running Pendragon Forms.[51]

Microsoft® Access: introduction

If you've browsed bookstore shelves with books about databases, you know that many books about Microsoft® Access are weighty, their bindings several inches thick. Microsoft® Access offers thousands upon thousands of features. It is quite adjustable, especially because it allows you to write programming code to customize features and even to create new features. It takes a vast amount of cataloging and narrative to communicate all this information (knowledge?; see Chapter 5). I tell you this to temper your expectations about becoming a powerfully competent Access user ("power user") simply by reading the book presently in your hands. But I also do not want to intimidate you. What this book can do is accelerate your consolidating key ideas and skills for developing a database application to manage patient information.

Access is the most popular database software development platform for desktop computers.[48] It is part of the Microsoft® Office Professional program suite; readers may already have it installed on their computers, though they may never have opened it up before or knew it was there at all. Note that Access is considered a relational database management system (RDBMS), but Access itself is not a database. You can create a database using Access. After creating a database, you create the corresponding database *application*. A database application includes all the features you need to work with the data.

- Queries: to assemble the subset(s) of data you need or to update data in the tables.
- Forms: to enter the data into the tables, or to view or modify the data, or to navigate within the application.
- Reports: to present information, often printed on paper.
- Programming code: to control each of these features.
- Means to restrict access (not Access) to the data – security.
- A user interface: a user need not be tech-savvy to interact with the data.

A database application may include the tables that store the data or may be linked to tables that reside on a different hard drive (split database application).

Starting to work with Access

The first thing to do is *design* the data model, as described in Chapters 7 and 8. Only then are you ready to open Access and create the database. When you first open Access 2003, the main part of the screen is empty and a sidebar appears on the right. Select **Create a new file . . .** then **Blank database**. A dialog box next requests the location you'd like to store the new file. After you specify a location, a generic database window called db1 opens.

If you are working with Access 2003, you probably experienced difficulty getting to the point of the db1 window. Microsoft added macro virus protection to the 2003 version of Access and set the default level of this feature to open a warning dialog box when you start up. You can make this go away by modifying the list of trusted publishers (see Access **Help** about macro security) or by setting the security level to **Low** – do the latter provided you are running antivirus software that can check for macro viruses and you are sure that all the macros you use come from trusted sources (see Access **Help** about "Change the security level for macro virus protection").

Access tables

The database window with the default name "db1" represents an empty database. It has no tables and therefore has no data. Access provides several ways to create a table. You can create a table by explicitly specifying the details (via design view), have a "wizard" do it based on your answers to several questions, or you can just start entering the data you have into a blank table and Access will create the table design specifications from those data. Access offers lots of "wizards." I find some helpful, some not. The helpful ones create objects that still may require extensive modification, but even so, your

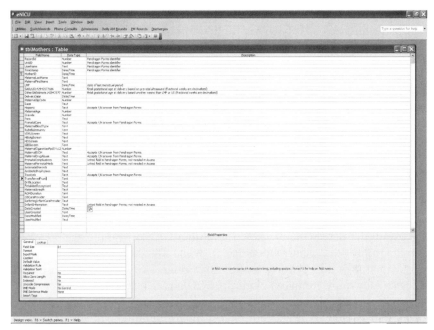

Figure 9.1 eNICU, tblMothers: design view.

starting point thereby begins farther along the path you must travel. You can also create tables and other database objects completely from programming code, but that is far beyond our scope.

Figure 9.1 shows the design view of tblMothers in eNICU. I explain the naming convention for database objects in Chapter 11. Design view allows you to

- set each field (attribute) name.
- set the type of data each field stores (to see your choices, click in the field).
- enter a description of the field (several authors strongly recommend you always fill this in; I tend to be remiss).
- identify the primary key field(s).
  After you highlight the desired field, click on the key button of the Access toolbar (imperceptible in Fig. 9.1).
- specify field properties – in the tabbed section at the lower left.
  Because eNICU is a dual platform application, for operational reasons, some field properties displayed in Access are set by Pendragon Forms rather than Access (this will make more sense in later chapters).

Is Access a good choice for our purposes?

Perhaps you have concerns about using Microsoft® Access to develop a patient information database application. You may have heard that Access is for "home use," not for serious data management; that it wasn't designed to handle a large amount of data or many users. Further, even if Access is suitable for your early training in data management, you may be concerned that you'll eventually outgrow its capabilities, to find that you've invested a lot of effort in something you can no longer use.

Access does have limitations you should be aware of, but they do not over-shadow the product's suitability for contexts to which this book is directed. Yes, performance slows when an Access database fills up with a lot of records. Authors vary on exactly what constitutes "a lot of records." When the database application resides entirely on one personal computer (PC) – in distinction to being client/server based, where the tables and their data are on a server computer and the other database objects are on the user's, the client, computer – then performance drops off around the time the application contains more than 100,000 records and simultaneously serves more than 10–15 users.[52] We have not reached that point in my NICU. Eventually, you may reach that point of diminishing performance. Therefore, we may ask: would a company like Microsoft® devote many years and substantial resources to develop Access into a possible blind alley? Of course, it would not. Access is said to be scalable with little or no rewriting.[52] Microsoft® offers a so-called enterprise-level (substantially more complex) platform, SQL Server, which is far less prone to such performance drop-off. With each new release of Access, it's becoming increasingly simple to move your Access application into SQL Server.

Pendragon Forms: introduction

Pendragon Forms is a mobile database development application that rests upon Microsoft® Access. It is PC-based but handheld-focused. The controlling software resides on the PC. Using Pendragon Forms, you create data forms that are distributed to a Palm OS® or Microsoft® Windows Mobile 2003™ handheld device (PocketPC™). (Dual platform form distribution first became available with Pendragon Forms version 5.0. My comments specific to this dual functionality reflect early experience with a prerelease beta version for developers. I thank Ivan Phillips for this opportunity.) You can download the Pendragon Forms manual and other support information.[51] The manual is also provided as a .pdf file that opens when accessing the Help menu of the eNICU Pendragon Forms application on the accompanying CD.

Typically, the data forms are distributed during a hot sync or ActiveSync®: synchronizing data via wire between a PC and a handheld device. You can then enter data into the appropriate form residing on the handheld device and that data is ultimately stored in a database on the PC (or network, if you've split the application). In the typical installation, Pendragon Forms creates its own tables that reside in the controlling PC software application and store the data you entered on the handheld. Because this arrangement offers little control over who can look at the data in those tables, I chose a more complicated, but secure, approach to storing the data for eNICU, as described in Chapter 17.

Using Pendragon Forms with either type of handheld device is fundamentally similar, so for brevity, my presentation mainly reflects Palm OS®

implementation. As you become more experienced using Pendragon Forms, you'll want to know about a few specifics that do vary for Microsoft® Windows Mobile 2003™ devices, including the following:[53]

- The PocketPC™ uses a Microsoft® SQL Server CE database (see comments about potential limitations of Access, in the previous section; note that the CE designation indicates this platform is shrunken, to work on a handheld device).

  As discussed in more detail later in this chapter, on either type of handheld device, Pendragon Forms does not behave as a true relational database.

- The database file is password-protected. Note that the Palm OS® additionally enables encrypting it (see Chapter 17).

- Options for Field View (single field occupies the entire screen) and Record View (up to 11 fields visible on the screen (common on the Palm OS® eNICU implementation) are unavailable on PocketPC™ .

  The alternative, Layout View, displays a variable number of fields per screen, depending on field design (e.g. how many words you use in the field title) and type of handheld device (e.g. screen size and option for landscape format). PocketPC™ users will see fewer fields per screen. I intend no value judgment: some users prefer more fields per screen, some fewer.

- VFS backup (Chapter 16) does not work on PocketPC™ . However, although not documented in the manual, the entire application can run off a memory card. This means that data otherwise stored on the PocketPC™ would be stored on the memory card. The company is developing security guidelines for this approach.

  Despite differences in handheld operating systems, in general, you can share data across either type of device. Palm™ and PocketPC™ users can coexist in the same eNICU environment.

Starting to work with Pendragon Forms

Figure 9.2 shows the opening screen for the eNICU application in Pendragon Forms. In the background is a standard Access database window with the Tables objects highlighted, showing the list of tables that Pendragon Forms created to store the data collected by each form. In the foreground is the Pendragon Forms Manager, showing the list of Form Designs in eNICU.

The Forms Manager is the main control panel for the application. If you highlight a form name and then click the **Properties** button, you see the FORM_ID number corresponding to one of the tables in the Access database window in Fig. 9.2. You also see information about whether a design was frozen – the term for having settled on the design and created the corresponding table to store the data. Freezing a form design imposes significant modification restrictions. To create a new form design, click the **New** button. To review a current design, click the **Edit** button. Highlight the Mothers form, then click **Edit** to see a screen resembling the one shown in Fig. 9.3.

The Form Designer is in the foreground of Fig. 9.3. This is where to specify the details for each field in the form. The details are grouped according to the

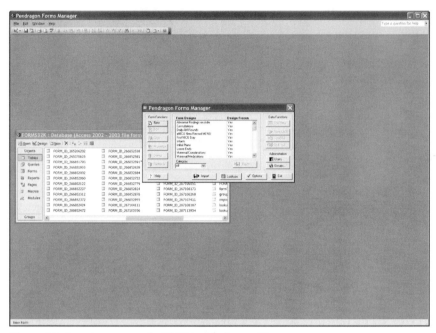

Figure 9.2 Opening screen of eNICU in Pendragon Forms.

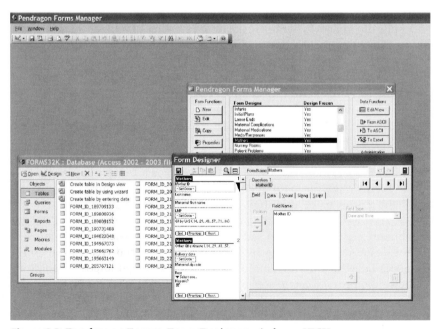

Figure 9.3 Pendragon Forms, Form Designer window: eNICU.

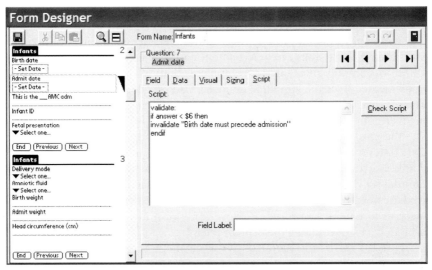

Figure 9.4 Script tab selected in **Form Designer** window.

tabs, visible in Fig. 9.3. You can customize behavior via programming script, accessible on the **Script** tab. In Fig. 9.4, program code alerts the user to an error if the NICU admission date precedes the date of birth.

Pendragon Forms: hierarchical model vulnerabilities

As already mentioned, Pendragon Forms is not a relational database application. Although it is an Access application, the handheld device is unable to support a relational model. Refer again to Fig. 7.5: tblMothers has a one-to-many relationship with tblInfants. Pendragon Forms gives you the "feel" of this relationship but does not conform to Codd's rules. You can create a "parent/child" form relationship, but it corresponds more closely to what is called a hierarchical model than to a relational model.

A hierarchical model uses a system of pointers that explicitly connects a particular parent record to a particular child record. These explicit connections always exist. You may think of parent and child records in a hierarchical DBMS as being "hardwired" to each other. Relational models don't require these explicit connections to always exist among individual records. Instead, the relational operations performed upon the tables create "virtual" connections, existing only in association with running a query. After that, they're gone. If you save the resulting table, you do not save the connections that obtained the subset of data. If you save the query, you save the instructions for reestablishing the connections that obtained the subset of data. If the data change before rerunning the query, then the same connections will obtain different data. A hierarchical database management system must continually maintain all those links. And the "hard wiring" of the links imposes performance constraints. You'll notice that handheld device performance speed slows perceptibly as the number of records grows large.

A hierarchical model can and does allow "bad" or "dead" links to occur,[50] and because those links are a permanent part of the database, a hierarchical DBMS is generally more prone to problems than is a properly designed and implemented RDBMS. I prefer to denote a "bad" or "dead" link as an "orphan" record, that is, a child record whose link to the correct parent record was inadvertently not created, or has been corrupted, or otherwise broken. This was the most common user problem I dealt with in the course of developing eNICU. It is often insidious. As you enter data, you may think you've created a link. However, at hot sync time, the hot sync log (see the Palm™ Desktop Manual provided with your Palm OS® installation) informs you of problems. And the next time you look for the child record from within the parent record, it seems to have disappeared. However, the form in which you entered the orphan data still contains the orphan record.

Figure 9.5 shows the hierarchical arrangement among some of the forms in the Pendragon Forms component of eNICU. This figure also helps you understand the way that forms may be nested on the handheld. Data entry on a child form entails opening a new record of the child form from within a parent record. The idea is similar to the traditional Russian doll that contains another smaller doll within, and that one contains another.... When you're finished entering data on the most subordinate child form, you tap the **End** button of that one and then the **End** button of each successively higher-level form, until you arrive at the parent form. Tapping the **End** button there finally closes the record and returns you to the main screen (this is illustrated in detail in Chapter 13).

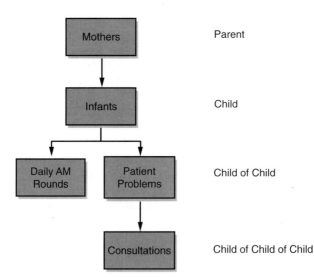

Figure 9.5 A portion of the hierarchical arrangement of eNICU in Pendragon Forms.

Mother

Mother ID	5/7/042:08 pm
Last name	....
Maternal first nam	....
LMP	–No Date‾
GA by U/S (.14, .29	....
Other GA estimate	....
Delivery date	–No Date‾
Maternal zip code	....
Race	↓White
Hispanic?	☐
Maternal age	....

End ◆ ◀◀ ◀ ▶ ▶▶

Figure 9.6 Mothers, screen 1.

A brief look at the eNICU Pendragon Forms implementation

Figures 9.6 and 9.7 show the first and last screens of the Mothers form. Recall the notion of a form from the beginning of this chapter: an object for entering and reviewing data without risk of direct damage to the tables or their contents. The key symbol next to the MotherID field label in Fig. 9.6 indicates this field is the primary key in the table that receives the data entered in this form. The symbols to the right of the Infant information field label in Fig. 9.7 indicate that the field is a subform link (child form); it takes the user to the Infants form. Tap the link symbol to open a screen similar to that shown in Fig. 9.8. Tap the **Add** button to see a screen resembling Fig. 9.9. Notice there is also a key symbol next to the InfantID field. If you neglected to enter an identical value

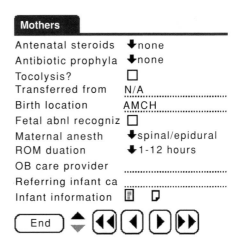

Mothers

Antenatal steroids	↓none
Antibiotic prophyla	↓none
Tocolysis?	☐
Transferred from	N/A
Birth location	AMCH
Fetal abnl recogniz	☐
Maternal anesth	↓spinal/epidural
ROM duation	↓1-12 hours
OB care provider	....
Referring infant ca	....
Infant information	▤ ▯

End ◆ ◀◀ ◀ ▶ ▶▶

Figure 9.7 Mothers, final screen.

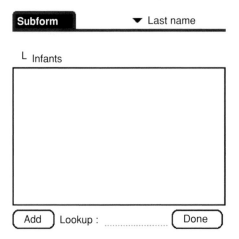

Figure 9.8 Infants subform manager screen.

for MotherID in the Infants form as the value of MotherID in the record you started in the Mothers form, the link that you thought was created between parent and child records would not actually occur. The infant record would become an orphan record, not connected to a parent record. The problem has nothing to do with the primary key in the Infants form. The problem rests with MotherID in the Infants form serving as a foreign key, pointing to the matching record in the Mothers form.

There are ways to minimize such risks. Primary key fields can, and should, be set as required fields, so you can't leave the form until the required field is filled in. In addition, eNICU automatically fills in the correct value of the foreign key when a new child record opens (see the chapter on subforms in the Pendragon Forms manual). Nonetheless, well-intentioned users still occasionally find ways to create orphan records. At the end of a hot sync,

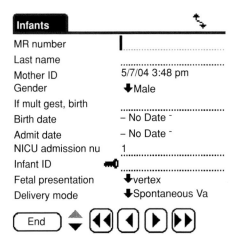

Figure 9.9 Infants subform.

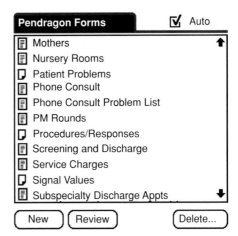

Figure 9.10 Screen capture, Forms list.

any problems with downloading data from forms to their respective tables on the PC are described in the hot sync log. A message that begins **Unable to append...** tells you an orphan record probably lurks on the handheld. To track that record down, review the records for the form named in the message: on the list of all handheld forms, highlight the form name, then tap **Review** (Fig. 9.10). Pendragon Forms points you to the offending record(s) by a bold arrow on the line of the problem record(s) to show you where to look for the problem.

CHAPTER 10

Integrity: anticipating and preventing data accuracy problems

The importance of data integrity

Dictionary definitions of integrity are apropos to our context: completeness, honesty, incorruptibility. Data integrity refers to the lack of errors in data within a database or to processes intended to prevent errors in that data.[46] It's intuitively evident that we want to have accurate data in our database, but it's also worth considering more explicitly why this is important. Bear in mind, one of the main reasons that clinicians turn to computers to manage patient data is because there's so much of it, much more than an unaided human can handle.

Imagine a database that stores data about 1500 patients from a busy NICU. Consider three possible database scenarios:

(a) A manually maintained database (not computer based): 95% of the data about each patient are accurate. Is this number realistic? Often such a project is handled by data abstractors, who are not clinicians and may have trouble recognizing when information is incorrect.

(b) A computer-based relational database: 99% of the data about each patient are accurate.

(c) The same database as in scenario b, except the data about each patient are a bit more accurate, 99.9%.

Using our imaginary database, we aim to answer questions (queries) about NICU-level performance that on average reflect our experience with 200 patients. [To emphasize the point of this exercise, assume that the average and median number of patients reviewed for the query is the same, the dispersion of values is narrow, any inaccurate value matters, and any attribute within a record has an equal chance of being inaccurate. Note that data that are x% accurate do not produce answers that are x% accurate; rather, they produce answers that are y% accurate, such that y becomes increasingly small to the degree that x departs from perfect accuracy ($x < 100$). Thus, each record may be correct or not, with a probability as assigned in scenarios a–c. The outcomes may be represented by the binomial probability distribution. The probability of a correct query answer, after simplifying combinatorial expressions, reduces to the probability of accurate data to the power of the number of patients reviewed for the query (see Chapter 22 for an overview of problem setup and computation).] We arrive at the following probability estimates for a correct query answer in each of the above scenarios:

(a) $0.95^{200} = 0.000035 = 0.0035\%$

(b) $0.99^{200} = 0.13 = 13\%$

(c) $0.999^{200} = 0.82 = 82\%$

Wow! The point is clear: we need the greatest possible proportion of accurate data in the database – and we must aim for perfection – in order to be maximally confident that any information we get out of the database is also accurate. Thus, we want to make it difficult to enter erroneous data in our database.

How to compromise integrity and how to protect it

Three ways exist to create a problem with the integrity of the data in one or more fields and one way to create a problem between tables in a database.[46]

Mistake 1: We can make a mistake entering a unique value in a single field. For example, if the MRNumber is a primary key field and we enter "90876" when we meant to enter "98076," unless "90876" is already in the database, the DBMS won't identify a problem. This kind of error occurred roughly once every other month during the early stages of using eNICU at my institution. *Solution*: in your copy of eNICU, examine the Pendragon Forms script in the InfantID field of the Infants form. Before concatenating MRNumber and hospital admission number, the program asks the user to double check that the correct data was entered. Although this is not a fail-safe method, the incidence of this error has dramatically fallen since I added that script.

Mistake 2: We can make a mistake entering standard data within a field. For example, we erroneously enter "MnSO4" instead of "MgSO4" in a maternal medication field. *Solution*: selecting a choice from a drop-down list helps prevent this sort of error. eNICU offers many such drop-down lists, both to help prevent this integrity problem and to speed data entry. Out-of-range values, such as an Apgar score of 11 (allowed range: 0–10), illustrate another instance of this problem. Both Pendragon Forms and Access allow you to specify *validation rules* that prevent the program from accepting nonconforming data and alert the user. For eNICU, this feature must operate mainly at the handheld device level. It would be annoying to the user if eNICU waited to complain about a value until the time of hot syncing – the first time the PC component "sees" the data. Figure 10.1 shows the script screen for the APGAR 1' field of the Infants form and Fig. 10.2 shows the corresponding data screen. If in Fig. 10.2, I had entered 0 as the minimum value and 10 as the maximum value, I could have achieved the same result by the built-in validation rule feature as by writing the code shown in Fig. 10.1.

A database application entirely within Access – relying on no Palm OS® handheld intermediary – offers the option to specify a data input validation rule at either the table-, form-, or query-level. As a general rule, you achieve the greatest degree of data integrity protection and lowest amount of maintenance work by applying the validation rule at the table level. If you set rules

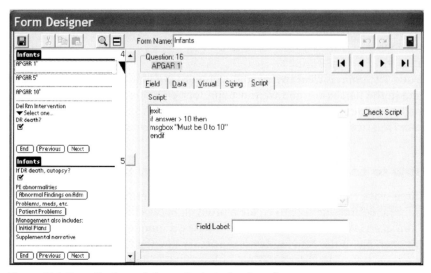

Figure 10.1 Form Designer, Infants; **Script** tab selected.

for a particular field at some level higher than the base table, then you must respecify those rules for every instance of that field in every form or query that it appears.

Mistake 3: We can make a mistake that creates a conflict in data integrity between different fields. For example, we enter a hospital admission date that precedes an infant's date of birth. *Solution*: in eNICU, examine the Pendragon Forms script in the Admit date field of the Infants form. Figure 9.4 shows the code that prevents admitting a patient before birth occurred. This check to prevent integrity errors occurs at the form level, comparing Birth date with

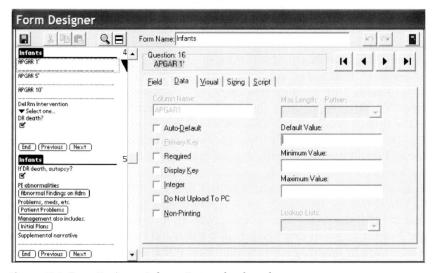

Figure 10.2 Form Designer, Infants; **Data** tab selected.

Admit date. But even for an entirely Access-based application that is the level at which you'd need to check for this type of compromise.

Mistake 4: We can make a mistake when establishing a link between tables, a mistake in what should be a common value for the primary key in one table and the foreign key in another table. This is called a problem with referential integrity. *Solution*: there are three basic rules to observe.[54]

1 To save a record in a subordinate (child) table, the value of the field that serves as the foreign key for the relationship must match the value of a primary key field in the superior (parent) table.

2 To delete a record, no related records in another table may remain such that the foreign key values in the remaining records no longer have a match with the value of the primary key field of a related table.

3 To change the value of a primary key field, no related records in another table may remain such that the foreign key values in those remaining records no longer match correctly with the value of the primary key field.

For example, in eNICU some attributes about a mother are stored in records in the tblMothers table, and some attributes about that mother's infant(s) are stored in the tblInfants table. To compose a chart note reflecting all the information requires a common value in the MotherID field in each table (the primary key in tblMothers and the foreign key in tblInfants).

Recall that the Pendragon Forms hierarchical DBMS has no inherent method to prevent "orphan" records. Referential integrity in Pendragon Forms must therefore be procedurally enforced. That is, the user must enter and delete data according to the correct procedure. The application itself recognizes a violation and stops it only at the time of a hot sync. At that time, Pendragon Forms places an **Unable to append...** message in the hot sync log, to inform the user that an orphan record exists. In contrast, in the course of establishing relationships in an Access database you can directly instruct the RDBMS to enforce referential integrity.

Implementing relationships in Access

You tell Access how a table is related to another table by designating key fields and joins. Recall that the primary key is the field(s) in a table that serves to uniquely identify each observation (row), and the foreign key is that same field inserted into the related table, linking the row in that table to the related row in the first table. You create the primary key field(s) when working with the table in design view. You identify the foreign key when creating a join.

Access provides a relationship window for working with joins. When the database window is in the foreground, find the toolbar button shown in Fig. 10.3. Click this button and the Relationships window opens up. In eNICU,

Figure 10.3 Relationships toolbar button.

Figure 10.4 Show Tables... toolbar button.

the tables are already there. Otherwise, to add a table(s) to that window, click the toolbar button shown in Fig. 10.4 to open the **Show Tables...** dialog box. Alternately, you can right click the mouse from an empty part of the Relationships window and accomplish the same task.

In Fig. 10.5 focus on tblMothers and tblInfants. In tblMothers the MotherID field is in bold font, indicating Access already knows this field is the primary key for this table. To establish a field(s) as the primary key for a table, open the table in design view, highlight the desired field(s), then click the toolbar button that has the image of a key on it (Fig. 10.6). Returning to Fig. 10.5, notice the line connecting the MotherID field in each of the two tables. To draw it, I left-clicked the mouse while the cursor was over the primary key MotherID field and then dragged the highlighted field over to the MotherID field in tblInfants. After I released the mouse button the line appeared. This process tells Access to consider MotherID in tblInfants as the foreign key for this table join. Place the cursor on the line indicating the join and double click with the mouse to open the **Edit Relationships** dialog box, also shown in Fig. 10.5. Notice the first box that can be selected, **Enforce Referential Integrity**. If you select this box and the two tables already contain data, Access will figure out the type of

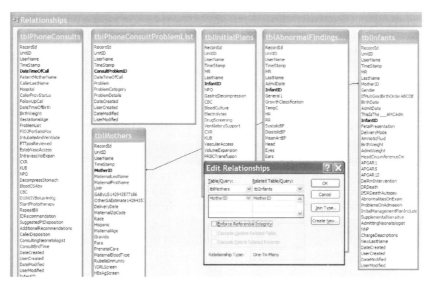

Figure 10.5 A portion of the eNICU relationships window, including the **Edit Relationships** dialog box.

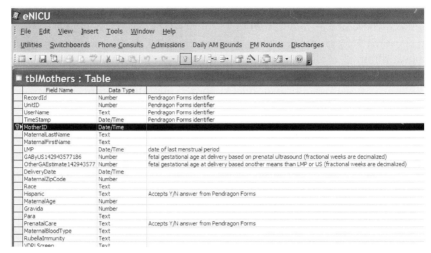

Figure 10.6 tblMothers, Design view; primary key toolbar button highlighted.

relationship and put a "1" or "∞" at each end of the line representing the join, to indicate a one-to-one or one-to-many relationship (see Fig. 7.5). If the data in the tables violate referential integrity, then Access will complain and require you to clean up the offending records before it establishes the relationship.

Join terminology

Some terms associated with joins might be confusing because the same words are used in the context of hierarchical models. Relational models, too, have parent/child relationships between tables. For example, in Fig. 7.5, tblInfants is parent to tblDailyAMRounds, the child. The parent table is said to own the child, or subordinate table. The parent is also said to be superior to the subordinate table. A parent table may also be a child to a yet superior table. Thus, tblInfants is also subordinate (child) to tblMothers. Joining tables establishes a dependency via the foreign key(s). Also, some child tables may have a relationship with more than one parent table. For example, tblProcedures/Responses has a foreign key dependency to tblInfants (via InfantID) and to tblPatientProblems (via ProblemID).

Cascading a change along a relationship

As mentioned, one important advantage of working with relational databases compared to hierarchical ones is the minimal "overhead" associated with keeping track of linked records. Recall that tables and fields are explicitly connected in a hierarchical DBMS, so as the number of records increases so does the complexity of keeping track of all related records. In contrast, adequately normalized tables that generally conform to Codd's rules require minimal "overhead": the relational algebra achieves the same end as explicit linking without the work of maintaining the connections. This is what the options in the **Edit Relationships** dialog box in Fig. 10.5 deal with, two of which appear dimmed and unavailable.

Once Access accepts your instruction to enforce referential integrity it prevents such violations. For example, suppose you entered information about a mother and her infant, and just as you finish the infant's symptoms completely clear. You want to cancel the admission and delete the information (we only consider database management theory here – not whether you should actually ever do this). If you begin by deleting the mother's record, then the Access RDBMS will complain because that would leave one or more child records containing foreign key values with no corresponding primary key value in the parent table. If you select **Cascade Delete Related Records** on the **Edit Relationships** dialog box, then Access finds all the dependencies and automatically deletes them.

Similarly, if you select **Cascade Update Related Records**, then Access finds all the dependencies and automatically updates them. For example, suppose you discover that the value for InfantID was incorrect for an infant you admitted last week. One week of record creation can result in many fields to be updated. If you simply try to change a primary key field like InfantID, Access complains that this would violate referential integrity and not allow the update – unless you first select the **Cascade Updates** feature. Then, when you change the primary key value in tblInfants or in an associated (Access) form, the change will propagate to all linked records. Of course, be sure that indeed you do want the change to cascade to *every* child table. These two cascade options, which appear unavailable in Fig. 10.5, become available after choosing to enforce referential integrity.

Sometimes, you might not want to delete or change some of the records. Instead, it might be preferable to keep the old data along with the new. In that case, you need a different solution to the problem of updating entered data. For example, suppose that an infant's last name changed after admission to the NICU. You might find it useful to be able to search the database using either name even though you want documents to indicate the new last name. For this reason, eNICU has a NewLastName field in tblInfants and on the Infants handheld form. Adding just another field seems pretty straightforward, but getting the particular name we want on the printed output is another matter. The details are given in Chapter 12. We must learn more about queries, forms, and reports before we learn to control exactly what these objects do via programming code.

CHAPTER 11
Queries, forms, and reports

In Chapter 9, I introduced the concept of a database application: a collection of objects for storing data, asking questions of the data, controlling data display and entry, presenting the answers to questions, and navigating among these various features. We now return to this concept to examine more closely those objects that are involved with manipulating the data and navigating among features. Let's begin by considering a way to name these objects that makes the developer's intent relatively transparent.

The Leszynski and Reddick naming convention

Various types of database objects appear on the left side of the Access database window: tables, queries, forms, reports, pages, macros, and modules. I name instances of these objects by a convention that uses a prefix suggesting the object type and no spaces within the name. A consistent approach to naming database objects is helpful both for developing an application and for administering it.

When you create new database objects in Access you might use an Access "wizard" to help you along. Often, the wizard provides a list of data sources that includes queries and tables on the same list. It can be difficult to choose the data source you want from such a list unless you've named each object so it tells you what it is and what it does. To produce a report like a discharge summary requires many database objects to interact. Coordinating this interaction is much easier when each object's name indicates what type of object it is and its role. You appreciate such a naming convention all the more when you create a new database object long after you created the objects that will populate it with data.

The naming convention I use is based on a system developed by Leszynski and Reddick in 1993.[55] This system is also referred to as Hungarian notation, to acknowledge the nationality of Charles Simonyi, who first described this naming method. Table 11.1 summarizes the "tags" (prefixes).

Tags are always written in lower case, so that the eye easily passes over them to find the first upper case letter that begins the base name. I use "camel caps" for the base name; no space between words (or abbreviations) and each word capitalized, because spaces within a name can cause errors with programming languages unless the names are specially set off. Most programming languages consider a space as a delimiter between items, not as a logical part of a single

Table 11.1 The Leszynski and Reddick naming convention

Database object type	Tag
Table	tbl
Query	qry
Form	frm
Report	rpt
Module	bas
Subform	fsub
Subreport	rsub
Label (on a form or report)	lbl
Text box (on a form or report)	txt
Command button (on a form or report)	cmd
Chart (on a form or report)	cht
Special prefix to precede tag	**Prefix**
Denotes a database object is still under development; a leading underscore sorts to the top of the list in the database container window; remove underscore when ready to use the object in the application (e.g. "_qryLooseEnds" while you're getting the query just right, "qryLooseEnds" when you're ready to use the query in the application.	_ (underscore)
Denotes a database object is no longer used in the application that you still want to keep in case it might serve some future purpose. The zz prefix will ensure that all such objects sort to the bottom of the list in the database container window, where they're "out of the way," e.g. zzqryLooseEnds.	zz

item. If a name just calls out for a space, use an underscore (_) instead. The base name should describe the object. Although often abbreviated, the name should remain informative.

In addition to these rules, Access specifically imposes some naming restrictions:[56]

- Total number of characters ≤ 64.
- No periods, exclamation points, brackets, or grave accents.
- First character may not be a space.
- No double quotation marks for applications running in SQL Server.

Queries

A query is the database object that asks a question of the database, such as "Which patients were in the hospital on 16 March 2004?" or "For how many days was the patient with InfantID = *xyz* exposed to supplemental oxygen?" To obtain their answers, queries select records from one or more tables, sometimes modifying or deleting data in those records if that is what you want. Unless your queries are complex or you choose otherwise, Access can keep

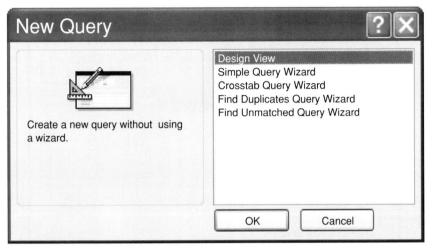

Figure 11.1 New Query dialog box in the Access portion of eNICU.

you at a distance from the underlying relational algebra operations. We shall look at queries from both the graphical – more "user friendly" – and programming perspectives. We consider them further in Chapters 12 and 20.

In the eNICU Access application, select the **Queries** object from the list on the left side of the database window, and click **New** in the upper portion of the window. A **New Query** dialog box opens (Fig. 11.1). Let's explore setting up a query graphically in **Design View**. I leave query wizards to other Access references, and point out that you may never need the simple query wizard after you understand what follows.

With **Design View** selected, click **OK**, and the **Show Table** dialog box (Fig. 11.2) opens in front of the graphical query design tool. You can ask questions of tables and of the results of other queries. We shall set up a query that asks questions of data in tblMothers and tblMaternalComplications.

Scroll down the list to see tblMothers, highlight it, then click **Add**. Do the same for tblMaternalComplications. The lists of fields in each of these tables now appear in the upper portion of the query design tool (Fig. 11.3). Separate the table lists a bit by dragging one. Next, place the cursor exactly on the right border of each field list: the pointer changes to a double-headed arrow. You now can drag the margin of the field list to the right so that the complete table name is displayed. Next, look for the split line just below the horizontal scroll bar in the upper portion of the design tool. Bring the pointer there and it changes to a double arrow with a split line through the middle. In that state, you can drag down to enlarge the upper portion of the design tool (the lower portion may be analogously enlarged). Now you have more room to expand the field lists vertically by doing to the bottom border what you did to the right border. The query design tool should now resemble Fig. 11.3.

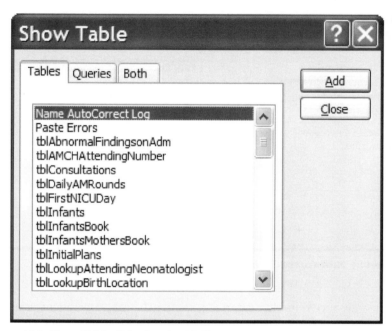

Figure 11.2 Show Table dialog box in eNICU.

Notice in Fig. 11.3 that Access indicates the relationship between these two tables by the line indicating a one-to-many relationship between tblMothers and tblMaternalComplications. Primary key fields are displayed in bold font, so you might wonder why the foreign key field in tblMaternalComplications, MotherID, is bold. It also happens to be part of a compound primary key. Scroll down that field list to find another field, MaternalProblem, in bold.

We're ready to set up our query. Suppose we want to know a particular mother's pregnancy complications. This information appears in the maternal complications section of the admission note and discharge summary in eNICU. We might set up the query as follows: Assume you know the mother's last name and delivery date. You'd have the query identify the set of records with values that match the maternal last name and delivery date you know. As you see in Fig. 11.4, the primary key in tblMothers is MotherID, so you

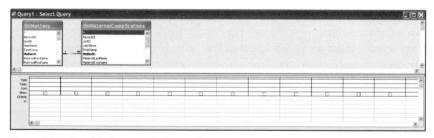

Figure 11.3 Graphical query design tool, eNICU.

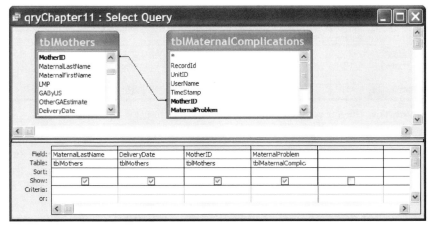

Figure 11.4 A query to provide a list of a particular mother's complications.

need to include it to discriminate among mothers who share a last name and delivery date. The information about pregnancy complications is stored in tblMaternalComplications, where MotherID is the foreign key. So drag each of these fields into one of the empty fields of the topmost row of the query design tool (Fig. 11.4). The selected box in the row labeled **Show:** indicates that those field values will appear in the answer table. What remains is to specify mother's last name and delivery date. We enter that information in the appropriate field of the **Criteria:** row. If you specify more than one criterion that must always apply, enter each in the appropriate field of the **Criteria:** row. When either one criterion or the other applies, enter the first in the **Criteria:** row and the other on the **or:** row in the appropriate field.

Figure 11.5 shows how the query design tool would look if we wanted to find the pregnancy complications for a Mother Brown who gave birth sometime

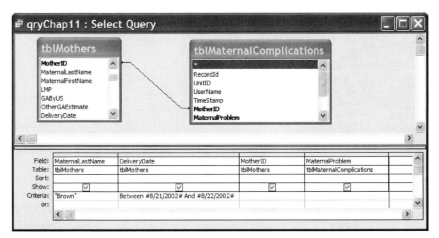

Figure 11.5 A specific instance of the query in Fig. 11.4.

qryChap11 : Select Query

MaternalLastName	DeliveryDate	MotherID	MaternalProblem
Brown	8/21/2002	8/21/2002 2:33:40 PM	High blood pressure (chronic)
Brown	8/21/2002	8/21/2002 2:33:40 PM	Pre-eclampsia

Record: ◄◄ ◄ 1 ► ►► ►* of 2

Figure 11.6 The answer table produced by the query in Fig. 11.5.

between August 21 and August 22, 2002. To run the query, select **Query** from the menu, then **Run**. Figure 11.6 illustrates an answer table; of course, the values depend on the data in the base tables.

SQL: what goes on backstage in a query design grid

Access doesn't actually use the query design grid directly to produce the answer table. The instructions provided to the RDBMS (also called the database engine; in Access, it's called the Jet engine) are passed on as program code. The specific programming language used for queries is Structured English Query Language, usually abbreviated as SQL (some authors tell you to pronounce it "Es-cue-el," others tell you to say it like the word "sequel"). Access converts the specifications you enter in the query design tool into SQL code. To look backstage, click on the leftmost icon on the toolbar (see Fig. 11.7) and select **SQL View**. The query design grid changes into a window that shows the SQL code your graphically designed query was translated into (Fig. 11.8). When you know some SQL you can compose or edit in this window.

It is via SQL that the relational algebra operations to produce subsets of the whole database are implemented. You can get a sense of how this works by studying the code displayed in Fig. 11.8. Each field is identified by the table name followed by a period followed by the field name, to avoid confusing fields with the same name but in different tables. The code says to SELECT MaternalLastName (in tblMothers), DeliveryDate (in tblMothers), MotherID (in

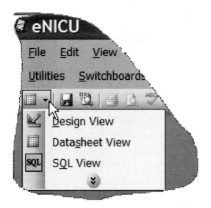

Figure 11.7 The **View** toolbar button.

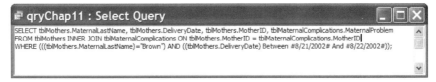

Figure 11.8 SQL view of the query in Fig. 11.5.

tblMothers), and MaternalProblem (in tblMaternalComplications) FROM a set of records in tblMothers and tblMaternalComplications that are linked (INNER JOIN) on the basis of sharing a common value in the MotherID field (tblMothers.MotherID = tblMaternalComplications.MotherID), such that (WHERE) the value in the tblMothers.MaternalLastName field is "Brown," and the value in the tblMothers.DeliveryDate field is between 8/21/2002 and 8/22/2002. In plainer English, the code instructs the Access Jet engine to find a subset of records consisting of the fields enumerated in the SELECT part of the statement that results from linking the records in the two tables on the basis of a common value for MotherID (primary key and foreign key) and choosing only the rows (records) that have Brown as the MaternalLastName and DeliveryDate between August 21, 2002 and August 22, 2002.

Query types

We may categorize queries as follows:

1 Select Query selects records from a table or query based on criteria you specify when you create the query.
2 Parameter Query, in its most basic form, when the query runs asks the user to provide selection criteria via a dialog box. We soon examine a more subtle approach to obtaining selection criteria at run time.
3 Range Query, a special case of a select query; specific range of values as the criteria.
4 Aggregate Query
   (a) summarizes data and
   (b) cross tabulates data.
5 Action Query
   (a) updates field values,
   (b) appends new records to a table,
   (c) deletes records from a table, and
   (d) makes or deletes an entire table.

We shall examine examples of various query types in Chapter 12.

There are a number of good introductions to implementing queries using the graphical design tool and writing queries directly in SQL.[46,50,57–59] Make use too, of Microsoft's Online Help, particularly the topics "Creating and Working with Database Objects," "Working with Data," and "Queries I: Get answers with queries."[60] Once you feel you basically understand these topics, you might want to look at an online chapter on relational algebra.[61]

You will want to save the queries that support permanent features of a database application. Other times, you may only need a one-time answer to a question about data in the database. You could simply run the query at the time you need the answer. However, if the query was not straightforward to create, it would be better to save it. Afterwards, right click on the saved query database object in the database window, select **Properties**, and write a description of the query. Referring to problems that you solved in the past might help you with future query tasks.

Updatable queries

Often you can edit data in the answer table for a query or in the fields on a form that are populated by the answer to a query, and those changes will propagate to the base tables that contain the source data. In this situation, we say that the query is updatable. However, when queries produce summary data (e.g. a count of records, a sum of values in a column) or data resulting from field-specific computations (e.g. finding the difference between two dates, where each of the two dates represents a value for a field in a table but the date difference does not represent a field in a table), the results are read-only. Changes to these fields won't propagate to the base tables because sometimes it's not possible to deconstruct the process so that the changes can be correctly allocated and other times relational integrity might be violated to do so.

Forms: overview

Forms are database objects for entering data, viewing data, and providing data to other database objects. Can't you use tables to do these things? Yes, but you may not want all users to have access to all the data in the tables. Or, you may want to work with a record that spans many tables. Forms are metaphorical windows that you design to *provide specific views* of data; views that *precisely control how data may be modified*. Forms facilitate entering and viewing data. To protect the primary data, database users typically do not get direct access to tables. Otherwise, a user may (inadvertently) change data or the structure of the table itself. Unlike tables, with their fixed field structure, forms also allow you to arrange the sequence of fields to reflect the logic of the task at hand. You can print the data that appear in a form, but the result tends to look rather cold and mechanical compared with what you can achieve with a report (see the next section).

Many eNICU forms reside in the handheld part of the application. For example, when you want to admit a new patient to the NICU, the first screen that opens after clicking on **Admit to NICU** is **Mothers** (Fig. 9.7). These forms are Pendragon Forms-produced forms that act as "remote" data gatherers, ultimately communicating with the respective table residing in the part of eNICU that is implemented in Access.

Figure 11.9 frmSearchNICUAdmits: a form to search among admission records.

Some forms in eNICU combine data entry and review, primarily to provide specific criteria (parameters) needed to run a query. For example, to create an admission note in eNICU, you specify the last name of the infant and select the correct InfantID number on frmSearchNICUAdmits (which opens after you click **NICU Admit Note** on the main switchboard (also a form), see Figs 11.9 and 13.25). In Fig. 11.9, the name that you enter doesn't go directly to a table; instead, it's used in a query: qryNICUAdmitInfantID. The answer to the query that runs after you enter the name appears for you to review the InfantID field. This is needed because some patients share the same last name, so several InfantID numbers may come up in the InfantID box. This multiple listing feature is called a combo box. You select the appropriate InfantID number from the list, and that choice, in turn, becomes a criterion in another query that runs when you click the button next to one of the three viewing or printing options. Thus, another function of forms is to serve as an interface through which the user can get the database application to manage data.

Forms: design details

The fundamentals of creating forms in either Pendragon Forms or Access are available in the Pendragon Forms Manual and the various Access references. The Pendragon Forms Manual is especially clear, so our focus here is on creating forms in Access. To illustrate, I refer to frmSearchNICUAdmits (Fig. 11.9).

Make the database window the active window (just click on any part of it), select frmSearchNICUAdmits, and in the top of the database window click on

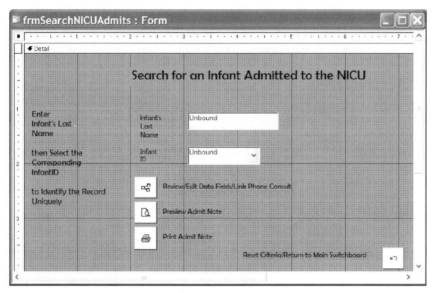

Figure 11.10 frmSearchNICUAdmits: design view.

Design (a little drafting triangle and ruler appear next to the word). [You may
have noticed that available menus and toolbars in eNICU change depending on
whether the main switchboard or the database window is the active window.
Your version allows both views, but application users shouldn't work with
design elements of the application. Most Access references tell you how to
limit display of the database window and specify which menus and toolbars
are visible.] The form opens but looks different (Fig. 11.10) from the way it
appears to application users. This is called design view. This is the developer's
working environment.

Each button, text area (label), or box to enter or review data is called a
control. When you left click on any of them, they become highlighted in a
special way that allows you to move them around, change their dimensions,
or change their characteristics. Access refers to any of the characteristics of a
control as properties. Database objects themselves also have properties. Access
displays the properties of a database object or a control in the corresponding
properties list. Figure 11.11 shows the same form as in Fig. 11.10, but now the
InfantID combo box is highlighted and its properties list displayed. Sometimes
the properties list automatically opens when you open design view for the
object. If not, select **View** on the menu, then **Properties** (Fig. 11.12), or click
on the **Properties** button on the toolbar (Fig. 11.13).

Returning to Fig. 11.11, look at the properties list and notice that the tab for
All properties is selected. Also notice the scroll bar on the right. If you plan
to modify eNICU or create your own database application you will need to
become familiar with object and control properties. Each control has lots of

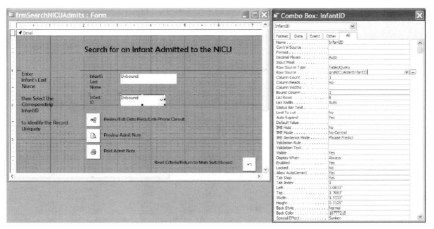

Figure 11.11 frmSearchNICUAdmits: design view along with property sheet.

properties and database objects may have many controls. Take lots of time to canvass these properties. Often, Access automatically enters information in a property field in response to your graphically manipulating the object. Other times, you must specify the information. Fortunately, you are often provided with a list of possible choices; you need not always know all the appropriate options. When a database object or control does not behave as you would like it to, the answer to your problem often lies in modifying one or more properties. Let's explore some of the properties for frmSearchNICUAdmits and its controls.

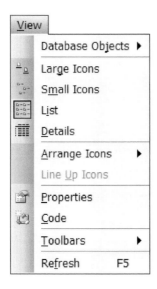

Figure 11.12 Drop-down menu offered after selecting **View** on the main menu.

Figure 11.13 Properties toolbar button.

Figure 11.11 shows the combo box associated with InfantID highlighted. We know this is a combo box because the properties list indicates this. What is a combo box? It provides the user with a list of choices appropriate for that field. It offers a drop-down menu. The Row Source property of a combo box determines what appears in the drop-down menu. In our example, entering (activating the cursor in) the InfantID control runs a query called qryNICUAdmitInfantID (look at the seventh line of the properties list in Fig. 11.11). To enter the control, you could left click in the empty box, or after entering a last name in the control above it, press the tab key to move to the next field. By the way, tab order is a property of a form; you can determine the order in which controls receive "focus." Now, let's examine the query that runs upon entering the InfantID control (Fig. 11.14).

This query (Fig. 11.14) contains some new elements. In the InfantID field, a sort order is specified. When you click in a field on the **Sort** row, a drop-down list of sorting choices appears. Typically, the infant you seek was recently admitted, and in many hospitals medical record numbers are incremented by one as each new patient enters. So listing the InfantID numbers in descending order will usually put the patient you seek at the top of the list. The other new element appears on the Criteria row and the row below, or (alternate

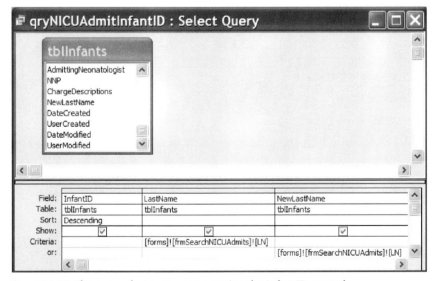

Figure 11.14 The query that runs upon entering the InfantID control.

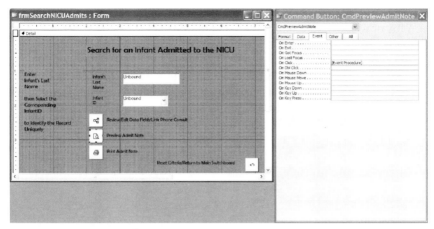

Figure 11.15 **Preview Admit Note** button highlighted and in its accompanying property list, **Event** tab selected.

criteria). The entry, [forms]![frmSearchNICUAdmits]![LN], specifies data in programming code. In plain English, look for a record with a LastName value in tblInfants that matches the value that appears in the control called "LN" (LN is the name of the control where the user enters the last name) that resides on the database object type forms, called frmSearchNICUAdmits; *or*, look for a record with a NewLastName value in tblInfants that matches the value that appears in the control called "LN" that resides on the database object type "forms," called "frmSearchNICUAdmits." After the query runs, a list of one or more InfantID numbers appear in the InfantID combo box for the user to make a selection.

At this point, the form contains data in two controls. Those data uniquely specify a patient. Suppose we want to review this patient's admission note before we print it. Click on the button beside the label **Preview Admit Note**. This button is another control, a command button. Figure 11.15 shows the form with this button highlighted, and its accompanying property list; this time with the **Event** tab selected. Only one event property contains information, the **On Click** property. When a user clicks this button an event procedure is triggered. The event procedure is specified in programming code. The programming code here is Visual Basic® for Applications, commonly called VBA. Why do we need another programming language besides SQL? SQL runs queries. VBA may be considered a master language for the RDBMS. VBA tells the various database objects what to do. Although we don't explore it in this book, VBA code may contain nested sections of SQL code when the instructions to database objects entail selecting a specific subset of data.

Some Access wizards automatically write VBA code for you. Even if the code isn't exactly what you want, it is often faster and better to modify the wizard's product that to start from the very beginning. We take a quick look at VBA now, and explore it in more detail in Chapter 12.

A first look at VBA

In Access, you work with VBA code in the integrated development environment (IDE). One way to enter this "environment" is to set the focus in the property containing the event procedure of interest, for example, in Fig. 11.15, the On Click Event Procedure. A button containing an ellipsis (...) appears to the right of the property field. Click this button and a busy new world opens (Fig. 11.16). This is the VBA IDE. The code relating to the control that had the focus appears in the active, top window in the IDE. Figure 11.17 enlarges the top window in Fig. 11.16, so you can read the code.

Much of the code in Fig. 11.17 was created by an Access wizard that asked me questions in the process of creating the **CmdPreviewAdmitNote** button shown in Fig. 11.15. To give you a sense of the VBA language study the following narrative description of the code:

> This is a procedure (Sub) that is restricted to this particular form (Private). This procedure is called CmdPreviewAdmitNote_Click().
>
> Should an error occur in the course of working through these instructions (On Error) go to the line that begins: Err_CmdPreviewAdmitNote_Click: and follow those instructions. Those instructions start further down the screen, with the line: Err_CmdPreviewAdmitNote_Click: and instruct Access to tell the user the error number that occurred (see a list of Jet engine error codes in appendices in Jones[59] and Saksena[58]), then to go to the line Exit_CmdPreviewAdmitNote_Click: which leads to instructions for leaving the procedure (exit Sub).
>
> If no errors occur when running the code, Dim stDocName As String tells Access to create a string variable (one that stores alphanumeric characters). Next, the value of that variable is set as the name of the database object called rptNICUAdmitNote1a. DoCmd.OpenReport stDocName, acPreview opens the report in preview mode.
>
> At this point, I added code to what the wizard wrote:
>   With Reports(stDocName).Printer
>   .Copies = 5
>   End With
> Once this report is open in preview mode, the first two lines above set the value of the property that determines how many copies the printer will print (in my office we need 5 copies of each admit note).
>
> Now we're finished, so we stop running this procedure (Exit_CmdPreview-AdmitNote_Click:).

Let's also examine the VBA code for the text box (another type of control) where the user enters the infant's last name (LN) and for the combo box that produces the related InfantID numbers (InfantID). Figure 11.18 shows the VBA code for the On Got Focus event of the InfantID control and for the On Lost Focus event of the LN control. The code instructs the drop-down property

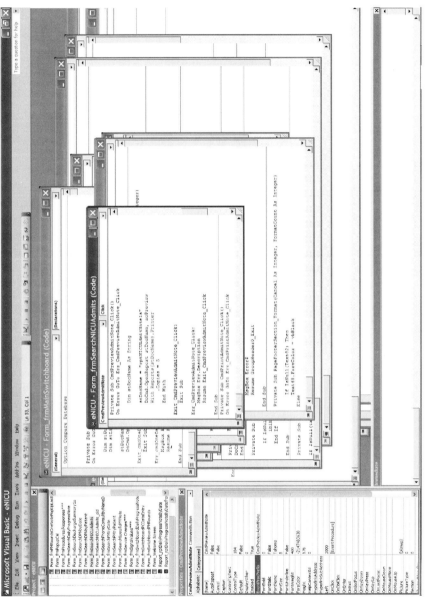

Figure 11.16 VBA integrated development environment (IDE).

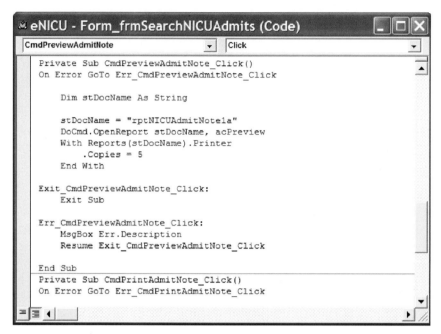

Figure 11.17 Enlargement of top window in Fig. 11.16.

of the InfantID field to activate when the user enters that field (control). When the LN field looses focus, a bit of error checking occurs. Note, lines of code that begin with a single quotation mark are considered comments (i.e, these explain the code but do not run). If the LN field was left empty (IsNull) then the user receives the message in quotes. The term "DisplayMessage" refers to a brief VBA procedure called basDisplayMessage (in Callahan[62]), which creates a message window to contain the specified message. Although I don't show the code here, basDisplayMessage is "public" rather than "private." That means it's available from anywhere in the application. Such VBA code is stored in a database object not yet discussed: a module object (look at the list of database objects on the left side of the database window).

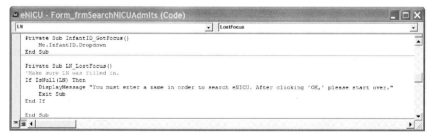

Figure 11.18 VBA code for the On Got Focus event of the InfantID control and for the On Lost Focus event of the LN control.

Access is not omniscient

Access is sometimes overconfident when it automatically fills in a property condition. To illustrate, I share an interesting problem a colleague recently encountered while using eNICU. One night, he admitted four infants, but he could get eNICU to assemble admission notes only for three of them. The following morning, I checked that the necessary data indeed appeared in the appropriate tables in eNICU; they did. Maybe we both made the same error entering the infant's last name in the LN (infant's last name) field of the search form (illustrated in Fig. 11.9). So, very deliberately, I entered the letters of the infant's name (suppose it was C, o, t, o, n) because these letters illustrate the point. Before tabbing to the next field I checked the spelling for accuracy; all was well. But the moment I pressed the tab key, the infant's name changed before my eyes!

Of course, I immediately concluded the computer was haunted. In searching for the mischievous spirit, we discovered that when I created the search form, Access had set the **Allow AutoCorrect** property to **Yes**. Whenever Access saw "Coton" in the last name field, (Access decided that we were poor spellers) it "corrected" the name to "Cotton" (Access decided that the name of a natural clothing fiber was misspelled). The take-away message: tedious though it may be, carefully check the properties sheet of the objects you create (particularly when Access helps you) to be sure that the features set are indeed those you desire.

Nesting forms

A form can be nested within a form. The subordinate form is called a subform. eNICU contains many examples. I use the concept to enter or display records involving one-to-many relationships, for example, to display the relationship between a patient problem and the medications a patient receives for that particular problem. To make sure the linkage is correct, the Link Child Fields and Link Master (i.e. parent) Fields properties of the subform must each be set to the same primary key/foreign key. The wizard often will do this in the course of creating the object or control. In eNICU, this key combination is commonly InfantID (as you can tell from the eNICU relationship diagram, Fig. 7.5). Access reference books provide straightforward instructions on how to implement a subform.

The toolbox

Access provides a "toolbox" to work with controls, subordinate forms, and reports. Initially, Access has it floating to the side of the main window, but I park mine at the top of the screen. If you don't see it, select **Tools** from the menu, **Customize...**, then click on the **Toolbars** tab, and make sure **Toolbox** is selected. Figure 11.19 shows the **Toolbox** toolbar. If the button with the magic wand (second from left) is selected, then pressing each of the other buttons activates the wizard for the respective control the button represents.

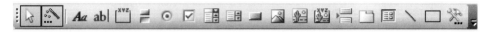

Figure 11.19 The **Toolbox** toolbar.

Reports: overview

The preferred way to present data is via a report. A report allows formatting options not available when printing a form or a flat table. Reports allow you to group and sort information according to several characteristics. I consider this capability a way of doing for text data what a graphical display can do for numerical and categorical data. Each can reveal patterns and trends in data otherwise not immediately evident.

Reports, like forms, can be based on tables or queries. Since queries usually include only the data required to answer the particular question, application performance is usually faster when you base a report on one or more queries rather than base tables. The tables where the required data reside usually include more fields than you need to answer the particular question, hence using tables as a data source entails unnecessary computation.

Access references do a good job explaining how to use wizards to create a basic report and also how then to modify it to reflect exactly your needs. By explaining some features of a complex report in eNICU, I hope to further illuminate what you read in those references. Let's begin by looking at what a report that's ready to print might look like. Figures 11.20a–11.20d show most of a discharge summary report produced from "dummy" data (I made it up; don't look for coherence among fields, the only aim was to illustrate features of reports).

There are several grouping levels here. At the highest level, the data are grouped by InfantID, that is, everything you see here belongs to the record with InfantID 1231231. Focus next on the problem list that spans pages 1–3. Problems are grouped by problem category, for example, pulmonary (notice that both pulmonary problems are included within one set of thick gray lines); and then by ProblemID (specific problem). Medications, procedures, consultants, etc., are also grouped by ProblemID.

Many different queries must run to provide the data for the many components of this report. Figure 11.20d illustrates a component almost never seen in traditional handwritten chart notes: a graphical display. In Access, it is called a chart object. A chart object also gets its source data from queries.

Reports: design details

Figure 11.21 shows this discharge summary report object in design view. Don't worry about identifying the details. Pay attention to the horizontal bars with titles like **Detail**, **Report Header**, **Page Footer**, and **Report Footer**, which appear throughout the image. The **Detail** bar toward the top of the figure, spanning the full width, demarcates the main part of the report. Subsequent instances of **Detail** bars and **Report Headers** identify subreports, that is,

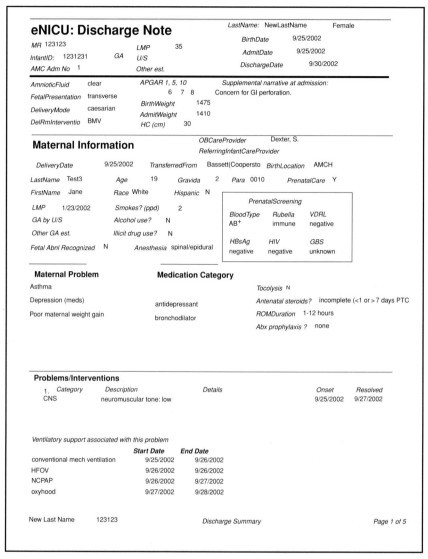

(a)

Figure 11.20 (a) First, (b) second, (b) third, and (d) fourth pages of illustrative discharge summary report.

reports nested within the main report and linked to the main report by a foreign key value identical to the primary key value in the main report. The **Page Footer** bar near the bottom of the figure sets off a space that contains fields that print at the bottom of each page. Look at the bottom of Figs. 11.20a–11.20d. The **Report Footer** contains items that print only at the bottom of the complete report. Note the Footer indicates the report contains 5 pages but

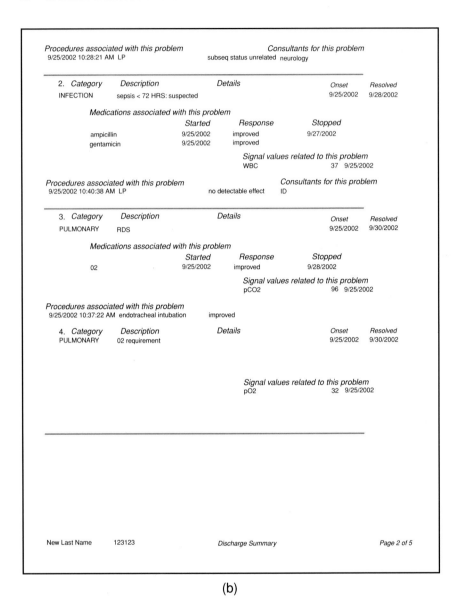

(b)

Figure 11.20 (*Continued*).

only 4 are shown (a Fig. 11.20e would only have contained this footer and so was omitted).

Obviously, the report design in Fig. 11.21 contains many subreports. The subreports are incompletely displayed. The whole thing is actually much more complicated than it appears in the figure. We examine the patient problems subreport in detail (Fig. 11.22) because it embodies many important design

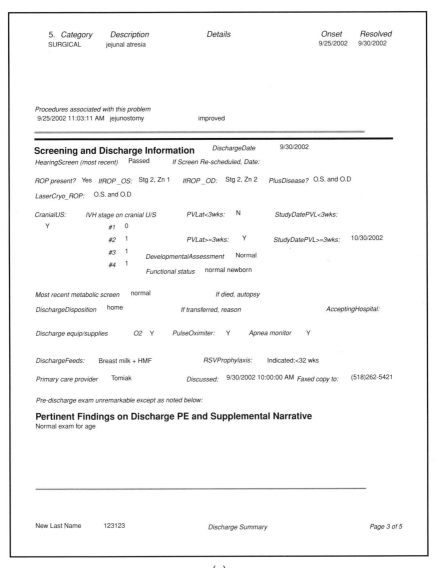

5. *Category*   *Description*   *Details*   *Onset*   *Resolved*
    SURGICAL   jejunal atresia   9/25/2002   9/30/2002

Procedures associated with this problem
   9/25/2002 11:03:11 AM   jejunostomy   improved

Screening and Discharge Information   *DischargeDate*   9/30/2002
HearingScreen (most recent)   Passed   *If Screen Re-scheduled, Date:*

ROP present? Yes   *IfROP_OS:* Stg 2, Zn 1   *IfROP_OD:* Stg 2, Zn 2   *PlusDisease?* O.S. and O.D

LaserCryo_ROP: O.S. and O.D

CranialUS: *IVH stage on cranial U/S*   *PVLat<3wks:*   N   *StudyDatePVL<3wks:*
   Y   #1   0

                                #2   1   *PVLat>=3wks:*   Y   *StudyDatePVL>=3wks:*   10/30/2002

                                #3   1   *DevelopmentalAssessment*   Normal
                                #4   1
                                             Functional status   normal newborn

Most recent metabolic screen   normal   *If died, autopsy*

DischargeDisposition   home   *If transferred, reason*   *AcceptingHospital:*

Discharge equip/supplies   O2   Y   *PulseOximiter:*   Y   *Apnea monitor*   Y

DischargeFeeds: Breast milk + HMF   *RSVProphylaxis:*   Indicated:<32 wks

Primary care provider   Tomiak   *Discussed:*   9/30/2002 10:00:00 AM *Faxed copy to:*   (518)262-5421

Pre-discharge exam unremarkable except as noted below:

Pertinent Findings on Discharge PE and Supplemental Narrative
Normal exam for age

New Last Name   123123   *Discharge Summary*   *Page 3 of 5*

(c)

Figure 11.20 *(Continued)*.

elements. Similar versions also occur in the eNICU Admission Note and Daily Progress Note. You cannot see the full extent of this or other subreports in Fig. 11.21 because I compressed the physical representation of each subreport in the main detail section. However, I set the "Can Grow" and "Can Shrink" properties of each subreport to "yes," so Access can adjust the actual size of each instance of the subreport to what the data require.

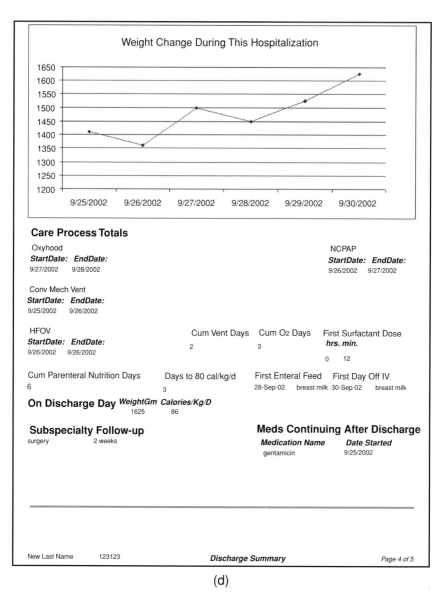

(d)

Figure 11.20 (*Continued*).

Our illustrative subreport, rsubDischargePtProblemsGrouped, is divided into three main sections.

• The (sub)Report Header contains only a label control.
  This control always displays only the words "Problems/Interventions."
  A label control is not linked to data in the database.

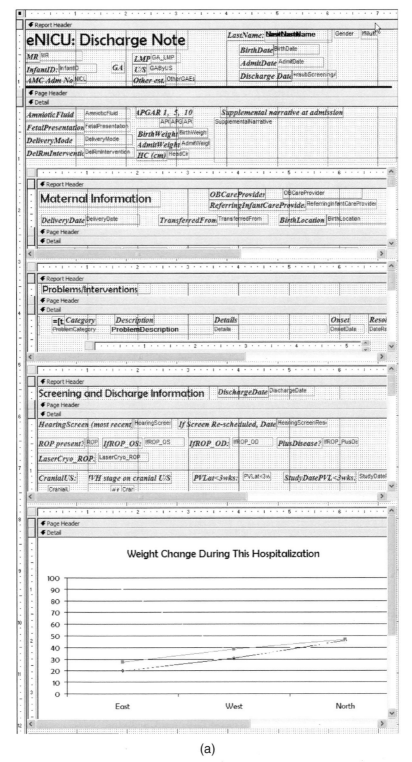

(a)

Figure 11.21 Discharge summary report object in design view.

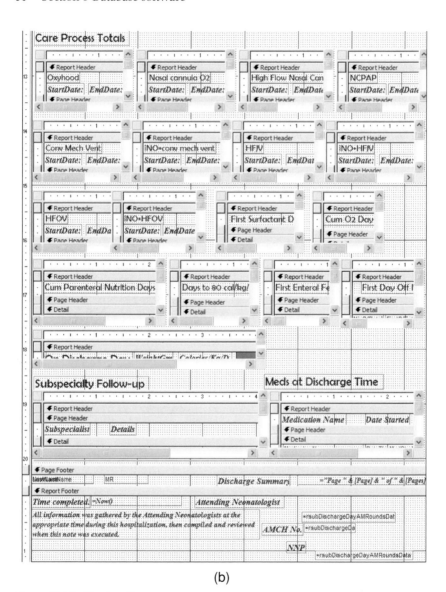

(b)

Figure 11.21 *(Continued)*

- The detail section contains, across the upper portion, labels and text box controls that describe each instance of a patient problem.
  The detail section also contains several additional subreports.
  Access lets you nest subreports within subreports.
- The ProblemCategory Footer appears near the bottom. The only object in this area is a gray line. By placing the line in this area, a line will appear at the end of each problem category grouping on the report (most evident in Fig. 11.20b).

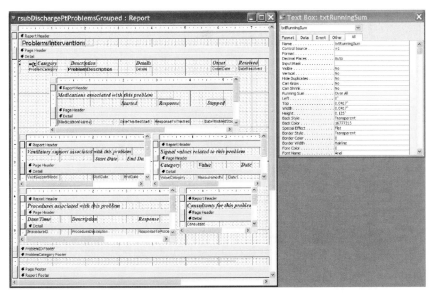

Figure 11.22 Patient problems subreport and property sheet for highlighted text box.

Grouping

How does the application group the information according to desired criteria? You can specify these things via a **Sorting and Grouping** window that may be opened when you work with a (sub)report in design view. Select <u>**View**</u> from the main menu, then **Sorting and Grouping**; or click on the **Sorting and Grouping** button on the design view toolbar (Fig. 11.23). Figure 11.24 shows the **Sorting and Grouping** window for the subreport shown in Fig. 11.22. When you enter a field under the Field/Expression column heading, a drop-down list of fields drawn from the source query for the subreport appears. Similarly, entering the field to its right allows you to select the sort order. As suggested by the presence of a scroll bar in this window, you may group by many more criteria than the two I used. (See the Operational details folder on the accompanying CD for a description of how I turned this subreport into a time-line by making the OnsetDate field the highest grouping level.) The topmost criterion you enter in this window becomes the overarching one, and the others function in progressively subordinate roles. For each grouping criterion you may specify the values for five properties that appear in the lower portion of the window. The choices you see in Fig. 11.24 determined the way the problems shown in Figs. 20a–11.20c are displayed.

Figure 11.23 Sorting and Grouping toolbar button.

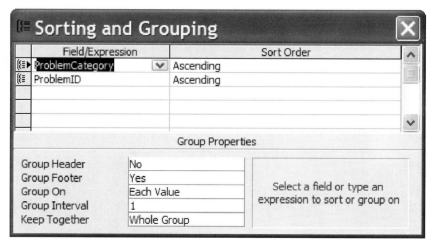

Figure 11.24 Sorting and Grouping window for the subreport shown in Fig. 11.22.

Less obvious in the upper portion of the detail section of Fig.11.22 are three controls that provide important data to the subreport, but are not themselves visible in the printed (or previewed) report. Look just below and to the left of the curved arrow next to the word Detail on the **Detail** bar. Do you see the little black square and the very thin rectangle below it? The very thin rectangle identifies two controls: the InfantID control (necessary to link data in the subreport with the main part of the report, but visually redundant) and the ProblemID control (necessary for the query and subreport, but the user generally wants to know only the problem category and problem description, so it too is not visible). The little black square marks a control that I highlighted, so that you could see the associated Property List, shown on the right side of Fig. 11.22. Controls that provide data necessary to the report (or form) but that the user does not need to see can be compacted, as I did here.

The highlighted and compacted text box is named txtRunningSum. This control and the control immediately to its right, also compacted, but not so much that you can't identify "=[t", together perform a neat trick. They provide sequential numbering of each patient problem, in ascending order. Here's how it works: Look at the Control Source property (second on the list): =1. This tells Access to set the starting value of the control to 1. Now look at the Running Sum property (eleventh row down the list): Over All. Access will update the value of this text box control by noting how many problems there are in the entire subreport ("Over All"; other choices include "Over Group" – to reset the counter for each problem category, and "No" running sum at all), computing the running sum as it moves down the list (see the result in Figs. 11.20a–11.20c).

I said that txtRunningSum was not visible. Indeed, the Visible property (sixth item down the list in Fig. 11.22) is set to **No**. So why do we see the enumeration shown in Figs. 11.20a–11.20c? The answer lies with the control to the right of txtRunningSum, the control that shows the =[t characters in the figure. This is another text box, named txtNumber. It's Control Source property is: =[txtRunningSum] & "."; meaning for every distinct ProblemID value concatenate (combine) the current value of the txtRunningSum control and the period character ("."). This is why you see "1." through "5." to the left of the category label for each instance of a problem enumerated in Figs. 11.20a–11.20c.

Macros

You probably noticed macro objects on the database objects list that appears in the Access database window. Some readers may have experience using macros in one or more Microsoft® Office applications. I avoid using them in eNICU.

Macros automate certain application features without requiring the developer to write program code, but macros are not the same thing in all Microsoft® Office applications. Unlike the situation with other Microsoft® Office applications, in Access, macros are not fundamentally VBA routines. This makes Access macros more limited in scope and flexibility than VBA solutions.[63] Also, Access considers macros as separate objects from the database objects they automate. VBA code is attached to a database object, but macros are stored separately from the object to which they're associated. This makes administration and updating more difficult.[56,63]

If you have created macros in Access (because you learned about them elsewhere) you can convert them to VBA by saving them as a module. This is also a way to learn some VBA code. Anyway, if you have an application that was using macros and you've now converted them to VBA, you also want to update the information attached to the event on the property list that triggered the macro (see Ref. 64 for details). We explore macros no further here because Microsoft® is backing away from this object's role in Access.

CHAPTER 12

Programming for greater software control

What constitutes a database application?

Haven't we already considered this question? In previous chapters we explored query, form, and report database objects, but primarily as discrete objects. We now consider how these objects can work together as a system. It is when objects are viewed from this perspective that the need for programming code to customize details of their behavior becomes more apparent. Formulated in terms of database objects, a database application is a package of features that tie together the database objects needed to achieve defined system goals. Figure 12.1a illustrates how database objects interact. Bear in mind, it portrays a single-platform application, such as one developed entirely within Microsoft® Access. Figure 12.1b shows the interaction between handheld-based forms and PC-based tables that occurs in eNICU. For both figures, pay attention to arrow directions.

Many of the interactions displayed in Figs. 12.1a and 12.1b occur via programming code. In Chapter 11, we saw how a VBA event procedure instructs objects to do something in response to a particular event (such as clicking a button on a form). In this chapter, we more broadly examine programming within each of the eNICU development platforms. For more details about scripting refer to the Pendragon Forms Manual[51]. For more about VBA start with Ref. 62; after that, try Ref. 63. For SQL, start with Ref. 50, then Ref. 65. Ref. 66 is handy for fine tuning SQL code already largely worked out.

Pendragon Forms script

Writing script means writing a relatively short program. Customizing Pendragon Forms often entails writing script. To supplement the useful illustrations in the Pendragon Forms User Manual,[51] here are a couple of examples from eNICU. I encourage you to write and run some code. Even a small success can be thrilling, and it reinforces your appreciation for thinking precisely about data management.

A script entails at least one event procedure (Pendragon Forms nomenclature differs from an Access VBA "event"). An event procedure is composed of an event procedure label – a word that specifies when the procedure should run – and one or more statements that specify what should happen when the procedure runs. Figure 12.2a shows the Form Designer for the Mothers

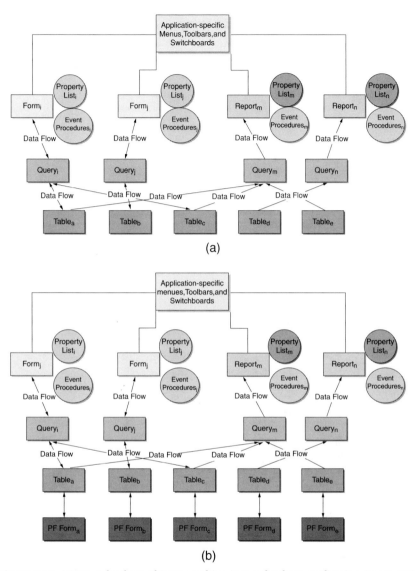

Figure 12.1 (a) How database objects combine into a database application (see p. 300 in Ref. 59). (b) How database objects combine into a handheld- and PC-based database application (PF means Pendragon Forms).

form, at field 1: MotherID; the **Script** tab is selected. The **Script** box contains perhaps the shortest bit of useful code that you can write. The first line represents the event procedure label. By definition, the initialize event procedure runs only one time: when you create a new record. The second line of code says to insert the current date and time as the value for that field. This is a

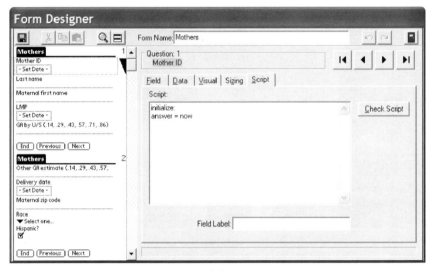

(a)

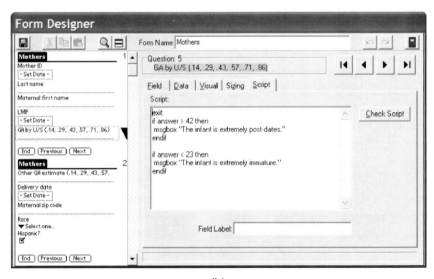

(b)

Figure 12.2 (a) Form Designer for the Mothers form, at field 1: MotherID; **Script** tab selected. (b) Form Designer for the Mothers form, at field 5: infant's gestational age, in weeks (decimalized fraction), based on prenatal ultrasound assessment; **Script** tab selected.

convenient way to enter the primary key value for each new maternal record. Even if several users simultaneously admit patients, it's extremely unlikely that any two will create a new record at precisely the same instant.

Figure 12.2b illustrates field 5: the infant's gestational age, in weeks (decimalized fraction), based on prenatal ultrasound assessment. The **exit:** event procedure runs when the user leaves this field for one with a higher number on the field list. When the event procedure is triggered, the two conditional statements test whether the entered value is >42 or <23; if so, a message specific to each criterion is displayed. This provides a simple form of input validation. If the user entered an inappropriate value like 76 and mindlessly clicks the **OK** button after reading the message "This infant is extremely postdates," the value of 76 will remain. The point is to invite the user to reconsider the value and provide an opportunity to revise it.

Visual Basic® for Applications : overview

You can use Visual Basic® for Applications (VBA) to customize most database objects to a far greater extent than you can with the Access graphical user interface. Essentially, you specify objects' properties and event procedures in VBA code. These specifications need not be permanently set at the time you create the application. For example, you may need to change an object's property only if a certain condition is met. Otherwise, that property remains in its default condition. Imagine you admit an infant under her mother's last name and 2 weeks later, mother decides her baby shall have the father's last name. We shall shortly explore one programmatic solution to this problem; first, more background.

Application features that VBA can enhance include (for a good introduction to each point, see Refs. 62 and 63) the following:
- Customized menu and toolbar options.
- Hidden or locked controls based on defined conditions (e.g. based on user identity).
- Ways to
  usefully inform users of errors,
  confirm a task is successfully completely,
  navigate through an application,
  synchronize data among forms, and
  establish an audit trail (who did what, when).[67]

Recall the VBA integrated development environment (IDE) from Chapter 11. The IDE is the editor application in which you enter, test, and debug (fix errors in) code. One way to access this environment is to open a module object in the database window. Alternatively, click **View** in the main menu, then select **Code**; or click the **Code** toolbar button (Fig. 12.3); or press **Alt+F11** (press this combination a second time to return to Access).

Figure 12.3 Code toolbar button.

Refer again to Fig. 11.17, showing the IDE. You can configure it to suit your needs. Mine has four main areas:

1 The project explorer (upper left).
2 The property sheet (lower left; we shall not examine it further).
3 The main editor (the largest of the four areas).
4 The immediate window (below the main editor).

Click one of the objects listed in the project explorer to see in the main editor the code associated with that object. This works even if you first got to the IDE by opening a specific module or event procedure. At the top left of each code window displayed in the main editor window is a drop-down list with the names of all the component objects (combo boxes, buttons to click, etc.) that are part of the object you selected in the project explorer. The IDE brings the cursor to the portion of VBA code associated with the object name you selected from the drop-down list. At the top right of that window is another drop-down list. This one presents all the types of subroutines (particular instruction sets) that VBA allows you to use to customize the behavior of an object of the type you selected in the drop-down list to the left (Fig. 11.18). The immediate window enables you to type code and see the results immediately in the same window.

VBA procedure code may be of two types: functions and subprocedures. When a function runs, the result is a value. When a subprocedure runs, it makes something happen to an object within the application; it may open a report, for example. Access stores VBA procedures in database objects called modules.

VBA variables

Often in the course of a procedure running, you temporarily need to store data that you will use elsewhere in the same or another procedure. This is the job of variables. VBA variable types are often, but not always, specific for the kind of data stored:

- A Boolean variable stores yes/no data.
- A date variable stores date/time data.
- A string variable stores text characters, including digits that will not be mathematically manipulated (e.g. zip codes).
- The type of variable that stores numerical data depends on the size and precision of the number, for example,
  byte, for single, unsigned, 8-bit (1 byte) – binary – numbers: 0–255,
  integer, for 16-bit (2 byte) numbers: −32,768 to 32,767, and
  long, for signed 32-bit (4 byte) numbers: 2,147,483,648 to 2,147,483,647.

- A variant variable stores any type of data the procedure might generate. This multipurpose variable trades storage efficiency for flexibility.

A VBA statement to create a variable starts with the keyword Dim. For example, "Dim BirthDate as Date" creates a Date variable called BirthDate.

VBA objects and syntax

VBA has its own kinds of objects, different from Access database objects. One frequently used VBA object is the DoCmd object, which used to *do* something with an Access object. Each VBA object has a variety of methods it can perform. For example, DoCmd.OpenForm "frmSearchNICUAdmits" opens the Access form named within the quotes. The dot following DoCmd indicates that what follows is a method. If you write VBA code you must become familiar with the syntax for the method you want an object to perform. However, you need not memorize the syntax requirements.

The IDE provides a feature called Intellesense that prompts you with the appropriate syntax choices as you type. Try it out: select the modules objects in the database window, and then click **New** at the top of the database window. The IDE opens along with a new window in the main editor (Fig. 12.4). The first line, Option Compare Database, tells Access to use the same rules for comparing strings (text, remember?) as it does when sorting such data in the database itself. The second line, Option Explicit, represents an option you can set for the IDE (**Tools**, **Options . . .**, **Editor** tab, select **Require Variable Declaration**). It forces you to declare explicitly any variable you use in code. This tends to prevent problems stemming from a misspelled variable name. After those automatically entered lines, I typed the name of the subroutine:

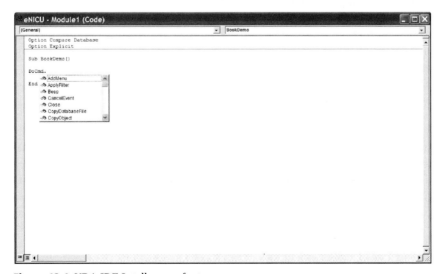

Figure 12.4 VBA IDE Intellesense feature.

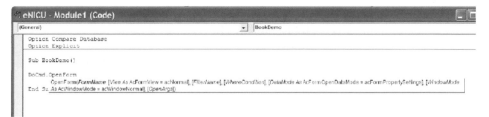

Figure 12.5 VBA IDE Intellesense feature.

BookDemo. I then pressed the **Enter** key: the last line of code shown in Fig. 12.4 (End Sub – partially obscured) was automatically entered too.

I next typed a VBA object name and a dot to indicate that the method followed. Immediately, the drop-down list in Fig. 12.4 appeared. Intellesense gave me the list of available methods for the DoCmd object. I scrolled down the list until I found the method I wanted (OpenForm in this case) and selected it. Again, Intellesense anticipated my need: it displayed the syntax and parameters to execute the OpenForm method (Fig. 12.5).

VBA code to change a property at run time

The preceding three sections provide something akin to taking a 60-second tour of London. Even so, you have learned enough to return to the programming problem set out earlier in this chapter: changing an object's property only if a certain condition is met; otherwise, that property remains in its default condition. In particular, how shall a database application handle a change in a person's last name? Let's examine how I solved this problem in eNICU.

tblInfants originally had one field to store a patient's last name: LastName. Rather than a name update entail information loss by replacing the old name, I decided the update should entail information gain. I therefore added a new field to tblInfants: NewLastName. All the reports, of course, already had a control to display an infant's last name. Adding a field for NewLastName addresses the data storage problem but not the data display problem. After a last name is changed, people working with a report may no longer care what the last name used to be.

In each report design, I created a NewLastName control and placed it directly over the LastName control. Look carefully at the upper portion of the Report Header section for the Discharge Note report in Fig. 12.6. You can easily read the LastName label control (in italics), but the text box control immediately to the right looks messy. The text box controls txtLastName and txtNewLastName (each in bold font) are superimposed. Let's take a moment to look at what this strategy achieves, because it will help you understand the rest of this exposition. Notice in Fig. 11.21a that the last name in both the header section and footer section reads "New Last Name." Remember, I said that I used "dummy" data to compose that report in order to demonstrate specific points. This "dummy" patient's original last name was "Test3." The first time I

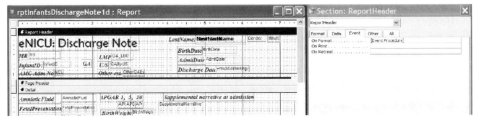

Figure 12.6 Discharge Note report header and property sheet.

hot-synced the original data about this "patient" and created a discharge note report, the last name in the header and footer read "Test3." I then updated this record on my handheld device by entering "New Last Name" in the "New last name" field of the Infants form. I hot-synced again.

Thanks to some VBA event-driven code, the patient last name displayed in the newly created discharge note report changed to "New Last Name." Figure 12.6 indicates this report contains an event procedure that is triggered by the On Format event for the Report Header. The On Format event occurs while Access identifies the data that will appear in the report section but before Access actually formats the section for printing or previewing on the computer screen. The Page Footer section contains a similar event procedure. Figure 12.7 shows the VBA code for each of these events in the main editor screen of the IDE. The code for the Page Footer is essentially the same, only I kept unchanged the name that Access gave to the text box control for last name when I created it with an Access wizard (Text109). Let's work, line

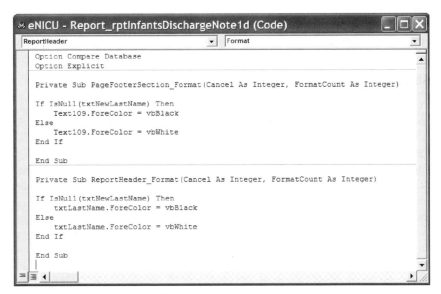

```
Option Compare Database
Option Explicit

Private Sub PageFooterSection_Format(Cancel As Integer, FormatCount As Integer)

If IsNull(txtNewLastName) Then
     Text109.ForeColor = vbBlack
Else
     Text109.ForeColor = vbWhite
End If

End Sub

Private Sub ReportHeader_Format(Cancel As Integer, FormatCount As Integer)

If IsNull(txtNewLastName) Then
     txtLastName.ForeColor = vbBlack
Else
     txtLastName.ForeColor = vbWhite
End If

End Sub
```

Figure 12.7 Code that deals with a change in name.

by line, through the code triggered by the On Format event for the Report Header.

1 **Private Sub ReportHeader_Format(Cancel As Integer, FormatCount As Integer)**   This is a procedure (subroutine) that is restricted to this report object. If code elsewhere called on instructions in this sub routine, the reference would be to the name of this sub: ReportHeader_Format. The words in parenthesis represent parameters, conditions for executing the routine. By the way, often a pair of empty parentheses appears at the end of a subname, as in Fig. 12.5: "Sub BookDemo()." Empty parentheses indicate no relevant parameters apply.

2 **If   IsNull(txtNewLastName)   Then   txtLastName.ForeColor   = vbBlack**   Check if txtNewLastName control contains data. If it is empty (IsNull), then set the ForeColor property of the txtLastName control to black (colors in VBA are generally set with a number, but VBA represents a few commonly used colors by names that are converted at run time to the correct number).

3 **Else**   Otherwise (i.e. if txtNewLastName contains data) **txtLastName. ForeColor = vbWhite**   Set the ForeColor property of txtLastName to white.

4 **End If**   We have arrived at the end of the conditional decision making routine that began with element 2, above.

5 **End Sub**   This subroutine is finished.

In summary, this VBA subroutine displays the letters of the original last name in white when the New Last Name field of a given record contains an entry. Conveniently, in my NICU we print discharge notes using black ink on white paper, so when the value of New Last Name is not null, *only* the new last name is legible on the report. Of course, when the value of New Last Name is null, no superimposition of data occurs on the report. I adapted this simple, effective method to preserve data and minimize confusion from Ref. 63.

SQL and queries

The graphical query design tool in Access generally does a good job translating your query matrix into SQL. However, occasionally answering a seemingly straightforward question is beyond what the Access query design tool can handle. Sometimes to get the answer table you seek, you need to run a query and input the result to a second query. An illustration follows soon. Other times you need to tweak the SQL code the design grid created. For example, suppose you want a list of all diagnoses made during a given year. In translating the design grid you set up, Access will probably create a SQL SELECT statement (see Select Query in the section following) that yields the information you desire but also probably includes repeat values: if 35 patients that year had BPD, then BPD appears 35 times in the answer table. The remedy is trivial: insert the word DISTINCT after SELECT, and the answer table will have no redundant values. The point is that you must broadly understand SQL syntax and execution to identify circumstances that require special constructions.

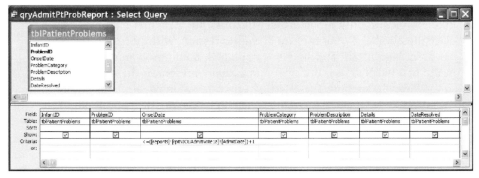

Figure 12.8 qryAdmitPtProbReport: design view.

Another reason to become familiar with SQL is that various software applications use SQL to transfer data. "Power users" of Pendragon Forms (or Intellisync MobileApp Designer,[68] formerly known as Satellite Forms – another database development application) know that the detailed instructions for data transfer during hot sync are written in SQL. The Stata[18] statistical software package that we work with in Part II of this book uses SQL code to create an analytical data set from one or more database tables.

Parameter queries

We now examine the eNICU query that populates the subreport displaying patient problems (rsubAdmitPtProblemsGrouped) on the NICU Admission Note (rptNICUAdmitNote1a). The name of this query is qryAdmitPtProbReport. Figure 12.8 shows the design view and Fig. 12.9 shows the SQL code created by the design tool.

This query is a basic select query with some sophistication in the selection criterion. The query doesn't specify a value for InfantID, because the subreport it populates is synchronized with rptNICUAdmitNote1a on the basis of the InfantID selected for rptNICUAdmitNote1a. The "Link Child Fields" and "Link Master Fields" properties are set to the same field, InfantID. Thus, Access supplies the value for the InfantID criterion at run time. The expression in the criteria field for OnsetDate accounts for the occasional need to print an admit note well after the infant was actually admitted. This selection criterion filters out patient problems with onset more than 1 day after admission. Let's examine this selection criterion:

<=([reports]![rptNICUAdmitNote1a]![AdmitDate])+1

This expression specifies the value in a control on a particular database object. It specifies a value less than or equal to the value of the AdmitDate field of

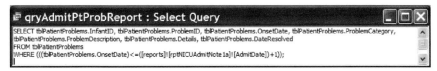

Figure 12.9 qryAdmitPtProbReport: SQL view.

the report object called rptNICUAdmitNote1a. If you prefer that the admission note enumerate only problems identified within 12 hours of admission, replace the number "1," at the end of the expression, with "0.5." Any selection cut-point is arbitrary and involves trade-offs. Some problems develop later in the first hospital day, but were not actually present at the time of admission. However, suppose the selection criterion value equaled AdmitDate. In the workflow sequence, this value gets entered before data about admission problems. Now, although the field is called AdmitDate, the data include time – with 1-second precision. Therefore, all admission problems occur after the value of AdmitDate and would be excluded. Further, some infants are admitted close to midnight and by the time you print the admission note it's the next day. This issue is but one example of why you must think about *exactly what it is you want to accomplish with an admission note, or any other report.*

Let's return to frmSearchNICUAdmits (Figs. 11.10–11.19 and associated text). In Chapter 11, we looked at how the form came up with InfantID values associated with the entered last name. Now we examine how a parameter query running within this form provides the selection criterion for the query that populates the admission note report (rptNICUAdmitNote1a). A basic parameter query asks the user at run time for selection criteria. For example, if the user is to specify a patient's InfantID value, enter the following in the appropriate criteria field of the design grid: [Please enter this patient's InfantID:]. When the query runs but before it can produce an answer table, it presents the user with the screen shown in Fig. 12.10. The query then uses the data the user enters in this dialog box as the selection criterion for running the query. In contrast, the kind of parameter query embedded in our form contains information about *where to look* for the criteria that are set at run time.

The query populating rptNICUAdmitNote1a is qryInfantsAdmitNote. A portion of that query design grid appears in Fig. 12.11. The query selects data from many more fields than are pictured; for our purpose we need focus only on one: InfantID. The selection criterion for that field: [forms]![frmSearchNICUAdmits]![InfantID] tells the query *where to look* to get the criterion value for running the query. The code says to use as the selection criterion the value currently entered in the InfantID field on the form object called frmSearchNICUAdmits. The user must still supply the selection criterion at run time. This approach, I think, represents most users' mental models of an automated information system, that is, users typically don't think in terms of

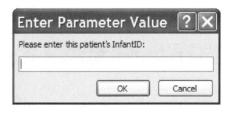

Figure 12.10 Parameter query user request.

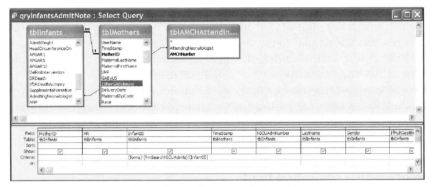

Figure 12.11 A portion of qryInfantsAdmitNote: design view.

queries, forms, and reports. More likely, they think "OK, here's the name of the infant I just admitted. When I press the button, print *this* infant's admit note."

Range query

Figure 12.12 shows a portion of qryDailyProgressNoteByDate. This query (obviously another parameter query) selects data to populate a progress note report for each infant that a physician visited on daily morning rounds. Focus on the field "Date: (DateTime1)." The selection criteria for this field is rather complicated: "Between

([forms]![frmSearchDPNbyDate]![ActiveXCtl14]) And

([forms]![frmSearchDPNbyDate]![ActiveXCtl14])+0.9"

Most of this notation you've seen before. ActiveXCtl14 refers to an "ActiveX" control. ActiveX controls are "goodies" (Access features not necessarily supplied by Microsoft®) that add functionality to an application. ActiveXCtl14 is what Access named the calendar control I placed on the search form that supports the parameter query populating the daily progress note report

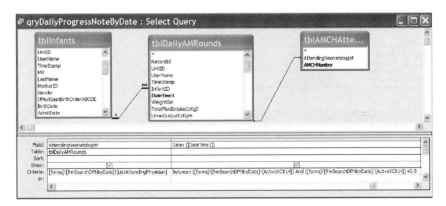

Figure 12.12 A portion of qryDailyProgressNoteByDate.

(rptDailyProgressNoteByDate). Ref. 64 provides details about how to work with this calendar control. For our purpose, you need only know that the user has set the calendar to the desired date (actually, it's programmed to display the current date as a default value, so usually the user doesn't need to set it at all). The "Date: (DateTime1)" field selection criteria instruct Access to select records with a value of DateTime1 that lies between the date indicated on the ActiveX calendar control and that date plus 0.9 days (another arbitrary cut-point). Range criteria start with the word "Between" and require the word "And" to demarcate the upper and lower boundaries.

Query with a computed field

Figure 12.13 shows a small portion of qryInfantsAdmitNote. GA_LMP is a computed field. A colon after the field name designates it as a computed field; the information following the colon specifies the computation. Computing (DateDiff("d",[LMP],[BirthDate]))/7 yields an infant's gestational age based on the date of the mother's last menstrual period ([LMP]). In discussing normalized database design (Chapter 8), I said you don't want a table to contain a field that can be derived from data in other fields. We do exactly that in a query with a computed field: derive a value we want from the necessary base elements. Let's examine the specific computational instruction, (DateDiff("d",[LMP],[BirthDate]))/7, step by step.

DateDiff is a SQL function that computes the difference between two date values. The parentheses contain the function parameters: "d" means express the result in days; [LMP] means use the value of the date in the LMP field as the quantity to be subtracted; [BirthDate] means use the value of the

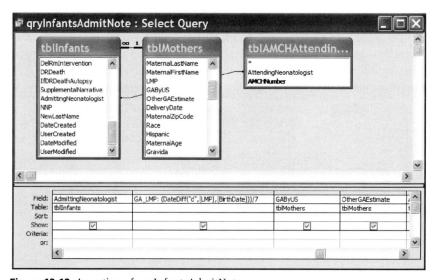

Figure 12.13 A portion of qryInfantsAdmitNote.

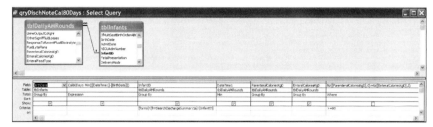

Figure 12.14 Aggregate query: first of two components.

date in the BirthDate field as the quantity from which to subtract the LMP value. Next, notice the parentheses enclosing the SQL expression (DateDiff ("d",[LMP],[BirthDate])) followed by: /7. This means divide the result of the expression contained by the outer parentheses by the number 7.

Aggregate queries and sequential queries

Here we examine an example of the two-stage query I mentioned earlier. The eNICU discharge summary report (rptInfantsDischargeNote1b) summarizes various care process exposures. One such element provides the answer to the question: "How many days elapsed after admission until the infant's caloric intake was at least 80 kcal/kg/day?"

Each component of the two-stage query (Figs. 12.14 and 12.17) populating this element is itself an aggregate query. Notice that the lower half of the design grid in Fig. 12.14 looks different from previous illustrations. The grid contains an additional row, Total, inserted between the Table and Sort rows. To convert a select query design grid to an aggregate query, click the **Toolbar** button shown in Fig. 12.15. Clicking in the Total field of a column activates a drop-down list of aggregation choices for the values of that field.

The rightmost column in Fig. 12.14 uses a computed field to establish the main selection criterion: Nz([ParenteralCaloriesKgD],0)+Nz([Enteral-CaloriesKgD],0) must be >80. This notation involves another SQL function, called Nz. The Nz function tries to resolve the ambiguity that null values create. A null value is not the same as a data value of zero; null means *no* data. If no data are entered in the field for ParenteralCaloriesKgD, that *may* mean zero, but perhaps the user simply forgot to enter the actual value. This is the point of setting fields to require a value be entered. Anyway, the parameters of the function specify the field upon which it operates and the value to substitute when it encounters a null value (0, in this case). Thus, this column instructs Access to select records if the sum of the parenteral and enteral caloric intake exceeds 80.

Figure 12.15 Aggregate query toolbar button.

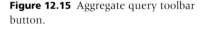

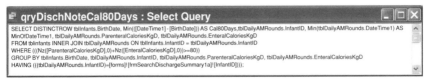

Figure 12.16 Aggregate query: first of two components (SQL view).

The second column from the left in Fig. 12.14, Cal80Days: Min(([DateTime1]-[BirthDate])), computes the minimum number of days before a patient met the criterion we just reviewed. You might think that running this query answers the main question: "How many days elapsed after admission until this infant's caloric intake was at least 80 kcal/kg/day?" But because of how SQL selects a subset, you haven't answered *this* question.

When you set up an aggregate query, Access sets the value in the Total row to **Group By**. A drop-down list in each row cell allows you to change the value to something else, but the other choices may not be suitable to your purpose. In Fig. 12.14, Group By ParenteralCaloriesKgD and Group By EnteralCaloriesKgD mean when the query runs it will create a cross tabulation, that is, a list containing the minimum number of days it took to meet the >80 calories selection criterion, *grouped by* ParenteralCaloriesKgD and by EnteralCaloriesKgD. Therefore, often the answer table will contain more than one value. Often the table will contain multiple values because the answer is grouped according to distinct values in these grouping fields. The question you *actually* answer with this query is, "For *each distinct* value of BirthDate, InfantID, ParenteralCaloriesKgD, and EnteralCaloriesKgD where the sum of parenteral and enteral caloric intake was >80, what was the minimum value of DateTime1 (i.e. the date the selection criterion was met)?" As an exercise, try to appreciate how the SQL code shown in Fig. 12.16, corresponding to the query in Fig. 12.14, specifies what I just tried to explain.

This is why we need a second query, that is, to reduce the first answer table to a one-row answer, representing the lowest (minimum) of the usually several values for the column, Cal80Days: Min(([DateTime1]-[BirthDate])). This time, we group by InfantID, for which there is only one value per patient (Fig. 12.17). This second query asks, "What is the minimum value of Cal80Days, grouped by InfantID, in the answer table produced by query qryDischNoteCal80Days?"

The point is that knowing the question you need to answer may be insufficient to get the query design grid formulation to answer it for you. By understanding how SQL goes about obtaining the answer set, you can identify situations that require you to decompose your main question into sequential components congruent with the SQL operational sequence.

Action queries

Action queries in eNICU operate primarily for data transfer from the Pendragon Forms application to the Access application during hot syncing. The

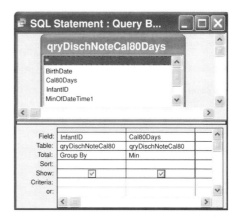

Figure 12.17 Aggregate query:
second of two components.

Pendragon Forms application takes care of this automatically, shielding you from direct involvement with the SQL code. To illustrate some aspects of action queries in Access, I created a couple of database objects in eNICU; these objects serve this didactic function only. In Chapter 11, we explored a way to handle a name change for an infant already entered in the database. Recall, a name update was to add data, not delete data (i.e.\ the old name); thus, a new field is added to tblInfants: NewLastName.

I share with you my first solution to the name change problem, one which I subsequently abandoned for using in eNICU. This solution entails updating the data in the LastName field by writing *over* the previous data, thereby losing it. To save development time, I started with a copy of the search form that I used to create an admission note, frmSearchNICUAdmits, to create frmInfant-NameUpdate (Fig. 12.18). The first two text box controls are the same as on frmSearchNICUAdmits. The third text box is new; here the user enters the infant's new last name. The command button below the new last name field also is new. Here is the VBA code that runs when a user clicks the button:

```
Private Sub cmdInfantNameUpdate_Click()
On Error GoTo Err_cmdInfantNameUpdate_Click

Dim stDocName As String

stDocName = "qupdInfantNameUpdate"
DoCmd.OpenQuery stDocName, acNormal, acEdit

Exit_cmdInfantNameUpdate_Click:
Exit Sub

cmdInfantNameUpdate_Click:
MsgBox Err.Description
Resume Exit_cmdInfantNameUpdate_Click

End Sub
```

Figure 12.18 frmInfantNameUpdate.

This procedure is similar to ones you've already seen. There are two new items:

1 In the fourth line of code, stDocName = "qupdInfantNameUpdate"; I use a new database object tag here: qupd, denoting an update query.

2 The DoCmd object uses a new method, the OpenQuery method; this does what it says.

Figure 12.19 shows qupdInfantNameUpdate. The criteria row instructs the query where to obtain the user-entered record selection criteria. In this case,

Figure 12.19 qupdInfantNameUpdate.

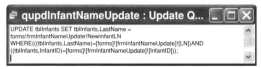

Figure 12.20 qupdInfantNameUpdate: SQL view.

the data are located in the LastName and InfantID fields of frmInfantName-Update. The **Update To:** row instructs Access to update the data currently in the LastName field of the record identified by the InfantID value specified in frmInfantNameUpdate, and replace it with the data currently in the NewIn-fantLN field of frmInfantNameUpdate. Figure 12.20 shows the corresponding SQL code.

Writing program code requires scrupulous attention to detail

I said that Pendragon Forms usually takes care of the action queries involved in data transfer during hot sync without the user's direct involvement. However, when I created the eNICU handheld form called Loose Ends, I did have to poke around in the SQL code controlling data transfer.

The Loose Ends form represents a "to do" list. To identify records that no longer need to remain on the handheld, the user selects the box in the **Done** field. This was the only form in the application that contained a check box completion field, and coincidentally, this was the only form that gave me an error message in the hot sync log:

> Pendragon Forms (v.3.2.00) synchronization started at 02/04/03 14:31:59 Unable to execute downlink SQL Form 'Loose Ends' (229100075) selectU-nitID,[TimeStamp],UserName,LastName,MRNumber,InfantID, IfMultGestBirth OrderABCDE,ItemID,Category,ToDoDetails,Done from tblLooseEnds where (Done = null or Done <> "Y") and UserName = 'Joseph Schulman' [Microsoft] [ODBC Microsoft Access Driver] Too few parameters. Expected 1. OK Pendragon Forms with 1 message(s)

Embedded in this message is a SQL string very similar to the one that follows, which I copied from the Advanced Mapping Properties window for the version of the Loose Ends form that has no synchronization problems:

> SELECTUnitID,[TimeStamp],UserName,LastName,MRNumber, InfantID, IfMult GestBirthOrderABCDE,ItemID,Category, ToDoDetails,Done from tblLooseEnds where (Done is null or Done <> 'Y')

One difference between the two SQL strings is worth a digression. The string in the error message concludes with: *and UserName = 'Joseph Schulman'*. I removed those words when I moved from a version that only I used to a version my colleagues also used. By including those words in the early version, only records in which the UserName field matched the handheld user name were sent to the handheld. In a multiuser situation, users could not share records. Deleting the UserName = ##USERNAME## statement allowed record sharing (see Pendragon Forms Manual).

Let's return to tracing the source of the error message in my hot sync log. It was rather subtle. Several dialects of SQL exist, of varying suitability for a particular database development application. Pendragon Forms created the SQL string in a dialect that recognized a completed check box by the letter Y (for "Yes") surrounded by *double* quotes. But my version of Access did not recognize the way the dialect used by Pendragon Forms handled a completed check box. My version of Access demanded the letter Y be surrounded by *single quotes*. Replacing Done <> "Y" with Done <> 'Y' eliminated the error message.

Microsoft's online help includes a three-tiered introduction to writing SQL code in Access. At least, have a look at the introduction to the topic.[69]

CHAPTER 13

Turning ideas into a useful tool: eNICU, point of care database software for the NICU

This chapter introduces you to working with eNICU, the database software application provided with this book. I tried to design this application so that learning to use it and working with it from a user's perspective would be largely self-explanatory. I agree with Donald Norman, a renowned design expert, who asserts that a product that depends on a large instruction manual is a design failure.[70] Likewise, a software application ought to contain in its user interface most of the necessary information to use it correctly. Following Cooper, I designed the application for intermediate level users rather than for beginners.[71] He argues that software applications should be designed like ski resorts, which optimize their facilities not for beginners but for skiers with intermediate skill levels. These people will find the prospects challenging, but with diligent effort can master the terrain. Otherwise, the application (or the slopes) seems trivial and boring to those who use it day after day.

Handheld use

I assume that you

1 use a device running Palm OS® 4.0 or higher, or Microsoft© Windows Mobile 2003™ or higher; I leave hot sync, device protection, and data encryption details to the documentation supplied with your handheld device.
   - For many forms, Windows Mobile 2003 devices show fewer fields per screen, but operate substantially the same. Please refer to Pendragon Forms documentation for specifics.
2 have already installed Pendragon Forms and the eNICU form designs on your computer (instructions on accompanying CD).

   Check that the upper right portion of the home screen on your handheld device displays the word **All**. Tap the Forms 5.0 icon; the graphical **eNICU New Record MENU** opens. It spans three screens, so scroll down to see Figs. 13.1–13.3. **New Record MENU** means that tapping on any category except **All Forms and Records** creates a *new* record, a new row in the corresponding database table. Tapping on **All Forms and Records** allows you to review a record previously created.

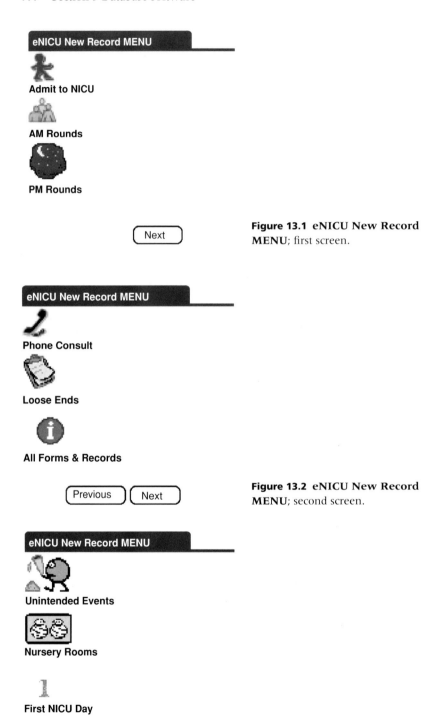

Figure 13.1 eNICU New Record MENU; first screen.

Figure 13.2 eNICU New Record MENU; second screen.

Figure 13.3 eNICU New Record MENU; third screen.

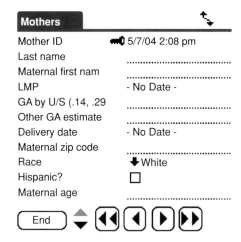

Figure 13.4 Mothers form; new record, first screen.

Skill: create a new record (admit a new patient)

We first examine how to create a new record and then how to review or modify an existing record. The method to enter data is similar for each type of new record; to illustrate, let's admit an infant to the NICU. Tap the screen over the text **Admit to NICU** or the associated icon.

The program creates a new record on **Mothers**, the parent form (Fig. 13.4). The double headed arrow at the upper right indicates this form is linked to another. Pendragon Forms considers the **New Record MENU** as a parent form (only temporarily, however); but in general the link will connect the displayed record to its parent record. Examples follow shortly. Anyway, tap in a blank field to activate the cursor and start to enter data. For date/time fields, tap where it says **- No Date -** to open a calendar (Fig. 13.5); tap the

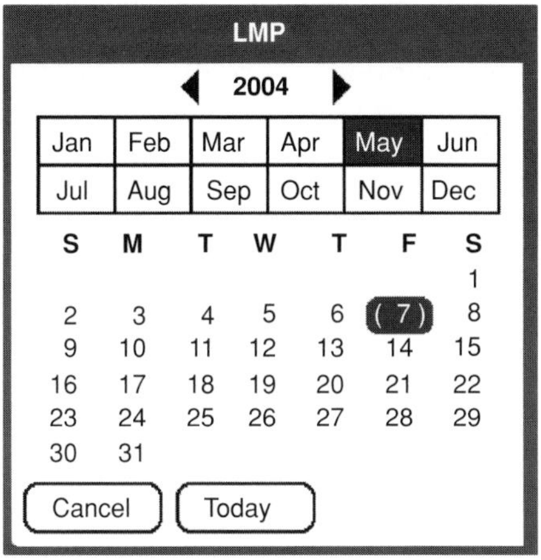

Figure 13.5 Date/Time field calendar.

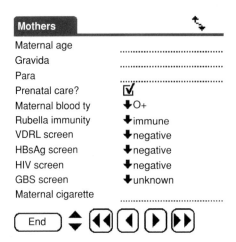

Figure 13.6 Mothers form; new record, second screen.

appropriate month and day (scroll to the desired year). Some field names exceed the allotted screen width. Tap the field *name* to switch to field view; now one field fills the entire screen. This is useful, for example, when entering gestational age by U/S (determined by prenatal ultrasonography); the decimal numbers in parentheses remind the user of fractional week equivalents. Also, for numerical fields like this one, using the displayed (in field view) numerical touch pad can speed data entry. A downward pointing arrow in a field denotes pop-up list choices. If one of the choices already appears, in the Race field, for example, then a default value was set. In eNICU, defaults reflect the most likely choice in the author's work setting. A check box field, such as "Hispanic?," means "no" if blank and "yes" if selected.

At the bottom of Fig. 13.4 notice the gray arrow pointing upward and the black arrow pointing downward, next to the **End** button. This indicates that no screens precede this one for this form, but one or more screens follow. Scroll down to the next screen (Fig. 13.6). Both arrows at the bottom of the screen are black, so continue to scroll (Fig. 13.7). Here you see two new field types. The symbols on the right side of the fourth field from the top, next to **Perinatal Complications**, indicate a subform field.

Subform fields

Tapping on the subform field opens an interface that allows you to (a) review existing child records (i.e. prenatal complications already entered, not records about children) in the subform **Maternal Complications** and (b) open a new linked **child** record in that subform. Figure 13.8 shows how this subform interface appears when no child records have been created yet. To create a new record (a maternal complication) tap the **Add** button in the lower left of the screen. A screen similar to that in Fig. 13.9 appears.

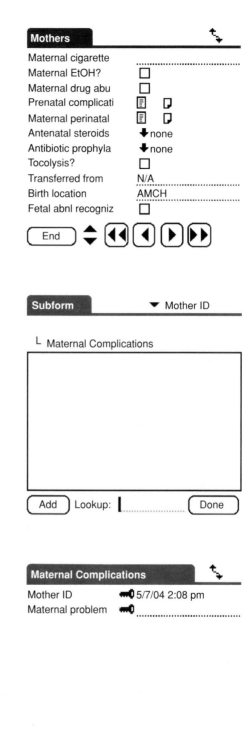

Figure 13.7 Mothers form; new record, third screen.

Figure 13.8 Maternal Complications subform interface when no child records have been created yet.

Figure 13.9 Maternal Complications (sub)form; new record.

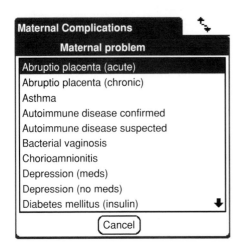

Figure 13.10 Maternal Complications look-up list; first screen.

Tap in the blank field and a look-up list appears (Fig. 13.10). (Thus, tapping in a blank field results in one of two responses. If it is a text entry field, a flashing cursor appears. If it is a look-up list field, the list appears. Note also, that some look-up list fields, like "Transferred from" or "Birth location" shown in Fig. 13.7, are set to display a default value when the new record opens. Simply tap the default value to see all the choices.) Tap the appropriate choice to return to the previous screen; your choice now appears in the field. For any look-up list field, if no item on the list is suitable, tap the **Cancel** button at the bottom of the look-up list display to return to record view, and then tap in the field name area rather than the data entry area. This will again open the look-up list, but now when you tap the **Cancel** button you go to a field view that allows you to enter exactly what you desire. Tap the **Record View** button to return to the screen display that shows up to 11 fields per screen.

After entering all your data, tap the **End** button at the lower left to return to the interface in Fig. 13.8. If you want to create another record (mother had more than one complication), tap the **Add** button again and repeat the procedure. After entering all the child records, tap the **Done** button in the lower right to return to where you left off in the parent (**Mothers**) form. At the bottom of Fig. 13.7, the downward pointing arrow is still black, indicating that more fields reside on this form. Scroll down to see a screen similar to that in Fig. 13.11.

In Fig. 13.11, the downward pointing arrow on the bottom of the screen is gray: you can scroll no further. *Important*: tap the **End** button only upon your *return* to this screen, *after entering data in all subforms subordinate to this parent form; including the subform(s) relating to this mother's infant(s)* (note the subform link, Infant information, Fig. 13.11). If you tap the **End** button before you

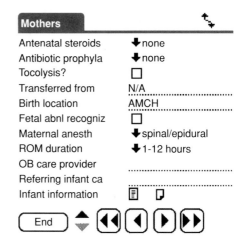

Figure 13.11 Mothers form; new record, final screen.

complete *all* data entry relevant to this record, to return to this record tap **All Forms and Records**, then tap **Mothers**, and locate your record. Tapping **Admit to NICU** will open a completely new record. If you accidentally do this, do not merely tap the **End** button; this only closes, and does not delete, the accidentally created record. To delete it, tap the **Mothers** tab at the upper left of the screen, then tap **Record**, and then tap **Delete**.

The interface for the **Infants** subform (child form) is analogous to the one we reviewed in Fig. 13.8. If this mother had a multiple gestation, after entering the data for the first infant and returning to the **Infants** subform interface screen, you would tap the **Add** button in the lower left to create another infant record – a real time saver when admitting twins, triplets, etc. In any case, after you tap the **Add** button you'll see a screen similar to that in Fig. 13.12.

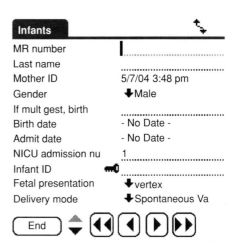

Figure 13.12 Infants (sub)form; new record, first screen.

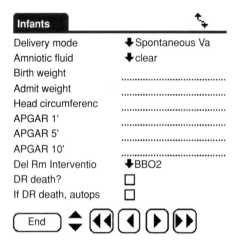

Figure 13.13 Infants (sub)form; new record, second screen.

   The first field of the **Infants** form asks for the medical record number; in my hospital this number serves as the unique identifier for a particular patient. The eighth field asks for the admission number (first admission = 1, readmission = 2 or higher). Tapping in field nine concatenates fields 1 and 8 to create Infant ID, the unique identifier for a particular *hospitalization*. A key icon appears to the left of the Infant ID value (you may have noticed this icon in some of the previous screens). This icon indicates a primary key field. Note that in what follows, field number refers to the position from the top of the displayed screen, not the sequential field number in the entire form.

   Figure 13.13 shows the second screen for the **Infants** form; no new field types here. Figure 13.14 shows the third screen.

   The fourth field in Fig. 13.14 is another subform link field, but this icon looks different from previously considered subform links. This new icon identifies a

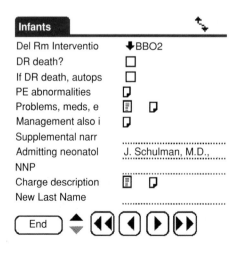

Figure 13.14 Infants (sub)form; new record, third screen.

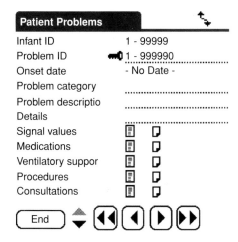

Figure 13.15 Patient Problems
(sub)form; new record, first screen.

"single subform" field, allowing you to create only a single child record. This is how Pendragon Forms implements a one-to-one relationship (Chapter 10). Since you can create only one child record, there is no need for the subform interface as in Fig. 13.8. Tapping on a single subform field takes you directly to the single linked child record, and tapping the **End** button in that record returns you to the parent record. The child record created via Field 4 records abnormalities on the admission physical exam.

The next field links to the **Patient Problems** subform. This important structure contains additional nested child forms. You first access the **Patient Problems** subform when admitting an infant, and continue to access the same structure when creating new records during daily rounds and when tying things together before discharge.

Figure 13.15 shows all but Field 12 in the **Patient Problems** form; Field 12 is near the bottom of Fig. 13.16. Field 4, Problem category, is a look-up

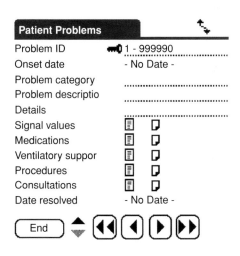

Figure 13.16 Patient Problems
(sub)form; new record, second screen.

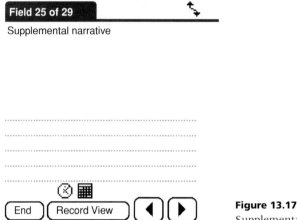

Figure 13.17 Field view; Supplemental narrative field.

list field. For each category you select in Field 4, a different set of look-up list choices becomes available to you in Field 5, Problem description. For example, if you select the Infection Problem category, one of your many choices in Field 5 will be "sepsis suspected, <72 hrs." Take some time to explore both of these lists. Field 6, Details, invites additional descriptive free text. The next field, Signal values, a (nested) subform field, takes you to a subform to record measurement values that signal the problem – or enter multiple values (i.e. create multiple records) to indicate this measurement's trajectory. The four fields that follow are analogous; they deal with Medications, Ventilatory support, Procedures, and Consultations. Each contains look-up lists with which you must become familiar. When a problem is resolved (typically, after creating the admission note; during subsequent daily a.m. rounds), remember to enter the Date resolved to ensure an accurate discharge note.

Let's return to Fig. 13.14. Field 7 allows a supplemental narrative. To write more than one line of text, tap the field name to switch to field view (Fig. 13.17). You can enter 250 characters here. The penultimate field, Charge description, takes you to a subform that reflects professional service charges in the author's practice setting. Finally, because sometimes infants' last names change, the final field allows you to record that information. That's basically all there is to collecting the data for a newly admitted infant.

Assign to specific room

My NICU is divided into several rooms; the **Nursery Rooms** choice in Fig. 13.3 takes you to a form to record which room an infant is in. This information is used to group patients on a sign-out summary report. Figure 13.18 shows the **Nursery Rooms** screen. To speed data entry, this and several other forms provide you with a list of patients to choose from. Tap in the Infant ID field

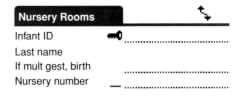

Nursery Rooms

Infant ID 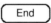 ....
Last name
If mult gest, birth   ....
Nursery number   — ....

Figure 13.18 Nursery Rooms form;   (End)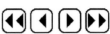
new record.

to see a list of Infant ID numbers stored in the handheld database. Select the appropriate one and the other fields automatically become filled with the corresponding information, leaving you only to enter the Nursery number (in my NICU, 1–7). This same look-up feature also operates on the forms for a.m. Rounds, PM Rounds, Loose Ends, Unintended Events, and First NICU Day.

First day data

The **First NICU Day** form (not shown) captures information for CRIB score risk adjustment[72] and time (# hours; # minutes) of first surfactant dose, as collected by the Vermont Oxford Network (http://www.vtoxford.org/, accessed May 11, 2004).

Additional menu choices

Referring to Fig. 13.2, **Phone Consult** is a form to record data about infants not (yet) on your clinical service, for whom you provide consultative support. **Loose Ends** is a "to do" list. You may access it from the rounds forms or directly. **All Forms & Records** takes you away from the graphical new record interface to the complete list of all 24 forms that constitute eNICU on the handheld. The list spans three screens and is shown in Figs. 13.19–13.21.

Skill: review an existing record

Form names with an icon beside them that looks like a page with some lines on it may be accessed either to review an existing record or to create a new record. Forms with an icon beside them that looks like a page with the lower right corner turned up may be accessed only to review an existing record, and not create a new one. This limitation ensures coherent record linkage. These limited forms are actually subforms, containing child records. You would not

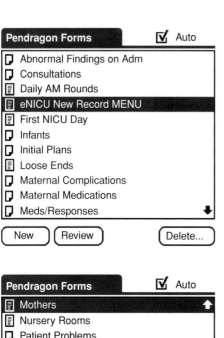

Figure 13.19 List of all forms and records; first screen.

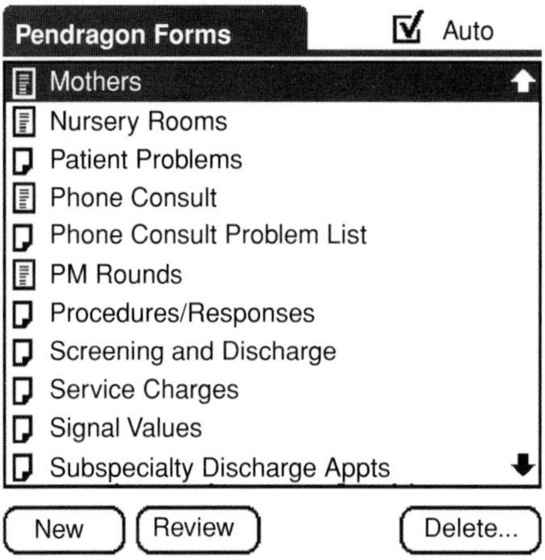

Figure 13.20 List of all forms and records; second screen.

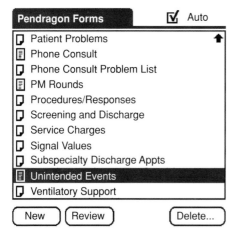

Figure 13.21 List of all forms and records; third screen.

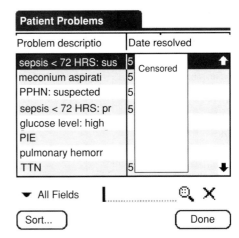

Figure 13.22 A list of patient problems with one accompanying field.

want to create a new record directly from one of these because it would be an "orphan," unlinked to a parent record. eNICU requires that a record on a subform be a child record to a record on a parent form.

Anyway, tap the **Review** button after highlighting a form name to see a list of current records on the handheld. Each form has been programmed to keep records on the handheld for a finite amount of time (see Pendragon Forms Manual[51]). For example, records on Infants are kept on the handheld for 180 days. Thus, when you tap in a field that looks up Infant ID numbers, you may see more records than just current patients, but only those in the past 6 months of use, not all patients ever admitted.

To help find the record you want, you'll probably need to adjust the field display. Figure 13.22 shows some of the **Patient Problems** records on my handheld. The first time I looked at this list, the display showed only the Problem description field. Often you want to see more than that. You may, for example, want to see which problems are still active. You can adjust the display to show you that. Notice in Fig. 13.22 the thin horizontal line below the **Patient Problems** header tab. When only one field is displayed, two very short lines project downward from this horizontal line, to the right of the displayed field name. Tap in that region to see a drop-down list of all fields on that form. The first time I tried this, I tapped on the Date resolved field and the display shown in Fig. 13.22 appeared. Records with no date are active problems.

Notice in Fig. 13.22 that just below the header there is still one small line projecting downward (above the "e" of the word resolved). I tapped in that area and selected the Infant ID field, and the display shown in Fig. 13.23 appeared. Now I could identify active problems for a particular infant. However, the Date resolved field now is too narrow. Place the stylus over the line demarcating two fields; drag it to change the field width (see Fig. 13.24).

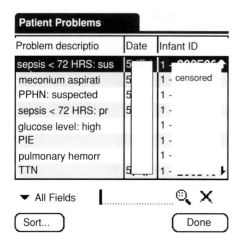

Figure 13.23 A list of patient problems with two accompanying fields (three fields total).

Skill: returning to the graphical MENU

How do you return to the graphical **eNICU New Record MENU** from the list of all forms? Simple: in the form list, select **eNICU New Record MENU** and tap the "Review" button. Unlike all other forms, you only need one record in this form, namely the graphical interface in Figs 13.1–13.3. This solitary record has no unique identifier. That is why the review screen displays one highlighted bar containing no identifying information. Tap the solitary highlighted bar to return to the graphical interface. Note that if after selecting the form name **eNICU New Record MENU** by mistake you tapped the **New** button instead of the **Review** button, you would create another record. Thus, if you see multiple bars in the review window for this form, you have inadvertently created unnecessary duplicate records. Since you need only one, delete any

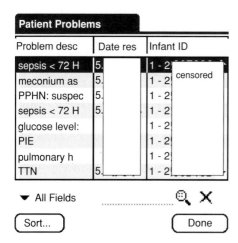

Figure 13.24 Changing the proportional size of the three displayed fields.

extras; in the review window, tap one of the extra bars, then tap the **eNICU New Record MENU** tab at the top of the screen, next tap **Record**, and select **Delete**; repeat until only one bar remains.

PC data management

In this section, I assume that you have collected data on your handheld device, synchronized the device with your PC, and have opened the eNICU Access application on your PC.

We have seen how to review eNICU data stored on the handheld device. However, the handheld device limits how much you can *manipulate* the data. Except for flexible sorting order, the data configuration you see pretty much is the data configuration you entered. Handhelds excel at *collecting* data at the point of care because these devices are quick to hand and highly portable. PCs excel at *managing* data: selecting and arranging the fields and records in the various tables to answer an enormous variety of questions.

eNICU's PC data management features center on creating reports for the patient record (admission notes, progress notes, discharge summaries). Once you become facile working with Access database objects, you have wide latitude to manipulate fields; you can do things you might not have thought about doing before. One such feature the software includes is an automated sign-out summary. Automated sign-out can do more than just save time: it can improve patient care.[73] eNICU's automated sign-out report groups patients according to their location in a multiroom NICU (if all your patients are in one room and you don't want to alter the software, simply assign them all to Nursery number 1).

Readers who want to add more functionality might create a summary report of professional charges. As provided, eNICU includes appropriate forms and tables (Service charges). You'll need to create the queries and the report.

It's simple to use the PC data management functions. The **Main Switchboard** form opens at start up (Fig. 13.25). Navigate throughout the application simply by clicking on the button associated with the task you wish to accomplish. Notice that one letter of the text associated with most buttons is underlined. Another way to run the code associated with clicking on the button is to press **Alt** and *underlined letter*. For example, **Alt + A** is the same as clicking on the **NICU Admit Note** button. Doing either opens the search form shown in Fig. 13.26.

In the topmost field of the form (Fig. 13.26), enter the last name of the infant of interest (Access is not case-sensitive, i.e. there is no need to capitalize the first letter). Next, either press the tab key or left-click in the Infant ID field. When this field "gets the focus," a query runs and results in a list of all infant ID numbers for patients with the last name you entered. Usually, the patient of interest is the one most recently admitted. InfantID numbers are sorted in descending order, so if your hospital assigns MR numbers in ascending order, then the first entry on the list will most likely be the patient you seek. After you

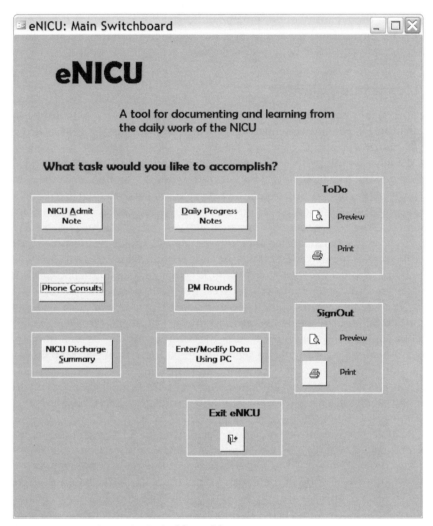

Figure 13.25 eNICU Main Switchboard form.

select the desired InfantID number, click the button next to the appropriate task description.

The topmost of the three task buttons takes you to a multipart form that allows you to review entered data, modify it, and link an admission record with a previously created phone consult record. This is the same multipart form that you also can access by clicking the **Enter/Modify Data Using PC** button. This is a very complicated form, in ways that an end user doesn't need to know about (many queries run to populate many fields on many forms); it takes at least 10 seconds to load. The various subforms are distributed among several tabbed sections of the main form. In the form header section is a button with an image of a telephone on it. Click this to link a previous phone consult

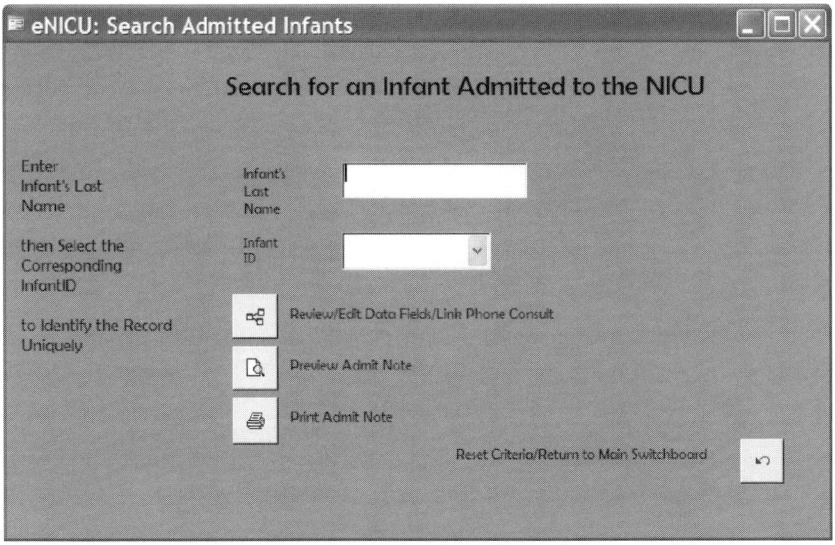

Figure 13.26 Form to select a record among admitted patients.

to an admitted infant's record. A form opens that contains phone consult records for all mothers with the same last name as that in the main form. At the very bottom of this form (or any of the others) is information about how many records are contained in the form. For a form containing more than one record, scroll through each record by clicking the right arrow to move forward or left arrow to move in reverse, until you locate the record you seek. When you have the phone consult record that corresponds to the infant described in the main form, enter the InfantID in the InfantID field (the conspicuous one, with yellow background and bold black outline). This places a foreign key value in the record in tblPhoneConsults, linking it with the corresponding record in tblInfants.

This multipart form for PC data review (discussed in detail in Chapter 14) synchronizes data in many subforms, to display a record that spans many tables. Before you use this feature to work with real patient data, make sure you thoroughly understand how forms and subforms work in Access. In the eNICU database window, the main form is called frmGlobalMother/InfantPC and frmGlobalMother/InfantPC_a, reflecting minor differences in opening it from either the admission switchboard or directly from the main switchboard. This feature is not integral to the rest of eNICU and its design and operation is beyond the scope of this book.

The middle of the three task buttons opens a preview of the admission note. To print what you see, click the printer icon on the toolbar or select **Print...** from the **Utilities** menu. If you need to modify what you see in the preview, you can change the data on the handheld device and repeat a hot sync, or do it directly via the **Review/Modify** form just discussed. After modifying the data, create the note once again in preview mode to make sure that it

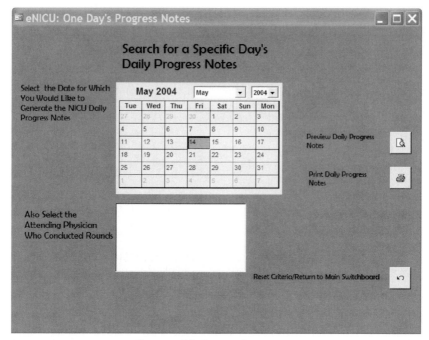

Figure 13.27 Form to specify a set of daily rounds reports.

now is correct. I rarely use the third button, to print the report without first reviewing it.

Figure 13.27 shows the form to specify a set of daily rounds reports. You set the date and identify the attending physician. Therefore, this form must display the appropriate names for your situation. In my institution, the white block contains my colleagues' and my names. Of course, you need to replace those. Here's how to do it.

Make the database window the active window. Click **Forms** in the Object list at the left of the database window, and then select frmSearchDPNbyDate. Open this in design view and click the **Design** button at the top of the database window. The area for physician names is blank, except for the word **Unbound** (Fig. 13.28). This is an unbound control – not linked to data in a table. And it is a list box control. Click this control to select it. If the associated property window is not already open, click the property button on the toolbar (Fig. 13.29). Figure 13.30 shows the property sheet for this list box. The property on the fourth row from the top is the Row Source. Some of the text is truncated in the image; the complete line reads: "D. A. Clark, M.D.";"M. A. Fisher, M.D.";"M. J. Horgan, M.D.";"Joaquim M. B. Pinheiro, M.D., M.P.H.";"U. Munshi, M.D.";"A. Rios, M.D.";"J. Schulman, M.D., M.S.". (My colleagues have kindly consented to this notoriety.) Delete or replace names needed; keep quotes around the names you use. When done, close the form by clicking the red **X** in the upper right. When asked if you want to save the changes you made, select **Yes**.

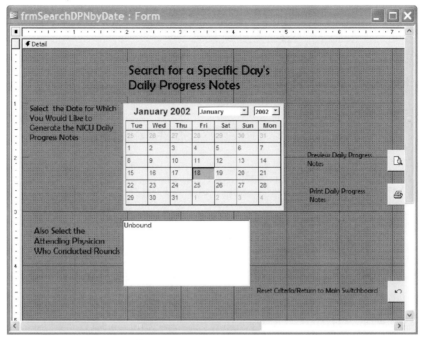

Figure 13.28 Design view of Fig. 13.27.

To check that all went well, open the modified form in form view (click the **Open** button at the top of the database window). The list should now display the names you just entered. Of course, you'll also want to change the look-up list of physicians for the handheld part of eNICU (see eNICU installation instructions on accompanying CD. Be certain that every character and space between the quotes containing each entry in the unbound field matches with those for the corresponding entry in the handheld lookup list).

With all this accomplished and appropriate infant data collected on the handheld and synchronized with the PC, you're ready to create daily progress notes. The calendar control (Fig. 13.27) is programmed to show the current date. For any other date, select the year, month, and date. Next, click the name of the physician that entered the data on the handheld, and then click the button either to preview or print directly.

Finally, the search form to create a discharge note has one more field than the search form for an admission note. After selecting the Infant ID, press the tab key or click the **Date/Time** field below it. A query runs, producing a

Figure 13.29 Property toolbar button.

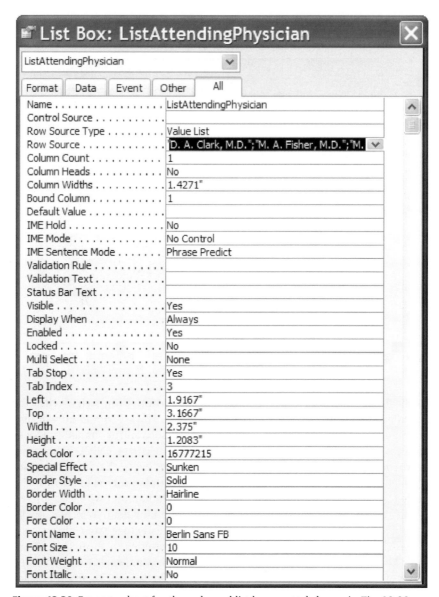

Figure 13.30 Property sheet for the unbound list box control shown in Fig. 13.28.

list of dates/times uniquely identifying a.m. rounds record. This information determines the discharging clinician(s) identified on the discharge summary. You'll usually choose the item at the top of the list, the most recent patient visit. Then either preview the document or print directly. If you forget to select the **Date/Time** of rounds that determine the discharging clinicians, a snippet of VBA code runs, reminding you.

CHAPTER 14

Making eNICU serve your own needs

Levels of conceptual focus

Even if you think eNICU is perfect, you will need to change it somehow, sometime. Software perfection is a moving target.[74] The context in which we use a tool changes; for example, new medications and procedures come along. If you want to use eNICU but you do not work in a NICU, you certainly need to modify it. So this chapter provides an overview of how to think about modifying eNICU. The possibilities for change are virtually endless. Plenty of references can help you implement specific application features.[51,52,56–59,64] What I have not found in those references is advice on how to *think* about database software problems and solutions. And you do need to think about these things, on several conceptual levels, including

- core concepts of database theory,
- data model,
- pros and cons of a specific development platform(s) for implementation,
- pros and cons of specific hardware,
- interaction of the latter two,
- exactly how to implement a feature detail in the software application, and
- database administration issues (discussed in Section 4 of this book).

If your experience resembles mine, the conceptual level at which you start to tackle an individual problem and a candidate solution will vary with the nature of the problem and the solution. Also bear in mind, the solution that first occurs to you may not be the best one to implement.[33] As you methodically consider the situation and as you observe how your solution works in the hands of other users, be open to revising your idea. To illustrate, I share some of my experience in developing eNICU.

I shall describe several specific challenges I've grappled with. Much of this chapter may seem arcane, until you actually work with this software and encounter similar challenges. My counsel: read what follows, so that you can connect back to it when the need arises, but don't worry if parts are unclear or boring. When the need arises, I think you'll find the material clear and spot-on. If not, or if you otherwise need a consultant, please contact me at schulmj@mail.amc.edu.

Dropping a Parent form: toward a generic eNICU

For patients beyond infancy, you probably have no need to store maternal information. You do not need the **Mothers, Maternal Complications**, and **Maternal Medications** forms on the handheld, nor the corresponding tables in the Access portion of eNICU. Deleting the parts of a report that contain unwanted data is straightforward; please refer to Access references.[48,52,56]

To delete a form design in Pendragon Forms, highlight the form name and click the **Delete** button on the **Pendragon Forms Manager**. Associated child forms, including **Infants**, in this particular case, do not automatically move up the hierarchy. If a form subsequently becomes the new parent form, you must explicitly change its subordinate status.

I explicitly designate child forms as such, by setting an option in the **Advanced Form Properties**. Highlight the form name, click the **Properties** button on the **Pendragon Forms Manager**, then click the **Advanced Properties...** button. Next, select the **Behavior** tab and look at the Subform section in the lower right. Selecting the first option ensures the form is displayed as a subform. [This way a user cannot start a new record by opening the child form directly. A user must start a new record in the parent form and proceed down the hierarchy. This restriction does not apply when reviewing existing records.] To elevate a child form to superior status, simply clear this subform option.

Unfortunately, in Pendragon Forms you cannot rename a form once "frozen." And to make a form design functional, you do have to freeze it. [If this doesn't make sense, please refer to the Pendragon Forms Manual.] So unless you want to continue calling the parent form by the name of **Infants**, you must copy it, rename it and modify it in any other appropriate way, freeze it, and if you work with a secured database, redo field mapping and synchronization parameters (as described on the CD accompanying this book). This is not necessarily just a nuisance, because you may also decide you want to drop or add some fields in your new **Parent** patient information form. In either case, you must go through the same procedure. Be sure to familiarize yourself with the different field types available in Pendragon Forms. I also recommend you not rush to implement your changes. I often reconsider the field type (also unchangeable after freezing the form design) or some other detail that becomes locked-in with freezing.

Anytime you add or drop a field in a form design copied from one previously frozen, remember to check that scripts continue to reference the correct field numbers. In Fig. 9.4, the script includes a line "if answer <$6 then"; here $6 means Field 6. If, as a result of adding or dropping fields in a revised form design, the previous Field 6 is now Field 9, the script will not execute as originally intended. A recent improvement in Pendragon Forms scripting allows specifying fields by name, obviating the need to revise a scripting field reference.

Lastly, you must modify the corresponding table in the Access part of eNICU. The handheld form must map to the Access table, so handheld form modifications may entail renaming the Access table (not crucial for field mapping, but important for clarity in the physical data model), renaming field(s), dropping or adding fields, and changing field properties. If you made drastic changes to the handheld form design, it might be easiest to import the table that Pendragon Forms created when you froze the new form design and use that as your starting point (look at the list of tables in the Pendragon Forms database window and select the one with the same FormID number).

Changing the data model

As you work over time with a physical data model (i.e. a data model actually implemented as database software), you may think of a better way to structure the data. Entering data day after day can provide fresh insight to the data structure that most accurately represents the daily work. You might appreciate the importance of explicitly linking data that presently is only implicitly connected, or not at all.

In an early version of eNICU, I entered data about ventilatory support in one field of the "Daily AM Rounds" handheld form. I thought this field satisfactorily represented this dimension of a patient's NICU care. Even so, during my teaching rounds I encourage staff to articulate exactly what patient problem we treat with the provided ventilatory support. Informed ventilatory management requires this explicit conceptual connection. Eventually, I realized that the database and the documentation should reflect this same thinking. In other words, I perceived that ventilatory support is not an attribute of "Daily AM Rounds." More appropriately, ventilatory support is an attribute of Patient Problems; analogous to Meds/Responses, Procedures/Responses, and Consultations. If this point is not clear, please review Chapter 7.

Next, I had to decide exactly how to model this new data relationship. If the relationship is one-to-one (one type of ventilatory support will pertain to any single problem), then I would only need to add this field to the **Patient Problems** form and tblPatientProblems. However, over the course of an illness an infant may require different types of ventilatory support. The patient may start on a conventional mechanical ventilator, then require high-frequency oscillation, then return to a conventional ventilator, and convalesce with intermittent oxygen supplied by nasal cannula. Clearly, the relationship is one-to-many. Ventilatory support data thus required its own table.

I created a new handheld form design **Ventilatory Support** (Fig. 14.1), and a corresponding table in the Access part of eNICU (tblVentSupport). In Fig. 14.1 you see the field list in the left side of the **Form Designer**, and on the right side the script for Field 3. **Ventilatory Support** is a subform of **Patient Problems**. I added a subform link field called Ventilatory support to the **Patient Problems** form (after copying the form design, deleting the former form design, and renaming the new one with the same form name minus the asterisk that Pendragon Forms automatically adds to the copied design name). In the tblVentSupport, VentSupportID is the primary key, InfantID is a foreign key (linked to tblInfants), as is ProblemID (linked to tblPatientProblems) (see

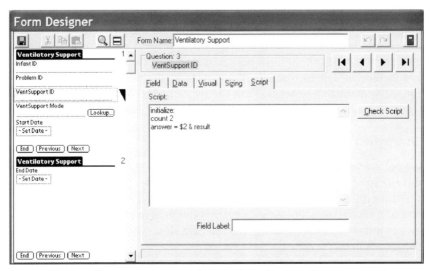

Figure 14.1 Ventilatory Support, Field 3: <u>S</u>cript tab selected.

the eNICU relationship diagram, Fig. 7.5). When executing, the script shown in Fig. 14.1 counts the number of records with a particular ProblemID value and concatenates that number with the ProblemID value itself. This method keeps track of various support modes provided for the same underlying condition. The VentSupport Mode field is a look-up list field. I prefer a look-up list to a pop-up list when list content is likely to change over time. You can't change a pop-up list in a frozen form. But you can change what is on a look-up list referenced in a frozen form (we examine how to modify look-up lists later in this chapter). The last two fields record the start and end date for each instance of a support mode. This model easily accommodates the common situation of a patient repeatedly going on and off different types of ventilatory support.

This section mainly illustrates how to implement a data model change to tables and forms. To refresh your memory about designing the model, please review Chapter 7. Identifying the changes to other database objects such as queries and reports derives from these preliminaries; implementing those database object changes generally is covered in Access references. Also remember that when you add a table to a database specify how it relates to the other tables. As you learned in Chapter 10, establishing relationships among tables is a necessary part of maintaining data integrity.

Hot sync (synchronization) problems after implementing a data model change

[This section may best support my earlier warning about the chapter seeming arcane, until you encounter similar challenges. Remember, the initial aim is simply to be able to connect back when the need arises. At that time, this material should at least point you in the right direction. Because the development experience I share was mainly with Palm OS® devices, I speak here of hot sync and not ActiveSync™.]

After changing a Pendragon Forms form design, don't be surprised if you receive an error message such as the following the first time you hot-sync. I direct your attention to key portions of the message by displaying them in bold font and show only output germane to our point.

HotSync operation started 4/7/2004 9:34:27 AM

Pendragon Forms (v.4.0, 4.0.1.17) synchronization started at 4/7/2004 9:34:29 AM **Unable to append record in Form 'Meds/Responses' (189808936)**, Field 10 select UnitID,[TimeStamp],UserName,InfantID, ProblemID,MedID,MedicationName,DateThisMedStarted,DateThis MedStopped,ResponseToThisMed from [tblMeds/Responses] where MedID = {ts '2004-04-07 09:42:46'}[Microsoft][ODBC Microsoft Access Driver] **You cannot add or change a record because a related record is required in table 'tblInfants'.**

Unable to append record in Form 'Patient Problems' (264606194), Field 15 select UnitID,[TimeStamp],UserName,InfantID,ProblemID, OnsetDate,ProblemCategory,ProblemDescription,Details,DateResolved from tblPatientProblems where ProblemID = '12345611' [Microsoft] [ODBC Microsoft Access Driver] **You cannot add or change a record because a related record is required in table 'tblInfants'.**

OK Pendragon Forms with 1 message(s)
 – Backing up db Saved Preferences to file C:\Program Files\Palm\...
OK System
HotSync operation complete 4/7/2004 9:34:36 AM

To figure this out, you need more information. At the time I tried this hot sync, the 'Infants' form ID number was 265206202: a higher number than the problematic child forms' ID number. Pendragon Forms creates a form ID number at the time you freeze a form. Recently created forms are assigned higher form ID numbers than forms created earlier in time. The hot sync process proceeds in ascending order of form ID number, so relational integrity rules in the Access part of the application were being violated. The hot sync process was attempting to populate (jargon for "enter data to") child tables with a record containing a foreign key value for which a record and primary key value in the parent table had not yet been established. This problem develops in the context of freezing a new (modified) version of a previously created parent form. The solution is to

1 copy the problematic form design,
2 freeze it, then replace the older design that was otherwise identical except for having a lower form ID number (find it in the upper right of the **Form**

Design property screen) with this new one (after making the copy, discard the older design, then rename the copy using the older design's name), and
3 field map and set synchronization parameters for the new child form (instructions are on the accompanying CD). The new child form will have a higher form ID number than the parent and therefore will synchronize *after* the parent form, eliminating the problem.

The foregoing procedure amounts to a lot of work, so first confirm your diagnosis. Before you change anything, try repeating the hot sync. You may no longer get an error message in the hot sync log. If you do not, during the first hot sync the problematic parent form eventually did synchronize its data, *after* the child forms tried to send theirs along. Since the parent record did get established during the first hot sync, on a second hot sync – even though the form ID numbers are still not in appropriate rank order – the child records will not violate relational integrity rules. Depending on how many layers of parent/child/child nesting your model contains, you may need to repeat the hot sync more than one time to get the tables populated. [If you have modified several form designs, then the situation becomes that much more complicated, but the same line of reasoning applies.] To illustrate, here's part of my hot sync log from the next time I performed a hot sync:

HotSync operation started 04/08/04 10:23:05

Pendragon Forms (v.4.0, 4.0.1.17) synchronization started at 04/08/04 10:23:08 **Unable to append record in Form 'Meds/Responses' (189808936)**, Field 10 select UnitID,[TimeStamp],UserName,InfantID, ProblemID,MedID,MedicationName,DateThisMedStarted,DateThis MedStopped, ResponseToThisMed from [tblMeds/Responses] where MedID = {ts '2004-04-07 09:42:46'} [Microsoft][ODBC Microsoft Access Driver] **You cannot add or change a record because a related record is required in table 'tblPatientProblems'**.

OK Pendragon Forms with 1 message(s)
 – Backing up db Saved Preferences to file C:\Program Files\Palm\...
OK System
HotSync operation complete 4/8/2004 10:23:14 AM

Look at the eNICU relationship diagram in Fig. 7.5. tblMeds/Responses has *two* foreign keys. The problem reported on the first hot sync try was that a corresponding primary key value for InfantID had not yet been established in tblInfants (**You cannot add or change a record because a related record is required in table 'tblInfants'**). The problem reported on the second hot sync try was that a corresponding primary key value for ProblemID had not yet been established in tblPatientProblems (**You cannot add or change a record because a related record is required in table 'tblPatientProblems'**). The third hot sync did the trick.

This sequence confirms the initial diagnosis: child form ID number > parent form ID number. I want to emphasize, the hot sync log provided important insight to the problem. Although a hot sync log may seem frighteningly unintelligible at first glance, it often provides valuable information to help you troubleshoot a misbehaving application.

Here's another example of an initially perplexing problem after modifying a form, which cleared in the light of reason.

HotSync operation started 4/16/2004 1:11:35 PM

Pendragon Forms (v.4.0, 4.0.1.17) synchronization started at 4/16/2004 1:11:37 PM
Unable to append record in Form 'Screening and Discharge' (267105952), Field 11 select UnitID,[TimeStamp],UserName,InfantID, DischargeDate,HearingScreenMostRecent, HearingScreenReschedDate, ROPPresent,IfROP_OS,IfROP_OD,IfROP_PlusDisease,LaserCryo_ROP,CranialUS,[PVLat<3wks],[StudyDatePVL<3wks],[PVLat>=3wks], [StudyDatePVL>=3wks],CranialUS1IVH,CranialUS2IVH,CranialUS3IVH, CranialUS4IVH, DevelopmentalAssessment,MostRecentStateMetabolic Screen,DischargeDisposition,IfTransferredToAnotherHospitalReason, AcceptingHospital,IfDiedAutopsy,GoingHomeOnO2,GoingHomeOnApnea Monitor,GoingHomeOnPulseOximiter,RSVProphylaxis,FunctionalStatus On FinalNICUDay,DischargeFeeds,PrimaryCareProvider,CalledPCPTime, FaxedDischSumTo,AdditionalNarrative from tblScreeningAndDischarge where InfantID = '1 - 161616'
Multiple-step OLE DB operation generated errors. Check each OLE DB status value, if available. No work was done.
OK Pendragon Forms with 1 message(s)
– Backing up db Saved Preferences to file C:\Program Files\Palm\...
OK System
HotSync operation complete 4/16/2004 1:11:45 PM

OLE DB is beyond our scope. Let's just say that OLE DB is a type of software technology for connecting a database to any type of data source, relational or not. If you want to know more, see Refs. 44 and 63.

Returning to the problem at hand, Thomas Roth and Ivan Philips (at Pendragon Forms), as they have done many times, helped me solve it. The Pendragon Forms company provides excellent technical support via email and telephone. Here's a list of candidate problems they thought might apply:

• Yes/No field on the handheld that did not have a default value. At hot sync, Access might object because it does not accept a null value in such fields on the corresponding table.
• Mismatched field type between handheld and database table.
• Field limitation in the table.

The last item turned out to be the culprit. The old **Screening and Discharge** form had fewer and different fields than the new one now giving me problems.

Field 11 was originally a Yes/No field. Data in this type of field is stored as a "Y" or a "N." In the old version of this form, I had set the default answer of "N" for that field. In the new version of the form, I entirely changed the question in Field 11 and provided possible answers on a pop-up list. I had made a copy of the old **Screening and Discharge** form to serve as a starting point for the modifications I planned. But I forgot to modify the field properties appropriately in the corresponding table in the Access part of eNICU. The old field size was set equal to one (1) character. But on the newly modified form, the shortest possible answer on the pop-up list was "No"; field size = 2. This was the field limitation that caused the problem (see Fig. 14.2). [Astute readers may have noticed that both highlighted fields of the two tables in Fig. 14.2 are of data type text, and not Yes/No. Field 11 on the old **Screening and Discharge** form on the handheld device was originally a Yes/No field, and collected answers as a "Y" or a "N." However, it didn't matter that the data storage type for the field being populated on the corresponding table was text.]

One way to prevent this kind of problem is always to import into the eNICU Access database the table that Pendragon Forms creates when you freeze a form design. You can subsequently modify the table design as appropriate, certain that data types and field limitations start out matched.

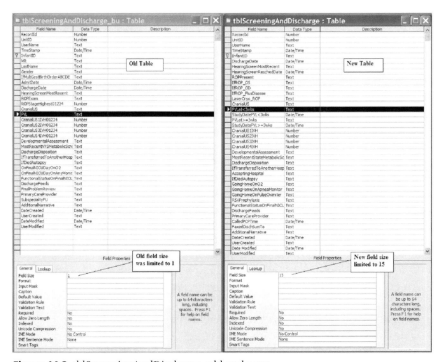

Figure 14.2 tblScreeningAndDischarge, old and new.

Working with the data via forms on the PC

In Chapter 13, I cautioned you to delay using frmGlobalMother/InfantPC with patient data until you are comfortable developing forms and subforms and synchronizing records among them. To help you reach this comfort level, explore this "mega-form" in conjunction with reading about forms in the already cited Access references. To complement what you read there, we shall examine how several component subforms of frmGlobalMother/InfantPC work. This material also paves the way for modifying the hardware configuration for using eNICU, in that this "mega-form" enables data review, and even data entry, without using the handheld device.

Specifically, we examine how to add another subform feature to frmGlobalMother/InfantPC: a subform linked to tblVentSupport. Figure 14.3 shows the design view of the tab page dealing with an infant's problems, meds, etc.

You probably know that you can move objects around a form by highlighting and then dragging them to where you want them. I did that for several labels, subforms, and fields, to make room in the upper right portion for the new subform. To create the new subform, use the subform wizard on the toolbox toolbar (fourth button from right; see Fig. 14.4).

The wizard will either create a new (sub)form from scratch, based on a table, or use an existing form. Either way, the wizard speeds your specifying which field(s) on parent and child forms should be synchronized. We first create the form, and then use it as a subform.

Activate the database window, select **Forms** objects, and then click the **New** button. In the dialog box, select **Form** wizard and also select the table upon which to base the form: tblVentSupport, and then click **OK**. The next dialog box asks you to select the fields you want to appear on the form. You need foreign key and primary key fields, and others that contribute to what you want this subform to achieve. The > button transfers one highlighted field at a time to the Selected fields list, the >> button transfers all the fields at once.

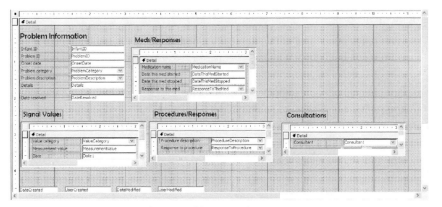

Figure 14.3 Design view: infant's problems, meds, etc.

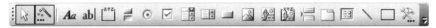

Figure 14.4 Toolbox toolbar.

Select the following: InfantID, ProblemID, VentSupportID, VentSupportMode, StartDate, EndDate, DateCreated, UserCreated, DateModified, UserModified. In the next dialog box select **Columnar** layout, and on the screen following select **Standard** style. In the final dialog box, name the form (I called it frmVentSupportPC) and then choose the radio button, **Modify**. You've just created a form!

This new form needs more work. We should remove unnecessary labels, rearrange control locations, and resize some controls (some need to be there for linking purposes but need not be visible). Controls that must be present but not visible may either be made tiny or have their visible property set to No. Figure 14.5 shows frmVentSupportPC in design view after I finished these modifications and added some background color (refer to the property list for the detail section).

A brief but important digression: the four text box controls dealing with **...Created** or **...Modified** are a way to keep track of who changed data and when. Each table in eNICU contains these fields (modeled after Ref. 67, pp. 247–252). Look at the details in the design view for each table.

Now we establish this new form as a subform. Click the subform button on the toolbox toolbar; over the empty area you cleared earlier on the tab page of the main form (see the upper right portion in Fig. 14.3) click and drag the cursor. This activates the subform wizard. Select the name of the new form. When asked about linking criteria, I usually prefer not to leave the choice to Access. For this subform, we link parent and child forms by InfantID and ProblemID. After you finish with the wizard, adjust the location of the subform and create a label for it (also using the toolbox); your product should resemble Fig. 14.6. Look closely at your text box control for VentSupportMode; it should not look exactly like its counterpart in the figure. The control in the figure has a downward pointing arrow at the right; it is a combo box – a control that provides a drop-down list of choices to select.

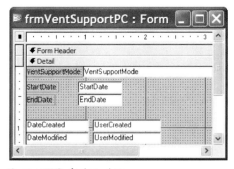

Figure 14.5 frmVentSupportPC: design view.

Next, we convert your text box control to a combo box that is linked to the same table used for a similar purpose in Pendragon Forms. Highlight the VentSupportMode text box and then right-click on it: select **Change To >**, **Combo Box**; now the control will look like the one in Fig. 14.6. However, they may look the same, but they are not the same. Your combo box lacks data to display. Look at this control's property list. The seventh item from the top is Row Source. Ultimately, Row Source will contain the name of the table that lists the choices you want this combo box to display. We first must create the table. Our table will be linked to the same file that archives what is in the corresponding look-up list for the corresponding field on the **Ventilatory Support** form residing on the handheld.

Activate the database window and select **Tables** from the list of database objects. Next, on the main menu select **File**, **Get External Data >**, and then **Link Tables...** Look on the accompanying CD for a folder called eNICU Lookups. *Important*: at the bottom of the dialog box, make sure you select **File type:** Text Files (*.txt; *.csv; *.tab; *.asc). Open the file **Ventilatory Support**. In the next dialog box, activate the **Delimited** button, and in the following dialog box, the comma delimiter. Accept the default field titles, and then name the linked table (I call mine tblLookupVentilatorySupport).

Now activate the Row Source field of the property list for your combo box (click within the field, to give it "focus"). Click the arrow at the right of that field, scroll down to find the name of the linked table you just created, and select it. Now the Row Source property indicates this table name. If the table configuration needed to import data into look-up lists in Pendragon Forms was the same as that for Access, we'd be finished. However, Pendragon Forms

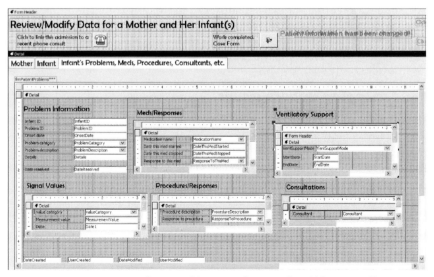

Figure 14.6 Design view: infant's problems, meds, etc., after adding **Ventilatory Support** subform.

requires some additional data, which have nothing to do with the choices you want to offer the user, to be present in rows at the top of each table stored as a .csv file. This additional data helps the Pendragon Forms application import a look-up list from the .csv file.

To keep that data from being unnecessarily displayed in your combo box, we turn the Row Source information into a query. Activate the Row Source property field again. This time, not an arrow but an ellipsis (. . .) appears at the right of the field. Click the ellipsis: a query design grid appears. Drag Field1 from tblLookupVentilatorySupport in the upper portion of the design grid into the first query field and insert the following text on the Criteria row: Not Like 'LIST*'. This eliminates from the combo box display the first three rows of the linked look-up table: LISTTYPE, LISTEXPORT, LISTSORT. Not Like 'LIST*' specifies the query not include any records beginning with the string fragment LIST, followed by any other letters (* being a wildcard character). Close and save the query; you are finished. To see how this subform, and the rest of the "mega-form," works, open it after the source tables contain your patient data via the main switchboard (you must specify a patient).

Pendragon Forms look-up lists

Pendragon Forms allows you directly to modify a look-up list via the Forms Manager. However, this feature doesn't allow you to insert an item anywhere in an existing sequence, nor does it allow you to access the lists from outside Pendragon Forms. I prefer the much greater flexibility obtained by keeping a library of lists outside of Pendragon Forms. This entails saving each look-up list as a .csv file (comma delimited text file, an option in Microsoft® Excel). The Pendragon Forms manual explains how to export existing look-up lists in this file format, and to import when you want to create or modify an existing look-up list. eNiCU-specific instructions for working with look-up lists appear in the eNICU installation instructions, on the accompanying CD.

Field mapping update issues

Field mapping is the process of explicitly mapping a field on a handheld form with a corresponding field in a database table. It plays an important role in protecting the confidentiality of patient information, by redirecting data incoming to Pendragon Forms via hot sync to the secured eNICU Access application instead. We look more closely at security issues in Chapter 17. For more explanation of field mapping, see the Pendragon Forms Manual[51] and the CD accompanying this book. Many of the changes you make to a handheld form will require that you reestablish field mapping to the corresponding table.

Modifying the graphical eNICU Main MENU

If eNICU table names are added, deleted, or modified, then the graphical Main MENU will also need to change. This is relatively uncomplicated to do once you have the images you need. The Pendragon Forms user manual clearly explains the process.[51]

Words of encouragement

I used to experience an unpleasant emotional reaction when my software misbehaved. I used to fear that troubleshooting and making incremental improvements to eNICU risked destroying what I had accomplished to that point. With increasing experience, I learned that even if a problem seems intractable at first, ultimately it almost always surrenders to analysis. "Almost always" because sometimes, after trying everything sensible failed, I simply rebuilt the object or rebooted the computer and afterward all was well. Perhaps I was oblivious to an error that existed in the original object but did not repeat that same error when I rebuilt it; rarely, the data constituting the object may be corrupted. And sometimes the data in the computer's RAM may be corrupted. *Solution*: simply reboot.

Data integrity is at risk when multiple users are at work

When you work with a document in a word processor, you might make provisions to share it with others involved in the project, but usually only one person at a time works with the source file. Databases on the other hand are often used simultaneously by various members of a group. The eNICU application as provided with this book reflects the author's NICU work environment. Typically, two attending neonatologists and two nurse practitioners collect and manage data each day. Our workflow patterns make it unlikely that two or more individuals need to hot-sync or manage the same data at exactly the same time. So the eNICU application does not incorporate features available in Access to deal with two or more users who attempt to work on the same record at the same time. In time, we expect to face this problem. Depending on your work environment, you may face it sooner. In any case, you should know something about performance considerations and database integrity threats posed by a multiuser environment.

Imagine eNICU is installed on your PC. Time goes by, and you find that workers are queuing up at that one PC. To improve the situation, you decide to install the file on your network file server. This is your institutional computer that supports several PCs connected to it; it's called a file server because it serves up the files you want. Now several workers can access this file from several PCs. Immediately, they start to add new records and work from various locations with existing records. Each PC accesses the eNICU application installed on the server. In Windows®/Microsoft® Access jargon, eNICU is an .mdb application (file type), meaning each PC must run the Access application installed on its own hard drive in order to open the eNICU.mdb file on the PC after retrieving it from the server. That is, eNICU is a discrete database application that runs within Microsoft® Access.

This arrangement stores the data on the file server, but still requires each PC to run all the application features (forms, queries, reports, VBA code). Importantly, this arrangement allows data sharing among users of the connected PCs. Therefore, the PCs should not operate independently of each other. The

PCs must communicate. To appreciate why, consider this scenario: suppose that shortly after the attending neonatologist leaves an intubated patient's bedside, this patient accidentally becomes extubated. The nurse practitioner assesses the patient and decides the patient could tolerate a trial of nasal CPAP. The practitioner, of course, updates the data on the Ventilatory support sub-form on her handheld device. By coincidence, both the neonatologist and the nurse practitioner each update the database (synchronize data between handheld and PC) at the same time and at different PCs. Some conflict resolution is built-in to the eNICU handheld synchronization instructions, so that in the event of conflicting data the most recently timed record is the one used for an update. Nonetheless, you can begin to appreciate the importance of understanding the general principles for protecting integrity in a multiuser environment.

If you have opened an unsecured version of eNICU or some other Access file from Windows® Explorer rather than from a shortcut icon, you may have noticed another icon next to the file icon while the application is open, or persisting briefly after you closed the application. This other icon represents a lock file. Notice the padlock that's part of this transient icon in Fig. 16.1. In this, Access stores information about who is doing what, when. If the nurse practitioner was the first to open the same record that the neonatologist wanted to work on, the neonatologist would receive a message that the record is in use. Fair enough, but what happens if the neonatologist opens the same record after the practitioner is done? Will the neonatologist's update replace the practitioner's data about the patient's extubation? This potential for error is why a multiuser database needs specific update rules. As provided with this book, eNICU keeps the most recently timed record – *based on the time it was created, not synchronized*. The Pendragon Forms manual discusses this issue in detail. We shall further explore record locking in Access shortly; first, we must examine database architecture.

Split database

When PCs are connected to a file server that stores the database application file including the data, as described above, the PC is called the front end. Although this arrangement allows multiple users to access the application, it makes for inefficient processing. For every query that runs, all the data must travel over the network from the file server to the PC. And the actual processing happens on the PC, so as the database grows, the more likely it is that you'll need to upgrade each PC. The arrangement may be acceptable, though, if your system has few "clients" (front ends) and the amount of data you store not very large. Whitehorn and Marklyn propose limits of 10 clients and 1 gigabyte (GB) of data.

Access offers a way to improve performance for this front-end/file server arrangement: splitting the database. Essentially, you create two .mdb files.

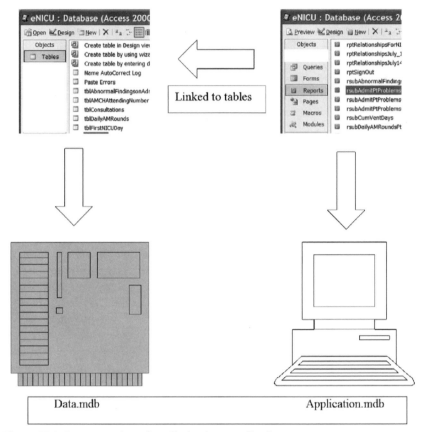

Figure 15.1 Representation of a split database application.

One file stores the data (tables) and resides on the network server. The other file stores all the other application objects (queries, forms, reports, macros, modules) and resides on each connected PC (workstation). Depending on the locking options (discussed below), now when one user is working with a record, another user may also work with it. Figure 15.1 illustrates the idea. To split an Access database application, select **Tools** from the main menu, **Database Utilities**, **Database Splitter**. But read about it in detail first.[56]

The price you pay for increased performance is increased work for the database administrator. Since the application file resides on the hard drive of each workstation, you must repeat the installation process for each workstation. You also must reinstall any upgrade you make, every time you make it. This last issue may be mitigated by making use of replication. I shall not expand upon it here, but remember to investigate the method when you get to this level of complexity in your system.

Database client/server

A client/server arrangement puts the user interface on the workstation, while the bulk of the data processing and the data itself reside on the server. The server is called a database server because it is dedicated only to running the database application. This improves performance but puts us in the realm of larger and more complex RDBMS platforms like SQL Server, Microsoft's heavy-duty database development platform. A split Access application does not technically qualify as a "client/server" arrangement.

Distributing the functionality of a RDBMS need not stop at a two-tiered arrangement. Web-based database applications often insert a web server between the workstations and the database server. My intent here is merely to introduce you to the notion of distributing a RDBMS among pieces of hardware (please refer Ref. 46 for more details).

Sharing and record locking options

Let's return now to the issues surrounding shared access to data. Microsoft® Access enables you to set a default mode for opening a database. A database may be used exclusively by the person who opens it or it may be shared. Exclusive use means that until the user closes the database file no one else can work with it. In shared mode, other authorized users can work with the database at the same time. To specify this, select **Tools** from the main menu, **Options . . .**, and select the **Advanced** tab (Fig. 15.2). The right side of this window contains an area to set the Default open mode. If you select **Shared**, then also specify the Default record locking option in the section below it. Here are the basic considerations.

Figure 15.2 shows the three record locking options. If you choose to lock **All** records the situation is simple: not just the record that a user is working on, but all the records in the underlying table are locked – the entire table – as long as the user is working with any records in that table. **No locks** does not really mean that no records are locked. It means that the edited record becomes locked only when it is actually updated. If you change data directly in the table, editing is the same as updating. But if you edit data in a form, the data in the underlying table does not change until you confirm the change, via an explicit feature designed into the form or when you close the form. This is precisely one of the advantages of using forms to work with data; it's safer to work with data in forms than working directly in tables. **No locks** is also called optimistic locking. **Edited record** locks the record the user is working on until the user is completely finished. This is also called pessimistic locking.

Here are some examples of how much detail you must attend to in designing and administering a large database application. Notice the **Refresh** interval specification in Fig. 15.2. This specifies how long to wait before automatically updating (refreshing) the data displayed in an open form. Suppose you look

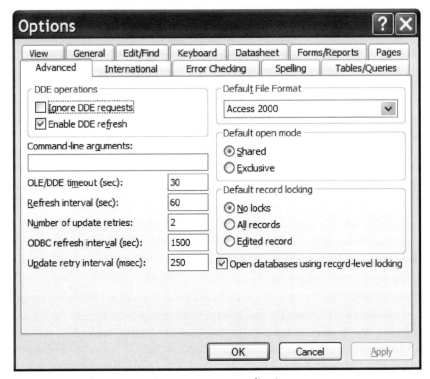

Figure 15.2 Database options in eNICU Access application.

at a record in a form while having lunch at your desk. Shortly after you open the form, another user updates the data for the record that you're looking at. Setting the **Refresh** interval to 60 means that if the data changed after you opened the form, the new data will be displayed within 60 seconds of when you opened the form. The **Update** retry interval, also visible in Fig. 15.2, determines how frequently Access tries to save a record you want to change, but that was locked because someone else was working with it. **Number** of update retries describes a similar idea. Individual forms have their own Record locking property that overrides the Access options, if they differ. If the need arises and you've become a skillful programmer, you can set this, and most other properties, at run time. For more details, see Refs. 43, 48, 52, and 59.

CHAPTER 16

Backup and recovery: assuring your data persists

A problem with data storage need not mean data loss

In data management, to back up means to make sure your work can continue to go forward, that is, to make a copy of your data.[75] You want to ensure that should a problem develop with your stored data it will not mean you have lost those data. This chapter provides an overview of this extensive topic and introduces you to the notion of a database recovery plan. Databases at the scale of a hospital system may experience special problems that are beyond our scope.

For general database security and protection advice, I rely primarily on *The Backup Book: Disaster Recovery from Desktop to Data Center*[75] and *Real World Microsoft Access Database Protection and Security*.[76] These sources also describe a variety of tools designed to protect important data.

Why do bad things happen to good data?

Bad things can happen to the place where you store data. Although unlikely, disasters hit buildings or rooms in a building, destroying the computers within them and the data they contain. Electric power is reliable, especially within hospitals. But electric power failure can make a hard drive crash, so you want to protect against surges and power failure.

Computer data storage devices will fail. Not can fail; *will* fail. The question is simply *when* failure will occur. Engineers rate data storage devices such as hard drives and CD drives by "mean time between failure rates."[75] The point is you *will* experience a disaster with your stored data at some time. Preparation cuts a disaster down to an inconvenience.

Software or data corruption can happen in myriad ways. The operating system that runs a computer tends to become less reliable over time, as users install more and more programs. The operating system is also a common target of computer viruses. Bits of data may vanish or become misplaced from the operating system, or an application file, or a document file as a result of or as an effect of an application freeze. Particularly at risk is a database application that was not correctly set up to handle record locking issues.[75] If you store a database on a network server and the server develops problems, the database can become corrupted.

Backing up an Access database file

Routinely backing up is an *essential* part of maintaining a database. We shall explore how to do it. For strategies and products oriented to general data backup, see Ref.[75] Our focus is on strategies and techniques to back up Microsoft® Access applications running on a PC and to back up Palm OS® applications.

I mentioned earlier that databases often require special backup methods. This largely reflects the risk of corrupting or losing data if you try to back up a database while someone is using it. Especially if the database resides on a network server, you don't want to rely on just "looking around" your facility to ascertain that all users are logged off. If someone is logged on while you back up, you'll have saved the database in an unstable state.[76]

You need a sure way to know that the database is not in use when you perform a backup. In the last chapter, I mentioned that Windows® Explorer displays an Access lock file icon when someone has an Access database file open. Figure 16.1 shows this padlocked icon. Notice that the locked file uses the .ldb file extension instead of the .mdb file extension used for Access database files. The file name preceding the file extension stays the same.

When you see this icon in the folder where your database file resides, usually someone is using the database. However, as you may know, if an Access database was open during a system crash or application program freeze, the lock file remains. So to be doubly sure about safely backing up your database, you could open the database in exclusive mode: open Microsoft® Office Access, select **File**, then **Open . . .** , and navigate to the directory containing the database. Select the .mdb file of interest; notice that the **Open** button in this window incorporates a drop-down list. By selecting **Open Exclusive**, you are assured no one else is logged on. Unfortunately, this method of double checking does not work for a secured database (see Chapter 17). You could try using Robinson's VBA tool to check if anyone is logged on.[76] For a secured database, you can also obtain this information via the VBA IDE immediate window by requesting current user names (type `Print CurrentUser` and then press **Enter**). Yet another approach to ensure no one is logged on to the database is via routine manual or automatic[76] shutdown at agreed-upon times.

Once you are convinced only you are working with the database, you can back it up. Access 2003 has a new menu command that facilitates the process. From either the **File** or the **Tools** menu select **Back Up Database . . .** and navigate to the folder where you want to save the backup file. As shown in Fig. 16.2, I backed up to the eNICU folder (on a removable disk in drive E). Access suggested the file name; it incorporates the current date. If you back up more than once a day Access will differentiate between each event. If you keep the application file on your PC, then store the backup file somewhere

eNICU.ldb
Microsoft Office Access Record-Lock...   **Figure 16.1** An Access lock file icon.
1 KB

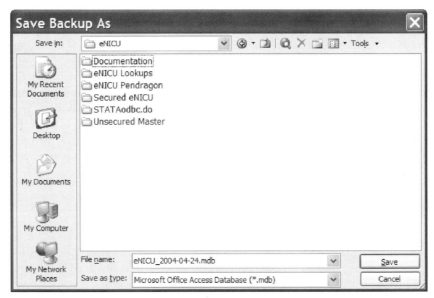

Figure 16.2 Save Backup dialog box.

else. The experts advise that you back up to an offsite location (in case your office floods or the building collapses).[75] If you split your database, remember to back up both the back end (the tables) and the front end (all of the other database objects). The backup frequency need not be the same for each. Back up the front end whenever you make a change to any of the database objects that constitute it.

Not only does Access back things up, but it also compacts and repairs the file. As you add or delete data or modify other database objects, the database file becomes fragmented; pieces of the file are stored in various locations in the hard drive. This increases the file size and decreases efficiency of data retrieval. Compacting undoes this fragmentation, so that file components abut in the same area on the hard drive. Additionally, as I mentioned earlier, files may become corrupted. Access can sometimes identify file corruption and repair it automatically. Indeed, between backups, if the application behaves unexpectedly, you can implement the compact and repair tool via the **Tools** menu, **Database Utilities**, **Compact and Repair Database . . . .**

Finally, you might want to keep a record of your database structure, object properties, etc. The Access Documenter, another of the tools available from the main menu, gives you a detailed report.[56] For additional references see http://www.vb123.com/map/bac.htm (accessed August 3, 2004).

A very important file to back up

Although we explore database security in Chapter 17, I must mention one security-related issue here because it involves file backup. For an Access database with user-level security (necessary to protect patient confidentiality) you also should back up the workgroup information file. The workgroup information file is a separate file that Access reads when it starts up an application that has user-level security. This file includes information about authorized users, including their passwords and what they may do with specific database objects. When you set up user-level security (instructions provided on the accompanying CD) you create a new workgroup for your secured database application. Otherwise any Access application would run from the same workgroup information file and that would compromise security. If the workgroup information file for your secured database is lost or damaged, you won't be able to start the application until you restore or rebuild it.

Backup is no help without recovery

Backed up files, safely stored in some secure and remote location, have no value unless you can use them to undo a data catastrophe. Windows® XP provides a recovery tool. Try it out regularly, so when you really need it to work, deploying it will be routine. Open the **Control Panel** from the Windows® **Start** menu and click **Performance and Maintenance**. Next, select **Back up your data**. Yes, this terminology is reminiscent of having to click the Windows® **Start** button to shut down your computer. Think "Back up *or* recover your data," because the wizard you launch actually does either. Remember to rename the backup file that the recovery process installs with the same name as the original database file. Doing so causes the backup file to overwrite the problematic file, thereby restoring things to the way they were when you made the backup. Of course, when you're just practicing the procedure you may want to choose a different name from the original database file. That way, if you made a mistake during your practice you won't overwrite the good file.

Backing up data on the handheld device

If you backup your database at 10 p.m. every day, and your system crashes at 9 p.m., you've lost 23 hours of data – right? Not necessarily, if you use eNICU. Palm OS® devices running OS 4.0 or later support virtual file system (VFS). VFS can write data to a memory card in the handheld device. You can tell Pendragon Forms to use VFS by setting an **Advanced Form Properties** option (Fig. 16.3). With VFS enabled, each new or modified record is also written to the memory card. This feature eliminates the between-backups problem above and gives peace of mind should the Palm™ device freeze. Refer to the Pendragon Forms manual for additional details and the procedure to restore records.

Imagine that after 3 hours into NICU rounds your handheld freezes. No problem: all the data you entered to that point are safely backed up on the

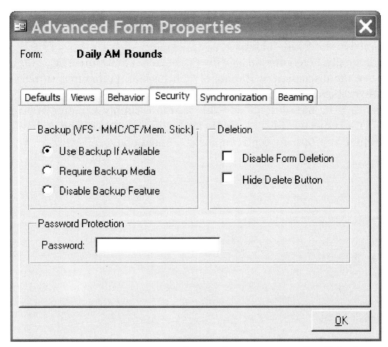

Figure 16.3 eNICU Pendragon Forms **Advanced Form Properties** dialog box.

memory card (see the Pendragon Forms manual[51] for a few common-sense caveats). Although I have never experienced eNICU freezing, until VFS came along, I used to live in fear that both the device and I would be tossed out the window should this happen to a colleague well along in morning rounds. VFS backup currently does not work on PocketPC[TM], but you can install and run the Pendragon Forms application from the memory card. The company is currently developing security guidelines.[53]

Backing up the Pendragon Forms application

The VFS backup protects *data* on the handheld. You cannot recover the Pendragon Forms *application* from the memory card or from the handheld itself. Therefore, you must also back up the Pendragon Forms file that resides on the PC. The company recommends backing up the entire application folder. Within that folder, the Forms32k.mdb file contains the source code and form designs (and data, if your application does not synchronize to an external database, as eNICU does).

Pendragon Forms automatically "backs up" your form designs. When you distribute a form design to a handheld device, Pendragon Forms places a copy of the form design as a .pff file in the PilotF folder. So it's a good idea to back up that folder because you could recover the application by reinstalling the program from the Pendragon Forms CD-ROM and importing the form designs contained in the PilotF folder.

Additionally, I recommend backing up the folder that stores the .csv look-up files. See the discussion in Chapter 14 of the look-up list files stored in the eNICU Lookups folder.

Restoring the files described in this section is simply a matter of placing a copy of the respective file or folder in its original location on the PC hard drive and, where appropriate, replacing the corrupted one.

CHAPTER 17

Security: controlling access and protecting patient confidentiality

Chapter plan

People who should not have access to your database may try to invade. They are far less likely to succeed if you implement some specific safeguards. A secured Access database contains safeguards that make it so time consuming or expensive for an unauthorized user to enter that it's not worth the effort. The security concepts we examine include the following:

- Diverting uploaded data using ODBC;
- Encryption;
- PDA security;
- User- and group-level security in Access;
- Additional application and operating system features to protect the database;
- Database security policy.

ODBC

Microsoft® created Open Database Connectivity standard (ODBC) as a way for a database application to connect to different data sources. The Access Jet engine uses ODBC software – drivers, provided by various software manufacturers and installed under Windows®, to connect to tables in a variety of back-end databases. Jet engine doesn't mean Access has wings and can fly through the air. Jet is an acronym for Joint Engine Technologies – the program application bundled with Access that performs the actual data management (it's also part of Microsoft® Excel and Visual Basic®).[59] For programming-level details about ODBC see Refs. 44 and 63. Through ODBC, Access acts as a client that communicates with the database server. The database server might be an application in one of the heavy-duty database platforms like Microsoft SQL Server or Oracle, but it can also be another Access database (the situation for eNICU).

As mentioned earlier, Pendragon Forms stores by default the data you collect on the handheld in tables that reside in the PC part of the application file. Even though Pendragon Forms is fundamentally an Access application, you cannot apply Access user- and group-level security to the Pendragon Forms application. That means obstacles intended to impede data access must be established outside Pendragon Forms. If Pendragon Forms is stored on a central server running a recent Windows® network operating system you could use

Windows® rights policies to establish which users have read rights to the Forms directory. A user requires such rights merely to see the Forms32k.mdb file in Windows® Explorer and certainly to open it.

I use ODBC to direct the data uploaded during hot sync or Activesync away from tables within Pendragon Forms and to a secured Access database, that is, the eNICU application. The procedure is provided on the accompanying CD. Of course, if you store your database files on a Windows®-based network server, it still makes sense to set user rights and achieve another level of security. (See Ref. 76 for details.)

Encryption

To encrypt a message is to disguise it. The *method* by which a message is disguised is called a cipher. Disguised messages are termed ciphertext. Undisguised messages are termed plaintext. The *process* of changing plaintext to ciphertext is called encryption. Decryption is the process of removing the disguise.

Modular mathematics and prime numbers underpin data encryption and decryption. To refresh your memory of modular (modulo functions) math, arithmetical operations based on 12-hour clock time involve mod 12. If we start at 12 o'clock and add 13 hours, we don't arrive at 25 o'clock, but we arrive at 1 o'clock.

Essentially, encryption algorithms convert letters and numbers to other numbers. Decryption algorithms apply a mathematical inverse operation that brings you back to where you started. If very large prime numbers are used in these algorithms, then it can take a very long time, even for very powerful computers, to break the cipher. The larger the number of bits in the algorithm, the harder it is for a "Black Hat" (an unauthorized person who tries to intercept data) to figure out what your data says. Two good books on this subject are *Cryptography Decrypted*[77] and *The Code Book*.[78] Also explore the U.S. Government Cryptographic Toolkit (http://csrc.nist.gov/CryptoToolkit/; accessed August 4, 2004) and a PBS site (http://www.pbs.org/wgbh/nova/decoding/textindex.html; accessed August 4, 2004).

You can protect patient data on the Palm™ handheld device by using locking and encrypting software that is part of the OS, or install a program like PDA Defense (http://www.pdadefense.com/products.asp; accessed August 3, 2004). Current algorithms are 128-bits, meaning extremely large prime numbers are involved. For Palm™ handhelds with this feature built-in, tap the **Preferences** icon on the home menu screen and select **Security** to activate this protection.

Since unencrypted Access database files may be readable by some text reading software, the procedure for securing the Access eNICU database (see the accompanying CD) includes a step that encrypts the database.

PDA security issues

The following guiding principles to protect data on a personal digital assistant (PDA) are derived from Ref. 79.

- Physical control: these devices are small; someone who shouldn't can easily walk away with one. Always keep the device with you or in a secure place.
- Encryption: if despite your best effort the device is lost, make it exceedingly difficult to retrieve the data on it. Note that for added security, Pendragon Forms version 5 encrypts the data stream during synchronization – a stronger encryption algorithm accompanies SyncServer (http://www .pendragonsoftware.com/syncserver/specifications.html; accessed August 3, 2004).
- Password: another security layer. Set your PDA to require a password when you switch on power and to reactivate after a pre-set time interval of no use.
- Data transmitted during wireless synchronization can be intercepted. For a Pendragon Forms application like eNICU, use the Pendragon Forms Sync-Server to encrypt data using a 168-bits algorithm. Alternatively, some devices support wireless transmission via a virtual private network (VPN); discuss this with your network administrator.

Workgroup information file: user- and group-level security

A workgroup is a defined group of database users. A workgroup information file describes the workgroup and is stored as an encrypted Access database file. After you first install Access, the setup program automatically creates a workgroup information file. It uses the User Name and Organization Name that you entered during the initial installation. If you do nothing more to this workgroup information file it will provide the Access security information for all additional Access applications for which you did not create a new, specific, workgroup information file.

Relying on a generic, minimally specified workgroup information file is an unwise state of affairs. An unauthorized user has only to guess the User Name and Organization Name that you entered at installation to gain administrative permission for your database. Administrative permission means you pretty much can do anything to the data and the database objects. To block this relatively easy way of breaching security, you can create a specific workgroup information file for each application you want to secure. In some cases, to secure your applications you might decide to use one specific workgroup information file other than the one created at initial setup. To secure a specific Access database file, for example, the unsecured eNICU.mdb file on the CD accompanying this book, use the security wizard as described in the instructions on the CD.

The security wizard will ask you about groups and users. A *user* is any individual who works with any part of the database. A *group* is a collection of users who have the same set of permissions for using data and database objects. The database administrator – the person to whom Access gives free reign of the database, that is, you, after you implement the security instructions provided on the CD – regulates what each person is allowed to do by granting *permissions* for each database object after setting up each user account. That means explicit authorization for using *each* table, query, form, report, and macro – modules are secured from within the VBA IDE – even for opening the database itself. These permissions control whether an individual can create a new database object, view it, modify it, or delete it. You may set permissions at the group level or the user level.

It is much simpler to manage group-level permissions than user-level permissions, so try to grant permissions only at the group level. When a new physician joins your organization, you simply need to set up a new user account, assign that user to the proper – already established – group, and set up a password. Assigning the new user to an established group automatically grants the new user the permissions previously granted to the group. You may assign a user to more than one group. In my local eNICU scheme I'm assigned to the Users group – the generic group to which belong all users; the Neonatologists group – a group to which belong all attending neonatologists; the Hot synchers group – a group to which belong all Palm OS® handheld devices authorized to synchronize with eNICU on the PC; and the Admins group – a group to which only I belong, the sole database administrator. *Important*: avoid granting any permissions to the Users group. Access puts everyone in that group by default. If you want all users to have certain permissions, it's better to assign those to all the groups you create. To block the application being changed without your knowledge or assent, you'll probably only assign permission to modify a database object to the administrator. Think too, about whether you want users to be able to delete a record once it's been entered. For more advice about configuring users and groups, see Ref. 67.

Once you have secured the database, the specifically created workgroup information file will be the only one the database will work with. If you split the database and keep the back end on the network server, you can either share the workgroup information file across the network or place a copy on each workstation.

I mentioned that at initial installation Access creates a default workgroup information file. In my experience, workgroup file assignments sometimes become confused. You should know that this default file is named System.mdw and it is always placed in the following path under Windows® 2000 or more recent Windows® operating systems: C:\Documents and Settings\<username>\ApplicationData\Microsoft\Access\System.mdw. Figure 17.1 illustrates the dialog box I see after I open Access (not the secured eNICU file), and select from the main menu **Tools**, **Security**, and **Workgroup Administrator**.

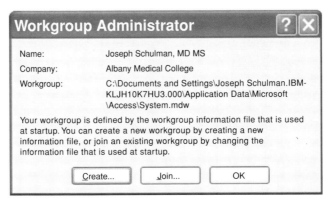

Figure 17.1 Workgroup Administrator dialog box.

Use the **Create** button (Fig. 17.1) when you want to bypass the security wizard (only an advanced user should do this), and use the **Join** button when you want to assign an existing workgroup information file to the database currently open. Although a typical eNICU user doesn't need to open the Pendragon Forms application that resides on the PC, suppose you want anyone who does open it, and therefore can work with the Forms Manager, to log in with the same user name and password needed to open the secured version of eNICU. This requirement blocks anyone but an authorized eNICU user from opening Pendragon Forms. To accomplish this, activate the Pendragon Forms Access database window (usually partially covered by the Forms Manager window) and the typical Access main menu appears across the top of the main window. Select **Tools**, **Security**, and **Workgroup Administrator** and you will see a dialog box resembling Fig. 17.1. Click **Join...** and browse to find the location of the secured workgroup information file for eNICU. If you accepted the wizard defaults when you set up user- and group-level security for eNICU, the file you seek is Security.mdw, contained in the Secured eNICU folder. Selecting that file joins Pendragon Forms to the same workgroup information file as your secured eNICU. Now when a user opens Pendragon Forms, the same log in as for eNICU will be required. If you change your mind about this arrangement, you can rejoin the default System.mdw. Return to the workgroup administrator window, click the **Join...** button again, and browse to the directory location specified in the previous paragraph.

To look inside a secured workgroup information file (.mdw database file), from the main menu select **File** and then **Open...**; at the bottom of the dialog box, in the **Files of type:** combo box, select **Workgroup files** (Fig. 17.2). You may be thinking, "What's the point of a secured workgroup information file that you can easily open?" Well, Access opens Security.mdw, but all you see in the database window is what you see in Fig. 17.3. Explore the queries objects to discover some data you can view. Fear not, you cannot see crucial data like passwords and we shall confirm this shortly.

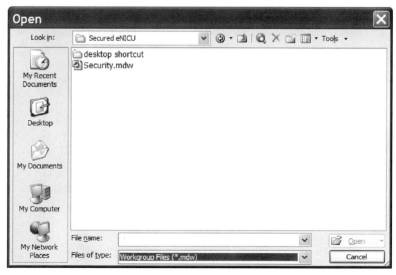

Figure 17.2 Open dialog box for viewing workgroup files.

Return to the list of Table objects in the database window. From the main menu select **Tools**, **Options . . .**, and then select the **View** tab. In the **Show** section, select the check box next to **System objects** and then click **Apply** and **OK**. The database window now resembles Fig. 17.4. The objects with the MSys tag are system objects, usually hidden, a fact symbolized by the dimmed

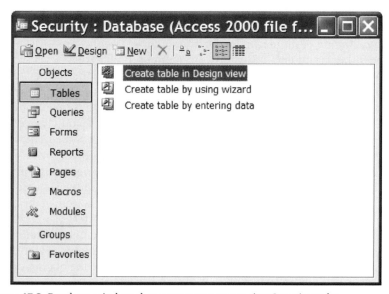

Figure 17.3 Database window that appears upon opening Security.mdw.

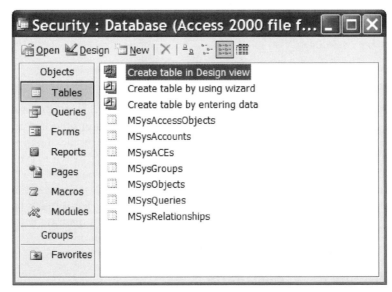

Figure 17.4 Database window that appears after choosing to view system objects.

icons. Open MSysAccounts. Figure 17.5 displays some user accounts. Good luck trying to figure out the passwords. When you're done exploring these objects, clear the check box next to **System objects** in the **View** options. Software programs exist to decrypt Access passwords.[76] So hide the workgroup file from database users: right click the **File** icon, select **Properties**, and select **Hidden**. When possible, use the operating system to limit who can look where.

To learn more about the topics in this section search Access **Help** for "Overview of Access security (mdb)" and look at the online Microsoft Knowledge Base Articles 289885, "Overview of How to Secure a Microsoft

MSysAccounts : Table

FGroup	Name	OLDSID	Password	SID
0	admin		祯□髢剩枭裂□	ã
-1	Admins			□□#□□□#□□□#
0	Creator			ђ
0	Engine			`
0	Hot syncher		I枭裂□剩枭裂□	揪□幄翻鏄搾弄
-1	Hot synchers			겻뒷짪娞酻뺩□
0	schulmj		I枭裂□剩枭裂□	▸□滄껟檂□嵒□□
-1	Users			Ǎ

Record: ◄◄ ◄ [1] ► ►► ►* of 8

Figure 17.5 MSysAccounts.

Access Database," and 305542, "Understanding the Role of Workgroup In-formation Files in Access Security" (http://support.microsoft.com, accessed February 18, 2004).

Protecting VBA code

Everything reviewed so far still does not protect the VBA code attached to pro-tected Access database objects. An authorized database user who has permi-ssion to view the database window can get to the VBA IDE by clicking the code toolbar button or pressing **Alt** + **F11**. To protect your code switch to the VBA IDE, from the main menu select **Tools**, then the concatenation of the name of the VBA project and the word Properties in eNICU, that is, **eNICU Properties...** (Fig. 17.6). Choose the **Protection** tab, select **Lock project for viewing**, and enter a password. From now on, upon opening the VBA IDE, no code will be available until the password has been entered.

Additional user constraints

Usually only the database developer needs to view the database window. Users navigate through the application by means of switchboard forms and custom

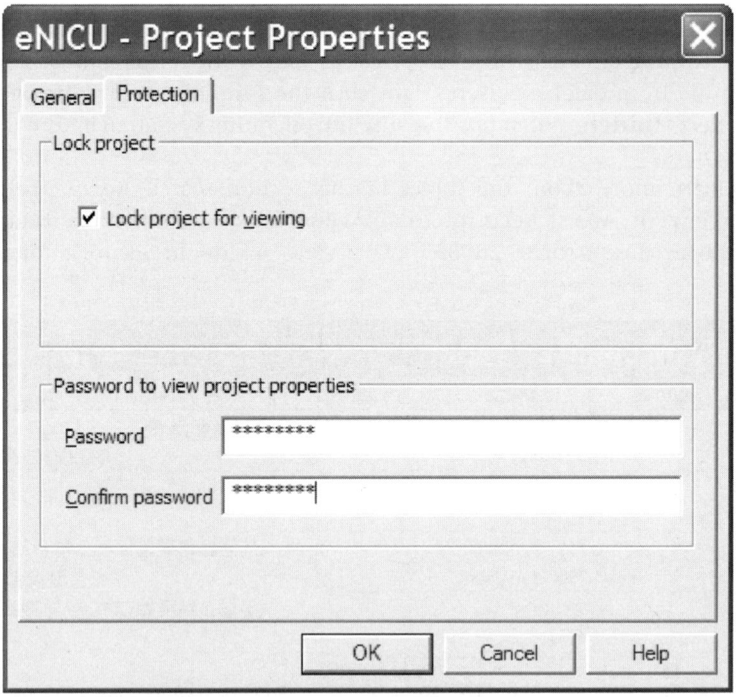

Figure 17.6 eNICU Project Properties dialog box.

menus and toolbars. Access references explain how to create these. You specify whether users can see the database window, and other options, via the **Startup** options dialog box.

From the main menu select **Tools** and then **Startup . . .** to see a dialog box resembling Fig. 17.7. Clear the following: **Display Database Window**, **Allow Toolbar/Menu Changes**, and **Use Access Special Keys**. However, Microsoft provides a workaround for these limitations. Search Access **Help** for **Startup** and read about "Ignore startup options." All anyone need do is to hold down the **Shift** key during startup to bypass the settings you specified in the **Startup** dialog box. Of course, most users don't know about this, but you should. This bypass feature may be turned on or off in VBA by setting the AllowBypassKey database property to True or False. Robinson provides a Form and VBA code to manage these things.[76]

After your development work is complete, on the version you distribute for users to do what they will, consider hiding most objects in the database window. It's easy: right-click the object, select **Properties**, look for Attributes:, and select **Hidden**. It's almost as easy to work around this, but most users do not. To restore hidden objects to the database window, from the main menu click **Tools**, **Options . . .** , press the **View** tab, and select **Hidden** objects. This makes the hidden objects appear in the database window, their icons dimmed. Now you can repeat most of the procedure used to hide the object, only clear the check box next to **Hidden**.

The general idea is that security entails building several layers of defense. Particularly in a network environment, you can use the operating system to create additional layers of defense. For more details, consult with your network administrator and also see Ref. 76.

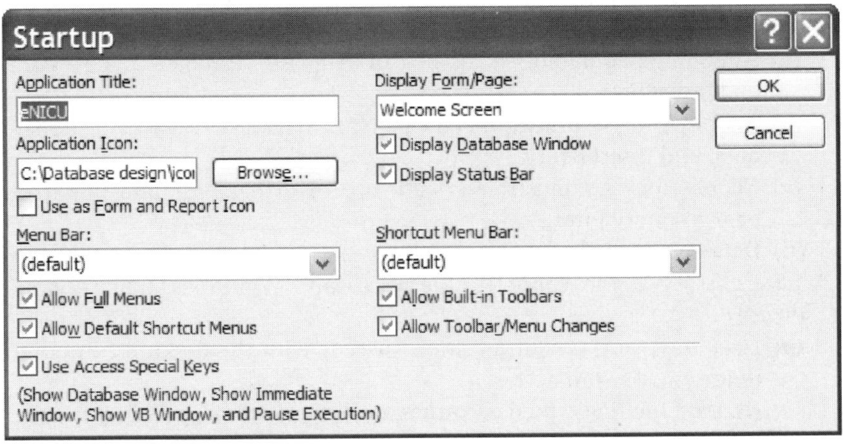

Figure 17.7 Database **Startup** options.

Establishing a database security policy

If you administer a patient information database, one of your duties should include writing a database security policy and making it known to all users. The following sample outline is based on Ref. 80.

1 What are we protecting?
   (a) Information about patients admitted to the NICU and patients at referring institutions whose physicians consult our clinical service by telephone.
2 Why are we protecting this information?
   (a) To protect the privacy and confidentiality of patients and to comply with Federal HIPAA regulations.[81]
3 Our information system inventory
   (a) Hardware
      (i) Handheld computer(s) (specify models and serial numbers): Palm OS® or Microsoft® Windows Mobile 2003™ devices that lock on power-off or no use after 3 minutes; the devices encrypt patient data and require a user password.
         • Physical restrictions: to be carried by care provider or kept in locked office.
      (ii) Desktop computer: Windows® PC (specify model and serial number) connected to institutional network server.
         • Physical restrictions: computer kept in NICU consultation room, only neonatology staff may access.
         • Protected by secure firewalls.
   (b) Software: Pendragon Forms 5.0 (Pendragon Software Corporation, Libertyville, Illinois), Microsoft® Access, and eNICU, which is a NICU database software application that runs in Pendragon Forms 5.0 on the Palm OS® or Microsoft® Windows Mobile 2003™ device and in Microsoft®Access on the desktop computer.
   (c) Data: NICU patient information.
4 Authorized data access
   (a) Attending neonatologists: open/run database, read data, update data, and insert data.
   (b) Neonatal nurse practitioners: open/run database, read data, update data, and insert data.
   (c) Neonatology administrative staff: open/run database and open/run backup query form.
   (d) Database administrator: administer.
5 Data entry (via the Palm OS® or Microsoft® Windows Mobile 2003™ device)
   (a) Data entry and synchronization (wired) with the desktop computer; requires password access.
      (i) Data files encrypted according to the respective operating system.

6 Data management on desktop computer
  (a) All users login with a user name and confidential password.
  (b) For any user terminating employment, user name and password to be deleted immediately by the administrator.
  (c) All patient data stored in encrypted format via Microsoft® Access.
7 Password guidelines
  (a) At least six characters long.
  (b) Alphanumeric combinations.
  (c) Avoid using a complete word.
  (d) Avoid personal statistics: birth date, anniversary, etc.
  (e) Consider connecting two words with a symbol or number between them, for example, penny4thoughts.
  (f) Store written copy of password in secure location.
  (g) Change password at regular intervals.
8 Data integrity and confidentiality
  (a) Only the database administrator can delete records.
    (i) Administrator obtains written authorization from chief of service before deleting a record that reflects an actual patient.
    (ii) Printed records are used only for the hospital record and the administrative office.
      • Office records are maintained in a locked file cabinet in a room that is locked when unoccupied.
  (b) All database users must log off Palm OS® or Microsoft® Windows Mobile 2003™ device and eNICU on desktop computer at end of each work session.
9 Audit trail
  (a) Tables are primarily populated with data coming from forms on handheld device. Each of these new or subsequently modified records includes the device owner name and date/time stamp.
  (b) Data modified via forms on eNICU Access application contain fields that document the logged-on user name and the date/time.
10 Data back up
  (a) Frequency: each week.
  (b) Data quality check: run query to count number of records in each table in database and in backup copy; check for matching number.
  (c) Media: network server; alternate: password-protected Zip® disk or flash drive with built-in encryption, stored in locked cabinet in administrative office.
  (d) Performed by: administrative personnel authorized by chief of service.
11 Backup documentation
  (a) Person performing the backup.
  (b) Date/time performed.
  (c) Total number or records in original database file (see item 10b).
  (d) Total number of records in backup database file (see item 10b).

12 How long do we store the backup media?

   (a) Two backup cycles.

13 How do we dispose of the backup media?

   (a) Erase data using proprietary data wiping software such as Cyber-Scrub (http://www.cyberscrub.com/cyberscrub/index.php; accessed January 19, 2005)

   (b) Reformat media before discarding.

14 Backup: front-end application (for split database)

   (a) Copy of the following, including any update, to be kept on password-protected Zip® disk or flash drive with built-in encryption, locked in administration office.

      (i) Pendragon Forms eNICU application.

      (ii) Secured and unsecured eNICU Notes Access application (no tables; no patient data).

     (iii) Workgroup information file for secured eNICU.

   (b) Paper copy of workgroup information is also kept locked in the administrative office.

Conclusion, Part I: Maintaining focus on a moving target

Van Der Meijden *et al.* reviewed publications between 1991 and 2001 that evaluated inpatient information systems requiring data entry and retrieval by health care professionals.[82] They found a plethora of studies extensively describing system failures, but could find no study that explicitly defined system success. Indeed, health information systems are rather prone to failing.[83] One fundamental for learning from an information system failure is to disentangle user resistance to change[84] from suboptimal technical solutions. Those who protest the changes now occurring in patient information technology must come to see that the real choice does not include the status quo.[13,15,19] Bearing in mind that user acceptance need not imply a problem successfully solved, you may want to see Ref. 85 for a review of individual and organizational factors that influence people to accept new information technology.

When you think about patient information technology, strive for clarity in

- how you determine what is the problem,
- how you articulate the problem,
- your candidate solutions,
- what you aim to achieve by your chosen solution, and why this matters, and
- how you will know when you have achieved your aims.

Wears and Berg warn that many clinical information system failures are doomed at the outset because the system model did not map the actual clinical work.[21] Further, "[software] systems cannot be adequately evaluated by their developers, a principle commonly overlooked in healthcare."[21] Users play a central role in evaluating a system and calibrating it to meet user needs.

What does it take to hit the bull's eye on the patient information system target? The target is large, so you might think that achieving even a near-success should not be very difficult. But the bull's eye is hard to discern. Our notions vary so much that we frequently can't agree on what constitutes the bull's eye.[10,83,86–88] Hitting the bull's eye

- may mean different solutions for apparently similar problems and aims that reside in different environments.
- requires realistic expectations: early iterations of a solution may produce only tolerable or promising results.
  It's just not possible to anticipate every issue that will arise after implementing new technology.

Let me expand on the bewildering, labyrinthine, indistinct, and protean nature of our information system target. We have yet to understand clearly what we do and aim to achieve. Here are some abstract examples; try to think of specific instances from your own experience.

- We confuse reporting information with interpreting information.
- We inconsistently learn from aggregate experience.
- We like to think patient records tell stories, but we have many different ideas of what these stories should be – content and utility vary widely.
- Too often, information systems have a singular target audience: health professionals.
- Although communication and interaction among providers, patients, and families is an integral part of care, operational particulars for these activities at the technological and organizational levels are underspecified[89]

Candidate aims for our systems might include the following:

- Minimum data sets for specific clinical contexts.
- Ensure clinicians interpret patient information by requiring that clinicians transform it to a useful category.

  Consider, for example, the differences between Na = 157, hypernatremia, free water deficit, and sodium excess. The first two are information, and alone, insufficient to guide clinical action. The latter two constitute knowledge, information you can use (Chapter 5), to guide clinical action.

- Facilitate both system-level and patient-level evaluation and learning.
- Protect patient confidentiality yet facilitate information sharing.
- Ensure capability to migrate to an alternate database management system.
- Ensure ability to communicate with other information systems.
- Integrally involve patients and their families in decision making.
- Recognize the communication space that is a regular part of health care; facilitate both the formal and informal social interactions that are a basic part of the daily work.[89]

  Broad evaluative criteria for solutions might include the following:

- Positive impact on duration and flow of daily work.

  Decreases work flow interruption associated with communication yet facilitates conversation – information sharing.[89]

- Decreased probability of error.[90]
- Identify unanticipated system problems by surveying the following:

  What do you need that you're not getting?

  What are you getting that you don't need?

  How did you decide each was the case?

- Agreed-upon attribute set is consistently populated for

  admission notes,

  daily progress notes,

  discharge summary, and

  sign-out summary.

- System consistently populates an agreed-upon attribute set that informs facility performance evaluation and specific research questions.
- Most table attributes can be readily queried.

- System includes elements aimed at patients and their families: information prescriptions that facilitate shared decision making, are based on current and high-quality evidence, reflect the patient's interests, and are easy to understand.[91]
- Improves operationally defined practitioner performance and patient outcomes.[92]

What do *you* think the target and bull's eye look like? See Ref. 93 for more perspective as well as specific suggestions for developing an information system strategy and designing formal methods of evaluation. For an excellent and succinct overview of the challenges in optimizing the interaction between clinical work and information tools, see Ref. 21.

Sharing the design and improvement work

I mentioned earlier that users, not software developers, are the best people to evaluate software products.[21] Any patient information solution must reflect user feedback because new technology changes the way the users do their work.[21,22,93–95] The work of health care is too complex and varied to rely on a but few people to give feedback about the effects of these changes and to calibrate the new technology. If our work is to achieve our aims yet vary little among us in each area of practice, then our information solutions must reflect wide-ranging consideration of those aims, tasks, and tools.[29,93] It is to encourage wide-ranging conversation, exploration, and innovation that eNICU is provided with this book. Product users increasingly are the source of product innovations.[96] However, we must also recognize that wide-ranging collaboration does not *guarantee* operational insight to mapping technology to the way we think. Ideas that appear good must be validated.

Voltaire observed that "the best is the enemy of the good." Our quest is for the best patient information system. But our task is to ensure we always work with a really good system among current alternatives. Rely not exclusively on others to point you to the bull's eye. To know that you hit the mark, develop an explicit evaluative framework that resonates with the fine structure of your work and its important aims.[33,93] But recognize too, that the target keeps moving and insight improves with reiterative study of our work.[20]

Part II
Learning from aggregate experience: exploring and analyzing data sets

Never try to walk across a river just because it has an average depth of four feet

Martin Friedman

SECTION 5
Interrogating data

CHAPTER 18
Asking questions of a data set: crafting a conceptual framework and testable hypothesis

Grounding experience in theory

Consider the MaternalEtOH field of tblMothers, in the eNICU application (Fig. 7.4). This is a check box field on the handheld, stored as a Yes/No, indicating a history of maternal ethanol ingestion during the current pregnancy. My colleagues and I routinely collect this information for each infant admitted to our NICU. But precisely what question(s) does this field answer?

1 Did this mother ingest any ethanol during this pregnancy?
2 Was this infant exposed to any ethanol during this gestation?
3 What is the association between a mother's admitting to using ethanol during pregnancy and phenotypic features of fetal alcohol syndrome in her infant?
4 Did this mother admit to any ethanol ingestion during this pregnancy?

The MaternalEtOH field answers only question 4. Other data are needed to answer questions 1–3. The point is that only after you have articulated the question you wish to answer does it make sense to identify the data elements you need.

In general, our questions are rooted in our experience. Recall, from Chapter 5, the notion of meaning as a context in which data are decoded. Therefore, professional experience has meaning to the extent that we consider the data we use in the contexts to which they correctly belong. And to this extent we work with information, but not necessarily knowledge. For meaningful professional experience to yield increased knowledge – information we can use – we must be able to connect one experience to other sets of experience. We must ground it in theory: a model that describes causal relationships. Indeed, it is largely by connecting disparate items of information to make predictions about system behavior that we establish our professional warrant for patient intervention (see Ref. 33, especially Chapters 9 and 10). How else can we justify doing things to a patient, if we do not understand how the information

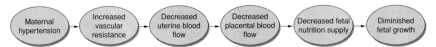

Figure 18.1 A theory of the relationship (causal pathway) between maternal hypertension and infant birth weight.

relevant to the patient's condition comes together? Be wary of doing analytical work that is atheoretical, that is, work that yields results you cannot connect to other knowledge.[97] Before you ever begin to think about data you need, formulate a theory about your subject of interest. It is upon this basis that you determine the variables and the analytical methods necessary to learn from your experience.

Imagine you're interested to know whether maternal hypertension affects birth weight (BW). In an atheoretical approach, you might compare BW of infants born to hypertensive mothers with that for infants born to mothers who are not so. Seems pretty straightforward, right? Suppose the comparison indicates that the group of infants born to hypertensive mothers indeed had lower BW. Well, *exactly* how do you interpret this atheoretical finding? If you do not relate the factors you studied to any associated factors or ideas – if your investigation was atheoretical – your interpretation is rather limited, isn't it?

In a theoretical approach, you might begin by reflecting on mechanisms by which maternal hypertension could affect infant BW. Figure 18.1 illustrates a simple theoretical approach.

Developing a conceptual framework from theoretical reflection

A theoretical approach to crafting a question employs a conceptual framework: a system of interrelationships among factors that may play a role in the suspected causal pathway. Each factor may be described by a variable (any characteristic that can be measured or placed in a category). The simplest conceptual framework contains two variables (Fig. 18.2): the dependent, or outcome variable (BW), and the independent, or predictor variable (maternal hypertension). At this simplest level, the framework is essentially atheoretical because it provides no basis to connect the findings to other knowledge.

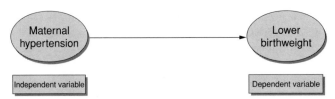

Figure 18.2 The simplest possible conceptual framework.

A conceptual framework grounded in theory might include some of the following additional considerations relating to the theory depicted in Fig. 18.1 (see Ref. 98).

- Preeclampsia includes hypertension and proteinuria.
- Preeclampsia may cause intrauterine growth restriction.
- Preeclampsia may cause premature delivery for maternal indications.
- Premature infants tend to have low BW.
- Multiple gestation is a risk factor for preeclampsia.
- Multiple gestation is associated with lower BW after 32-weeks gestation.
- Cigarette smoking decreases the risk of preeclampsia.
- Cigarette smoking is associated with lower BW (see p. 93 in Ref. 99).
- Women with chronic hypertension are at greater risk to develop preeclampsia, and when it develops, of greater severity.
- The diagnosis of preeclampsia may be confounded by the presence of other, unrelated conditions that also cause hypertension or proteinuria.
- Preeclampsia may also be associated with poor placentation.
- Poor placentation can affect fetal growth.
- Mild preeclampsia at term may have minimal neonatal effects.
- Lowering the blood pressure of a preeclamptic mother may decrease uterine blood flow.

To account for these additional considerations we must add to the simple conceptual framework of Fig. 18.2, covariates, that is, additional variables believed to influence the outcome variable.

Confounding

Some covariates represent confounding variables. George Bernard Shaw illustrated confounding this way (see p. 116 in Ref. 100):

> Thus it is easy to prove that the wearing of tall hats and the carrying of umbrellas enlarges the chest, prolongs life, and confers comparative immunity from disease; for the statistics shew that the classes which use these articles are bigger, healthier, and live longer than the class which never dreams of possessing such things. (Preface to "The Doctor's Dilemma" 1906)

A confounder is a factor that distorts the association between an exposure variable (also called an independent or predictor variable) and the outcome (also called the dependent variable). The distortion arises because the confounder is itself associated with both the exposure and the outcome. The effects of the exposure on the outcome are thus mixed with the effects of the confounder on the outcome, confusing – confounding – one's understanding of the true causal relationships. Figure 18.3 introduces cigarette smoking as a confounder of the relationship in Fig. 18.2. Note that a confounder may have either a positive or a negative effect on the outcome.

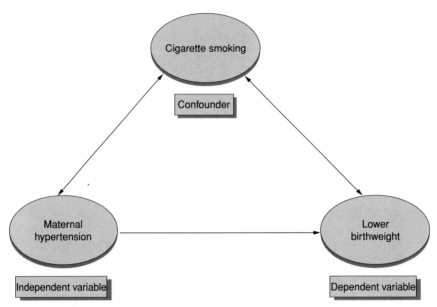

Figure 18.3 Cigarette smoking as a confounder of the relationship in Fig. 18.2.

Bias

Bias creates data that suggest a different relationship between an exposure and outcome than actually applies. Bias denotes some systematic error affecting the outcome data. This implies the outcome data describe comparison groups. One group is exposed to an intervention or something in the environment and another is not. Bias exists when the groups differ systematically in the way they are selected to enter the study or in the way data are collected, interpreted, or reported, and when *the difference is related to exposure status*. In other words, a biased study design allows other differences that affect the exposure–outcome relationship to systematically sneak in to one group more than the other. In the hypertension/BW relationship we've been considering, selection bias might occur if some groups were assembled from infants admitted to a NICU and others were not, because their mothers are more likely to have experienced multiple complications during pregnancy. Both selection bias and observation bias could creep in if the comparison groups were not matched on adequacy of prenatal care. (See Refs. 101–103 for additional discussion.)

Cohort and case-control studies[103]

There are two basic approaches to explore an association between exposure and outcome (Table 18.1). A cohort study examines the experience of a defined group of individuals during a specified period of time. A cohort, in ancient Rome, was a group of soldiers who marched together in time. Cohort

Table 18.1 Comparison of case-control with cohort study design

	Case-control study	Cohort study
Whom are we studying?	Subjects *selected on the basis of whether or not they experienced the outcome* of interest. We distinguish exposure status after entry to the study.	Subjects *defined on the basis of exposure status*. Only after entry to the study do we distinguish who experienced the outcome and who did not.
What are we comparing?	*Exposure prevalence* among those experiencing the outcome and controls – those not experiencing the outcome who were sampled from individuals at risk to be identified as cases if they experience the outcome.	*Outcome occurrence* among the different exposure groups.
How do we ensure the comparison is fair?	For all exposures but the study exposure, a control must have the same exposure prevalence as that of the population that produced the cases. A control is not necessarily the same idea as a randomly selected non-case.	Exposed and unexposed should have the same baseline outcome risk: groups should be alike in every other way besides the specific, defined exposure and its effect.
Strength	Suited for studying infrequently occurring outcomes.	Suited for studying infrequently occurring exposures.
Limitation	Prone to selection and other bias.	Rarely occurring outcomes require very large and expensive studies.

subjects also "march together in time." A cohort study distinguishes groups by their exposure, comparing the respective outcomes. The other approach, a case-control study, distinguishes groups by their outcome, comparing the exposure prevalence (proportion) among cases (individuals who experienced the outcome) with controls (individuals who did not experience the outcome and were sampled from the study base). The study base is all individuals at risk to be identified as cases if they experience the outcome during the same period of time in which cases are identified. [Including among controls all individuals at risk to be cases, regardless of whether they can be identified, can inflate the size of the group.]

In a cohort study, the exposed group should have the same *baseline* outcome risk as the unexposed group. Only then may we accurately account for any effect of the exposure. From the experience of the unexposed group we estimate the outcome occurrence that the exposed group would have had if they *were not* exposed. This way of thinking is called counterfactual reasoning; it may seem peculiar at first. The point is that exposed and unexposed ideally should be alike in every other way besides exposure, and quite possibly, outcome. If the unexposed group provides an inaccurate estimate of the baseline outcome risk then the cohort study is biased.

In a case-control study, the controls should have the same exposure prevalence as the study base (the population experience that produced the cases) for all exposures but the one under investigation. Only then may we accurately account for any effect of this study exposure. If the controls do not accurately reflect the study base then the case-control study is biased. Thus, we can't simply select controls at random from a geographically defined group, because we don't know that our study base, so defined, is congruent with the population experience the cases actually came from. The cases may have emerged from a study base that is a distinct subgroup within the study base we defined by randomly selecting individuals from the geographically defined group.

Analytical interpretation

Let's return to the list of considerations relating to maternal hypertension and lower BW. Figure 18.4 depicts a more detailed conceptual framework for

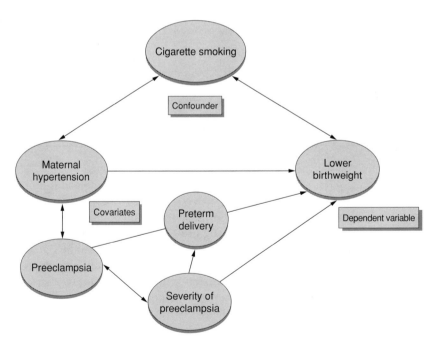

Figure 18.4 A more detailed conceptual framework for the association between maternal hypertension and lower birth weight.

the association between maternal hypertension and lower BW. Suppose you analyze the data in a manner (which we consider in later chapters) consistent with this conceptual framework and find an association between predictor and outcome. Several interpretive possibilities exist[101]

- The association is real.
- The association is influenced by bias. It may still be real, but the measure of the effect may be over- or underestimated.
- The association is distorted by confounding.
- The association appears simply by chance.

Statistical techniques enable us to evaluate the role of chance in associations that appear in our data. Statistical techniques also enable us to adjust the analysis for the contribution of known confounders and other covariates. In studies where confounders are unknown or difficult to identify for statistical adjustment, to neutralize their effects we try to distribute these factors equally among the groups via random exposure allocation. Statistical techniques do not reveal bias, although they can sometimes account for it once we recognize it. To recognize bias in a study, we rely on knowledge of proper study design and critical reflection.

Identifying the variables you need

A conceptual framework identifies the variables you need to include in a study, and those you need not.[104] The preterm delivery covariate in Fig. 18.4 appears in the causal pathway between preeclampsia and lower BW. It thus depicts an intervening variable, one in the causal sequence between the independent variable and the dependent variable. Including this intervening variable in the analysis adjusts to some extent for the antecedent exposure. By "adjusting away" the primary causal exposure you "adjust away" the relationship you are seeking to identify and you get the wrong answer from the analysis. Remember this when we consider multivariate modeling. A model that contains more covariates is not always a better model. A model containing multiple covariates that are part of the same causal sequence is overspecified: it obscures rather than reveals causal relationships.

Hypothesis

A hypothesis is a special type of statement derived from a broader – and often at the outset, vague – question. For example, the question "Do infants of birth weight <2500 g tend to have poorer outcomes?" might lead to the hypothesis that "Infants with birth weight <2500 g have a higher neonatal mortality risk than those of birth weight ≥2500 g." Your conceptual framework facilitates connecting to other knowledge your interpretation of such a hypothesis test. A testable hypothesis is one that attempts to describe an association or predict what will happen. The method by which a hypothesis is tested varies with the nature of the data (much of the forthcoming material explains the particulars).

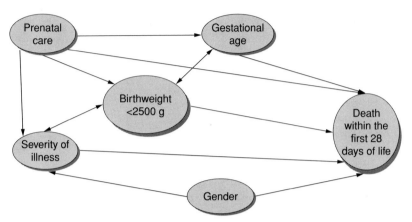

Figure 18.5 The conceptual framework underlying the hypothesis: "After adjusting for prenatal care, gestational age, severity of illness, and gender, infants with birth weight <2500 g born to Hispanic mothers at my medical center have a higher neonatal mortality risk than those of birth weight ≥2500 g."

A good hypothesis describes relationships among *plausibly relevant and clearly defined factors* that are *readily measured.*[105] The hypothesis "Infants with birth weight <2500 g have a higher neonatal mortality risk than those of birth weight ≥2500 g" comes close to meeting this definition of a good hypothesis. One factor not yet clearly defined is the population of interest. The answer to the hypothesis as presently stated may depend upon the population groups being compared and may vary quantitatively or qualitatively. Here is a good hypothesis: "After adjusting for prenatal care, gestational age, severity of illness, and gender, infants with birth weight <2500 g born to Hispanic mothers at my medical center have a higher neonatal mortality risk than those of birth weight ≥2500 g" (Fig. 18.5).

The null hypothesis

The null hypothesis is a special hypothesis. Often denoted H_0, it posits no difference among the groups you are comparing. The so-called alternative hypothesis, H_A, posits the contrary. It's that simple, except for the computation. For example, in comparing the average BW in two groups of infants, one group whose mothers had preeclampsia and one group whose mothers had no medical problems or pregnancy complications, suppose that the average BW in the latter group was 3265 g. The null hypothesis would affirm that the average BW of the group whose mothers were preeclamptic was not statistically different from 3265 g.

CHAPTER 19

Stata: a software tool to analyze data and produce graphical displays

Kinds of knowledge about Stata

Donald Norman distinguishes two kinds of knowledge: knowledge *of* and knowledge *how* (p. 57 in Ref. 70). Knowledge of – declarative knowledge – entails facts. Knowledge how – procedural knowledge – entails functional capability and increases with practice. The difference between the two is the reason that most people can't simply read a book about playing the piano and then play it skillfully. Besides knowledge *of* playing the piano they need knowledge *how* to play; they need to practice at the keyboard. It's the same, I think, for statistical analysis.

Stata[16] is a popular statistical software package for analyzing a data set. Although it's not essential for you to work with it as you read through the chapters to follow, doing so will enhance your analytical skill. Stata enables you to manage data, analyze data, and display tabular and graphical results. Stata will execute any valid command you ask of it, so don't be impressed with the output unless you are confident you've asked it to execute a procedure appropriate for the data and the question.

Stata comes in several "flavors," as the company calls them – feature packages. The "intercooled" flavor will serve you well. Among the 13 separate books constituting the Stata printed documentation, do read the *Getting Started* manual. Peruse both the *User's Guide*, especially Chapters 2, 3, 5, 7, 8, 14–16, 19, and 31, and the *Graphics Manual*, especially the introduction. Selecting **Help** from the Stata main menu leads to summaries of commands and syntax.

Figure 19.1 orients you to the Stata interface. Each line of code you type in the Stata command window – no matter how short or long – conforms to the following basic structure, or syntax:

```
[by varlist:]command [varlist][= exp] [if exp] [in range] [weight]
[,options]
```

- *varlist*: a list of one or more variable names.
- *command*: a particular Stata command.
- *exp*: some expression, typically in algebraic form.
- *range*: the values you want to be included.

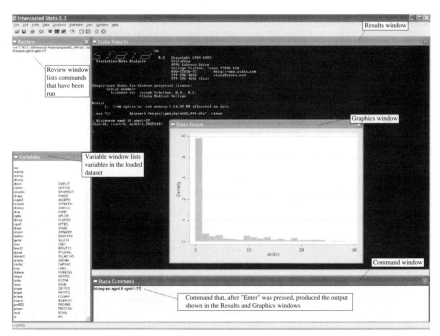

Figure 19.1 The Stata interface: after loading data, adjusting window proportions, and generating a graphical display.

- `weight`: some expression that describes how much weight the analytic item should have (other than unit value).
- `options`: special features (not optional elements), separated by a comma from the earlier part of the statement, that you select to be part of the computation or display.

The command appearing in the command window in Fig. 19.1 is relatively simple: `histogram aged if aged<=27`. The command does not begin with the optional `by varlist`:. If, for example, you want to see one histogram describing only males and one describing only females, you might begin the command with `by gender`:. Note that some variable lists, such as the one illustrated, exceed the confines of the variable window display size, so you must scroll down the variables window to see all variables in the data set. No other options appear in the illustrated command. If, for example, you want a histogram describing each gender, and containing 30 bars instead of the 21 shown: `by gender: histogram aged if aged<=27, bin(30)`.

I recommend three additional resources to help you become comfortable using Stata: *A Short Introduction to Stata 8 for Biostatistics*,[106] *Statistics with Stata*,[107] and the UCLA Academic Technology Services Stata website.[108] At a minimum, you'll find it helpful to refer to the latter resources and to Stata documentation regarding the illustrative analyses in the coming chapters.

CHAPTER 20
Preparing to analyze data

Getting the right data in the right arrangement

Stata needs its data served just so

Perhaps you have some experience working with data in a spreadsheet program like Microsoft® Excel. As described in any of the Stata resources mentioned in Chapter 19, it's easy to turn this into a Stata analytical file. You must convert data to Stata file format to analyze them, but that doesn't mean any Stata file is ready for analysis. Original data sources commonly are not ready for analysis. Although reformatted, the data may retain fundamental deficiencies. As I use the term here, format means a method of storing all the data in the electronic file. Stata data files are denoted by the file extension .dta. A data set in Stata file format is data plus metadata, which is data about data, such as variable names and labels, variable type and size specifications, and notes about the data.

An alternative meaning of the term format is the nature of the data constituting a variable. Analysis may require that we convert a variable's data format. For example, a variable that records a "yes" or "no" response might initially be coded as "Y" or "N," but computational algorithms require a "1" or "0." Characters may appear as numbers but in fact are formatted as strings, that is, alphanumeric characters that are not subject to mathematical operations. If you try to perform such operations on a string variable, Stata will complain until you convert the variable to a numeric format (see Chapters 15 and 26 in the *Stata User's Guide*[16]).

Dirty data

The jargon for fundamental deficiencies in an original data source is "dirty data": values may be improperly formatted, incorrect, or missing. Data can become "dirty" at any stage of their existence.

1 They may start out dirty, having been inaccurately entered.
2 "Clean" data may become dirty in the course of subsequent storage, manipulation, or moving the data, for example, into Stata.
   - Stata offers several commands to read data into the program, including `insheet`, `infile`, and `infix`. You must always check that the data set Stata has read into memory correctly maps to the data source. More or less apparent discrepancies are common.
   - They may become dirty in the process of creating the analytical data set from the source data.

(a) Errors may occur when you assemble one flat table for analysis in Stata from linked records in several tables; either by merging records using the Stata `merge` command or by queries that operate on a database.

(b) Errors may occur when you create new variables in the analytical data set. For example, a data set contains 1500 records of infants varying in birth weight between 460 and 4570 g. You want to explore the relationship between birth weight and neonatal death. It makes biological sense and facilitates interpretation to create a few categories of birth weight and explore how they relate to neonatal death, rather than compute the probability of neonatal death as a function of each 1-g increment in birth weight. Here's how you could do this. The birth weight variable is called BW; you could choose different categorical cutpoints:

```
generate BWcat=1 if BW >= 460 & BW < 500
replace BWcat=2 if BW >= 500 & BW < 1000
replace BWcat=3 if BW >= 1000 & BW < 2500
replace BWcat=4 if BW >= 2500 & BW < 4000
replace BWcat=5 if BW >= 4000 & BW <= 4570
```

I created a new variable called `Bwcat`, which takes on values 1 through 5, corresponding to hypothetical risk categories. You must check that the categories each contain the correct number of records and are correctly bounded (methods appear in later chapters.)

Checking data quality

When using a new data set, it is worthwhile to perform a few routine procedures to check the quality of the data. Check

- the number of records in the resulting data set.
  For example, some observations may be dropped because of record linking problems or because a variable type mismatch prohibited creating a merged record.
- that linkages indeed occurred on the correct variable (when merging two or more data sources).
- each variable for (the `codebook` command is very useful)
  missing values,
  appropriate values, and
  correct formatting or data type.
- record integrity for at least a sample of the data set, that is, within an individual record, the values of each variable should make sense individually and in the context of the values of the other variables.

Getting data into Stata using ODBC

Consider these situations:

1 Your data source contains 1750 observations, of which you wish to select only those with a particular postal code.

2 Your data source is composed of linked records stored in 23 different tables. Unless you are familiar with methods to import data into Stata, you could spend a lot of time searching for the desired data and moving it into your analytical data set. One very efficient approach is to run from Stata a query on the source database, creating an answer table to serve as your initial working data set. Stata (version 8) can run a command that includes SQL code, to open an ODBC data source (even one requiring a password), retrieve exactly the data you need, and create a Stata file from the answer table to the query. Before I show you how to do this, you may want to review the sections of Chapters 11 and 17 that deal with queries and ODBC; also, search Stata **Help** on ODBC.

Stata provides several ODBC commands that enable you to load, write, or view data that reside in ODBC sources. An ODBC-enabled software application can use a set of standardized functions that allow access to relational, such as Microsoft® Access, and non-relational, such as Microsoft® Excel, data sources. Here are some of the Stata ODBC commands:

- `odbc list`: Stata produces a list of data source names (DSN) to which it can connect. Here's the output I got when I ran this command on my laptop:

```
. odbc list

Data Source Name                    Driver
------------------------------------------------------------------
MS Access Database                  Microsoft Access Driver (*.mdb)
Excel Files                         Microsoft Excel Driver (*.xls)
dBASE Files                         Microsoft dBase Driver (*.dbf)
NICU Notes                          Microsoft Access Driver (*.mdb)
eNICU                               Microsoft Access Driver (*.mdb)
```

- `odbc query`: **is more complicated; the syntax is:** `odbc query` `["DataSourceName", connect_options]` **For a secured Access database,** `connect_options` **means you must specify the user name and password you would ordinarily provide when trying to gain access to the data. In the following command, NICU Notes is the DSN (NICU Notes is the predecessor of eNICU), user [name] is "myname," and password is "noneofyourbusiness":**

```
. odbc query "NICU Notes", user(myname) password(noneofyourbusiness)
```
retrieves a list of table names available from the data source's system catalog

```
DataSource: NICU Notes
Path      : C:\Database design\Secure NICU Notes\NICU Notes
------------------------------------------------------------------
tblAbnormalFindingsonAdm
tblAMCHAttendingNumber
tblConsultations
```

```
tblDailyAMRounds
.
. output omitted
.
tblSubspecialtyDischargeAppts
tblUnintendedEvents
```

- odbc load: **the syntax is:** odbc load [extvarlist] [if exp]
  [in range],{table("TableName") | exec("SqlStmt") }
  [dsn("DataSourceName") connect_options clear noquote lowercase
  sqlshow]. **For example:** odbc load, table("tblInfants")dsn("NICU
  Notes") user(myname) password(noneofyourbusiness) clear; **you
  could substitute** exec("SQL SELECT...") **for table. A second
  example:** odbc load InfantID LastName BirthWeight AdmitWeight,
  table("tblInfants") dsn("NICU Notes") user(myname) password
  (noneofyourbusiness) clear; **in this instance of the** odbc load
  **command, I identified particular fields as the only fields to load
  from the selected table.**

  The syntax for odbc load **enables you to choose either a**
  table **statement or an** exec **statement within the curly brackets**
  {table("TableName") | exec("SqlStmt") }. **This option (it's an
  option because it appears after the comma in the syntax model)
  enables precise specificity in selecting only the variables and
  records you need. The** "SqlStmt" **you would insert between the set
  of double quotes would specify in SQL the precise subset - the
  particular variables and records - you need. You could write it
  directly, if you're feeling capable with SQL, or copy and paste
  the SQL statement created by the Access query design grid, as
  described in Chapter 11.**

The analytical Plan

This part of the chapter is about the Plan, written with a capital "P," because it is
so important to *plan* how you intend to analyze your data before you actually
analyze them. Return to this section from time to time as you continue reading
Part II of this book. Some terms in this chapter are fully defined only later in
the book because they involve concepts whose foundations are not yet set.
Equally important, the planning suggestions gain traction as your analytical
experience increases. I present the Plan relatively early in the story so you
may fit the individual analytical techniques of the coming chapters within an
integrated and coherent cognitive structure.

Elements of an analytical Plan

To maximize the validity and interpretation of your analysis, develop a written
analytical Plan that explicitly states the following:

- The main hypothesis
  secondary hypotheses
- The outcome (response; dependent) variable(s)
- The exposure (explanatory; predictor; independent) variables
  possible confounders
  possible effect modifiers
- How you will check the variables for "dirty data"
- How you will explore the variables to understand the individuals you are studying (graphical displays, tabulations, cross-tabulations, etc.)
- The variables you think you will need to derive from the starting data set
- The univariate analyses you think will inform later multivariate analyses
- The appropriate type(s) of multivariate analyses
- Possible interactions among exposure variables and how you will explore these
- How you will ensure that your analytical work is both reproducible and understandable to you after much time has passed (log files, Stata .do files)

Such a plan guides you in conducting your analysis, interpreting the results, and reporting them. Such a plan also keeps you honest should you discover something unexpected. For example, suppose your outcome variable is categorical: yes or no for having received an incorrect medication; exposure variables include plausible predictors: month of year and patient turnover rate. You find no association between the outcome and your exposure variables. Although you didn't plan to examine this, you add patient gender to the model and discover a significant interaction. In reporting what you found, you ought to say whether you hypothesized this interaction or you discovered it unexpectedly among the data you collected to test another hypothesis.

Hypothesis precedes analysis

When analyzing a data set containing many exposure variables, you might lose sight of the central aim of the analytical effort – the test of the main hypothesis. Always write the main hypothesis to ensure you have a clear idea of what it is, to anchor your thinking about whether it is indeed "testable," and to check that the hypothesis you tested is the hypothesis you articulated. For similar reasons, also write the null hypothesis.

Distinguish the main hypothesis from secondary hypotheses. Particularly when the result of testing the main hypothesis is disappointing, it may be tempting to shift the focus to a secondary hypothesis that has emerged as more interesting or more conclusive.

The problems of *ad hoc* and *post hoc* hypotheses are important for guiding both analysis and interpretation. A pattern you find in data may confirm a hypothesis only if you formulated the hypothesis before you started to look at the data. As mentioned, any apparent association you find in data may represent a chance event, bias, confounding, or a real causal relationship. By specifying a hypothesis before you analyze the data, you focus on the probability of finding a significant difference between a *particular* set of variables. When you "find" a significant difference between groups, one you didn't suspect at the outset, you can't use the same analytical methods to estimate the probability of an effect of that size occurring by chance as you did when you specified the hypothesis in advance. If this difference you "found" was indeed a chance effect, it's unlikely you would find it a second time if you look at the same association, only in another data set. On the other hand, if the difference reflects a real causal relationship, you are likely to find it when you look for it anew in another data set. So when you "find" an association that you didn't originally set out to find, you should treat it as *a new hypothesis to test, using a different data set.*

Data checking

This part of the Plan helps prevent GIGO (garbage in, garbage out).[47] Once you're comfortable with it, Stata is a fun program to use. It's very tempting to jump right in and run the regressions, produce the multicolor graphics. However, to be confident the analytical results accurately describe your sample or population, you must also be confident the data you analyzed are accurate. "Dirty data" is very common; problems range from subtle to flagrant. Well-designed database software anticipates and tries to prevent these problems, but problems occur nonetheless. For example, accidentally add a terminal zero to an infant's birth weight of 3780 grams and the distribution of values is drastically changed. See what happens when you try that on the handheld portion of eNICU.

You might start checking the data by examining the distribution of values for each variable. A graphical display often allows you to identify a questionable value almost as soon as you look. Have an idea of the range that you expect most values to lie within, and look for "outliers." A frequency-distribution histogram requires only one Stata command line and can tell you a great deal about a variable.

Sometimes you encounter a problem as soon as you *try* to look at the distribution of values: the variable may not be correctly formatted for the desired analysis. Numerical formats depend on the size of the numbers and the desired decimal precision. Text formats are called strings. Date and time data get their own formats, as well. A common explanation for problems producing a frequency-distribution histogram is observations containing apparently "numerical" entries that are in fact formatted as string data. Although the data, to you, look like a number, they are not amenable to mathematical computation. For example, a medical record number is often stored as a string variable; you'd never add or multiply medical record numbers.

The codebook command is very helpful for several aspects of checking your data. Does the data set contain missing values? Stata can recognize missing values and report them to you. Here is output resulting from codebook *SAMPLEVAR*, mv:

SAMPLEVAR

--type: numeric

```
(byte)
range:    [2,2]                  units: 1            unique values: 1
missing .:   1573/1877
                   tabulation:  Freq.  Value
                                  304  2
                                 1573  .
```

The `codebook` command reports the data type, that is, format, range of values, measurement units, number of unique values, and tabulates the distribution of values; the `mv` option adds the number of missing values. Stata denotes a missing value as "." and in version 8 offers 26 additional ways to denote missing (beyond our scope).

Check that the number of records in the data set corresponds to the number of records that you should have. Running queries and input commands, manually entering data, and creating a derived variable, all can result in lost observations.

Check that within particular observations the entered values for the variables make sense and that they are consistent with each other, that is, tell Stata to `list` some observations. For example, if an infant has a gestational age of 41 weeks and a birth weight of 780 g, there's likely a problem with data accuracy – though not always.

Exploring the data set
Now that you've cleaned the data, look again at the distribution of values for each variable. Use both tabulations and graphical displays to settle any doubts that the data are clean. Once reassured, you can begin to understand the characteristics of the individuals in your data set.

Derived variables
Sometimes the variables you measured are not the appropriate ones for your analysis. Suppose you collected date of birth and your analysis calls for patient age. It's easy to derive age from date of birth: subtract date of birth from "today." Or you collected gestational age in weeks and you think that the informative exposure variable is gestational age category: ≤23 weeks; >23 and ≤27 weeks; >27 and ≤32 weeks; and >32 weeks. Here's one way to do this in Stata. The continuous variable describing gestational age is `gestat`. Generate a new categorical variable, GACAT, and assign it values ranging from 1 to 4, as follows:

```
gen GACAT = 1 if gestat<=23
(1526 missing values generated)

replace GACAT = 2 if gestat>23 & gestat <=27
(1029 real changes made)

replace GACAT = 3 if gestat>27 & gestat <=32
```

```
(396 real changes made)

replace GACAT = 4 if gestat>32
(101 real changes made)
```

You can sometimes simplify the process of estimating a risk relationship for a variable that has many possible categorical states. If one of the possible categories represents "unexposed" and all the others represent different degrees of exposure, treat as separate groups the "unexposed" and *any* type of exposed. In a maternal smoking variable, for example, values might range between 0 packs/day (nonsmoker) and 5 packs/day. You might create a nonsmoker variable (0/1) and a smoker variable, with categories that describe degree of exposure.

The choice of categorical cutpoints depends on statistical considerations and knowledge of the phenomenon under study. The GACAT categories I created above reflect known relationships with mortality risk. If you create many categories in relation to the number of observations, small categorical samples will make it difficult to obtain significant *P* values for differences when differences indeed exist among the source populations (we expand on this in Chapter 25).

Univariate analysis

Begin by exploring the association of the outcome of interest with various individual exposure variables. Univariate analysis can indicate early in the analysis where most of the "action" is going on. Which among all the variables subsumed in your hypothesis are most strongly associated with the outcome? Moreover, by comparing the effect estimate in the crude (unadjusted, univariate) analysis with the effect estimate for the same exposure variable in the adjusted, multivariate analysis, you appreciate the degree of confounding accounted for by the other significant exposure variables in the multivariate model. Univariate tabulations can also provide additional data quality checks. Knowing, for example, that for a particular univariate exposure/outcome association there were only a few outcome events, or a few observations with the particular exposure, might point you to a data quality problem.

Multivariate analysis

For our purposes, planning the multivariate analysis means thinking about what type of regression analysis is appropriate and which variables to include in the model. This planning reflects the conceptual framework we described in Chapter 18 and the material in Chapters 28, 30, 33–35.

Interactions

The regression models we examine that account for the effect of two or more exposure variables on an outcome assume independent effects of the exposure variables. Sometimes this assumption isn't valid. To explore whether the effect of one explanatory variable on the outcome depends on the value of another explanatory variable in the model, you add an interaction term to the model. An interaction term is a new variable that represents the product of the two variables you suspect may interact. Chapter 33 contains an illustration of the idea.

Documenting your analytical work

You must ensure your work is reproducible, by you and by others. When you execute a command in Stata you get an immediate result, but you do not get a permanent record. Stata operates in RAM memory; when you exit the program, all results are wiped from the computer's memory. Fortunately, Stata offers a log file feature: unless you use it you will lose your work. However, if you have experience working with a statistical software package, you know that a real analytical session does not flow without difficulty. You may enter a command and receive an error message. Or you may enter a command and get dozens of pages of output you never wanted. For these reasons, log files fill up quickly. To ensure your analysis is both reproducible and efficient, make a Stata .do file for each analytical task you have tested and refined. A Stata .do file often derives from an edited log file.

A Stata .do file contains all the commands, in the sequence you ran them, for your analytical task. Merely tell Stata to execute the file and your analysis and results reappear. The Stata manual clearly explains how to work with this feature. As an illustration, here is a .do file that opens a log file at the start of the session, uses ODBC to load data in Stata from a separate database, and closes the log file at the end. Explanatory comments not integral to the program appear between /* and */.

```
version 8
clear
set more off
cd "C:\Data"
log using "ODBC load.log" , replace

/*

Program name: ODBC_load.do
Programmed by: Joseph Schulman
Last update: 20 December 2004
Function: allow STATA to load data from NICU Notes
Note: Dataset: NICU Notes database; Task: load data from tables;
examples of commands appear below

*/

odbc list          /* list all odbc database in system directory*/
odbc query "NICU Notes", user(myname) password(noneofyourbusiness)
/*retrieve a list of table names available from the data source's
system catalog*/odbc describe "tblInfants", dsn("NICU Notes") user
```

```
(myname) password(noneofyourbusiness) odbc load, table("tblInfants")
dsn("NICU Notes") user(myname) password(noneofyourbusiness) clear
/*can substitute exec("SQL SELECT...") for table */odbc load
InfantID LastName, table("tblInfants")dsn("NICU Notes") user
(myname) password(noneofyourbusiness) clear /*select columns*/

/*end commands*/

log close
exit
```

SECTION 6
Analytical concepts and methods

CHAPTER 21
Variable types

Identical symbols may represent different information

Although data values may appear alike, they may represent very different kinds of information. Consider the variables – attributes, or fields, in database jargon – shown in Table 21.1. The value "0" for "Day of life" denotes age in days. The value "0" for "Prenatal care" denotes no prenatal care ("1" would denote prenatal care was received). The value "0" for "Gender" denotes male ("1" would denote female). And the value "0" for "CRIB score" denotes the lowest possible value in a gradation of severity of illness.

Table 21.1 Four variables, all taking on the value "0"

Variable name	Value
Day of life	0
Prenatal care	0
Gender	0
CRIB score (neonatal severity of illness)	0

Table 21.1 illustrates the notion of different variable types, and at the same time an idea from Chapter 5: Information = Data + Meaning. Recall that this relationship may be rearranged to state that data alone, just the plain symbolic representation, is *meaningless information*.

Variable types

Variables may be of different types; each type contributes particular meaning to the data. Common variable types:
• Categorical, of which there are a few types.
   1 *Nominal*: categories that have no particular order. The categories may be identified by a number but that number represents no information about order or magnitude, for example, race/ethnicity: Black – 0, White – 1, Asian – 2, Hispanic – 3, and Native American – 4.

Table 21.2 A list of patients and their gender

Patient number	Gender (0 = male; 1 = female)
1	0
2	1
3	0
4	0
5	1
6	1
7	0
8	0
9	1
10	1
11	1
12	0
13	1
14	0
15	1
16	1

(a) *Dichotomous*: nominal variable with two possible values, for example, male/female (0/1), or yes/no (1/0).

(b) Note that nominal values commonly are represented by numbers, but think carefully before you apply arithmetic operations to them. Consider, for example, Table 21.2. Out of 16 patients, 9 are female. Suppose we calculate the average value of the Gender variable: $(0 + 1 + 0 + 0 + 1 + \cdots + 0 + 1 + 1)/16 = 9/16 = 0.56$. What does this mean? The average patient is not 56% female. The proportion of all the patients that are female is 56%. On the other hand, if race/ethnicity is coded: Black = 1, White = 2, Asian = 3, Hispanic = 4, and Native American = 5, it is meaningless to speak of an average race/ethnicity of 2.6.

- *Ordinal*: categories for which order matters; for example, mild = 0, moderate = 1, and severe = 2. The interval magnitude is undefined; the categories could have been inversely coded. The coding scheme does not imply any relative scale: severe does not necessarily mean twice as bad as moderate and mild does not necessarily mean negligible just because it's coded by a zero.
- *Ranked*: this is typically a derived variable. Order matters, but ranked data entail arranging all the observations for a variable in order of relative magnitude and then assigning each observation to its place in the ordered sequence, its rank order. Ties share the same rank order. Rank ordering underlies a method of hypothesis testing that we examine in Chapter 31.
- *Discrete*: both order and magnitude matter. For the variable types discussed so far, numerical values represented labels for the actual values the variable

could assume (such as severe = 2, or Asian = 3). For discrete variables numerical values represent an actual measurement whose possible values are restricted, so subdividing an interval between two adjacent values is not possible.

1 For example, the number of patients admitted to the hospital in a month, and the number of children born to a mother. A hospital may not admit 36.7 patients in a month, and a woman may not have 2.3 births. Such values may occur, however, as the outcome of an arithmetic operation like computing an average. Thus, manipulating discrete data may result in data that is not discrete.

- *Continuous*: numerical values represent an actual measurement whose possible values are not restricted. Between any two possible values we may choose an arbitrarily small interval to insert another possible value.

1 For example, patient A may have a blood glucose value of 88 and patient B may have a blood glucose value of 88.1. Patient C could have a blood glucose value of 88.05 – assume meaningful precision.

2 Although arithmetic operations may be applied to continuous variables, such computations may yield results implying greater precision than is possible or meaningful. For example, you might round off an average blood glucose value of 88.0987 to the most meaningful unit, say 88.1.

Sometimes you care only about what broad group each subject belongs in, rather than each subject's particular value for a variable. For example, Chapter 20 illustrated how to convert BW (birth weight), a continuous variable, to BWcat, a categorical variable. The conversion collapsed many thousands of possible values (BW = 460 g, 461 g, ..., 4569 g, 4570 g) into only five possible values. Some might say that BWcat contains less information about each infant's birth weight compared to the BW variable. I think it's clearer to say that the cost of conversion was a loss of precision: BWcat describes each infant's birth weight less precisely than does BW. Nonetheless, this is sometimes appropriate because the categorical conversion can improve analytical efficiency.

Generally, you determine the appropriate type of variable to use by the nature of the characteristic you want to describe or measure, and by the question you seek to answer. As we shall see, the question you seek to answer and the types of variables you plan to analyze determine the appropriate analytical method.

CHAPTER 22

Measurement values vary: describing their distribution and summarizing them quantitatively

Random variable

For a random variable, the value of any observation is a matter of chance as described by a specific mathematical function. A discrete random variable has a finite number of possible values, so each one has a particular probability of occurring. A continuous random variable has an infinite number of possible values, so we divide the range of possible values into precise intervals in order to assign a probability of each interval occurring.

Data frequency distributions

For some variables, the frequency with which particular values or intervals occur may appear to have no pattern. In health care, patterns are common; often resembling a theoretical mathematical function termed as probability distribution. Our study of data distributions focuses on two common theoretical distributions: binomial distribution and normal distribution.

The binomial distribution

Patient data commonly fit the binomial, or Bernoulli, distribution. This distribution describes the possible outcomes of a dichotomous random variable as a function of the probability of the event occurring, p, and the number of observations, N. The particular outcomes might be heads/tails, lived/died, disease/no disease, male/female, etc.; the general is failure/success, with no attached value judgments.

To compute the probability of K successes given N trials[109]

$$\binom{N}{K} (p)^k (1 - p)^{N-k}$$

where $\binom{N}{K} = \frac{N!}{K!(N-K)!}$; $! = $ factorial, for example, $3! = (3) \times (2) \times (1) = 6$; and $p = $ probability of success. This method assumes that each observation, or trial, is independent and the probability of success is constant for each trial. Consider this when you analyze dichotomous data. For example, when analyzing survival data for a group of patients, are you sure that all the deaths were independent of each other? Following the first few deaths in a series, might some cascading events in processes of care alter the probability of subsequent deaths? Staff focused on a dying patient might inadvertently divert attention and resources from other patients. Clinicians might draw unwarranted inferences from one or a few cases in the past, biasing subsequent outcomes.

The factorial component $\binom{N}{K}$ describes the number of ways in which the number of successes, K, may occur given the number of trials, N. For example, to compute the number of ways 3 heads can occur among 7 coin tosses:

$$\binom{N}{K} = \binom{7}{3} = \frac{7 \times 6 \times 5 \times 4 \times 3 \times 2 \times 1}{3!(7-3)!} = \frac{7 \times 6 \times 5 \times 4 \times 3 \times 2 \times 1}{(3 \times 2 \times 1)(4 \times 3 \times 2 \times 1)} = 35.$$

Try writing out all the ways a head can occur; for example, if H = heads and T = tails, then the possibilities include: TTTTHHH, HHHTTTT, THTHTHT, THHTTTH...Now, to compute the probability of 3 heads ($K = 3$) among 7 tosses ($N = 7$), assuming a fair coin ($p = 0.50$), and reducing expressions:

$$(35) \times (0.50)^3 (0.50)^4 = 35 \times (0.125) \times (0.0625) = 0.2734375$$

Stata has a set of so-called immediate functions; one such function computes binomial probability: bitesti. Note that a command displayed in the Stata results window is preceded by a period. The answer we seek is given in bold.

```
. bitesti 7 3 .5, detail
        N     Observed k    Expected k    Assumed p    Observed p
------------------------------------------------------------------
        7          3           3.5          0.50000       0.42857
Pr(k >= 3)                 = 0.773438  (one-sided test)
Pr(k <= 3)                 = 0.500000  (one-sided test)
Pr(k <= 3 or k >= 4)       = 1.000000  (two-sided test)

Pr(k == 3)                 = 0.273437  (observed)
Pr(k == 4)                 = 0.273437  (opposite extreme)
```

Theoretical probability distributions are commonly displayed as graphs. Figure 22.1 shows the distribution for all possible outcomes of the coin toss scenario just discussed. To create it I used Stata. First, I computed the probability of each possible outcome, in the same way demonstrated above for 3 heads from 7 tosses. Next, I created a Stata data set by directly entering the data in the Stata editor. Figure 22.2 shows my **Stata Editor** after I labeled the two variables. Lastly, guided by advice in the Stata Graphics manual, I ran the following command. It should contain no carriage returns: although it may not fit on one line, I did not press the **Enter** key to continue the text on the next line.

```
graph bar Prob, over( Heads) ytitle("Probability")
title("Probability of Obtaining x Heads on 7 Tosses")
```

The distribution in Fig. 22.1 appears symmetric because $p = 0.5$. A dichotomous event with a different probability of success would produce a different

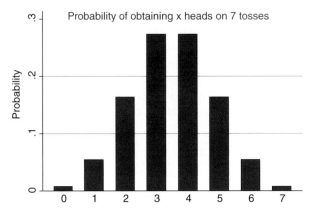

Figure 22.1 The probability of each possible outcome of 7 tosses.

distribution. Thus, if the probability for a woman to receive prenatal care is 0.71, then the probability distribution for x of 7 women to receive prenatal care would be as shown in Fig. 22.3. For any graph representing a discrete probability distribution regardless of the shape of the distribution, if the bar representing each possible value has width = one unit, then the sum of the areas (probabilities) represented by each bar = 1.

You can now answer this question: "Given the probability of a woman receiving prenatal care is 0.71, what is the probability that among 7 women 5 or more received prenatal care?" One simply adds the component possibilities: 5, or 6, or 7 women have received prenatal care. From Fig. 22.4, the answer is $0.318645 + 0.260044 + 0.090951 = 0.66964$.

Probability density function

As the number of possible values that a random variable may take on increases, the number of bars to represent the distribution must agree; thus, the width

Stata Editor

Preserve	Restore		Sort	<<	>>	

Heads[1] =

	Heads	Prob
1	0	.007813
2	1	.054688
3	2	.164063
4	3	.273437
5	4	.273437
6	5	.164063
7	6	.054688
8	7	.007813

Figure 22.2 The data that produced Fig. 22.1.

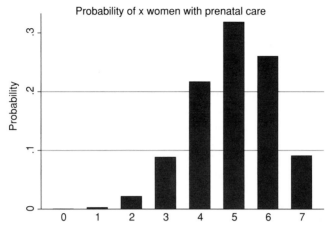

Figure 22.3 The probability distribution for x of 7 women to receive prenatal care when the probability for a woman to receive prenatal care is 0.71.

of each bar becomes correspondingly small. As the number of bars approaches infinity, the contour of the boundary approaches a curved line. This is how to think about the probability distribution for a continuous random variable. Such a smooth distribution function is called a probability density.

Because the curve describes the probabilities of all possible outcomes, the area bounded by the function, that is, the summed probabilities of each outcome, must add up to 1. Of course, if the number of possible outcomes was truly infinite, then the probability of a particular outcome would be 0. That is, the limit approaches 0 as the number of outcomes approaches infinity. In light of this, we focus not on a particular outcome value but on an appropriately small interval that contains the outcome value. We compute the probability

■ Stata Editor

	Women	Prob
1	0	.000172
2	1	.002956
3	2	.021713
4	3	.0886
5	4	.216918
6	5	.318645
7	6	.260044
8	7	.090951

Preserve | Restore | Sort | << | >>

Women[1] =

Figure 22.4 The data that produced Fig. 22.3.

of an outcome located between two specific values on the horizontal axis as the area of a vertical slice under the distribution curve bounded by those two specific values. This idea is illustrated in Fig.22.11 (ignore the axis legend for now).

Introducing the normal distribution

Figure 22.5 shows the distribution of birth weights for 161 infants. I aggregated the individual values into 50 "bins," Stata's word for bars. The distribution appears to have more than one peak: a bimodal or multimodal distribution (mode means most commonly occurring value). The data distribution reflects a biased sample because all these infants required neonatal intensive care. The well-baby nursery would probably yield a distribution more closely resembling the superimposed smooth curve: symmetric with a central hump. Such a distribution is called normal.

We shall explore the normal distribution in some detail because
- variables we deal with in patient care commonly approximate the normal, or Gaussian, or bell-shaped, distribution.
- the normal distribution plays a central role in analytical theory, including estimating population characteristics from a sample and hypothesis testing.

The normal curve in Fig. 22.5 has a different shape from either of the two normal curves in Fig. 22.6. Suppose Fig. 22.6 describes the distribution of birth weights for two groups of infants: the curve on the left shows the distribution of values for infants born to economically disadvantaged mothers and the

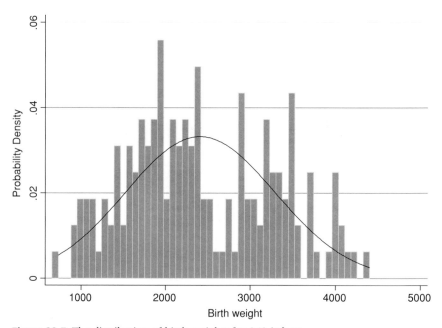

Figure 22.5 The distribution of birth weights for 161 infants.

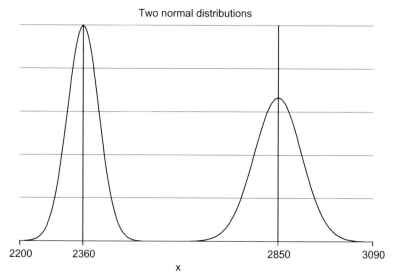

Figure 22.6 Two normal distributions (produced using zdemo2.ado).

curve on the right shows the distribution of values for infants born to mothers with some higher standard of living. The point is that probability distributions of a given theoretical type such as Gaussian nonetheless vary. We may describe how distributions of the same type vary through measures for summarizing a distribution. Summary measures describe two essential characteristics of the distribution of values for a variable. Measures of central tendency indicate where values tend to cluster—the hump in the curve. Measures of dispersion indicate the extent to which the values spread.

An asymmetrical distribution is called skewed. On an x-axis with values increasing to the right, a positively or right-skewed distribution has the longer tail (containing the outlier values) to the right; a negatively or left-skewed distribution has the longer tail to the left. Tail in French is *queue*: you can think of skew as *s(queue)* to remember that skew direction refers to where the tail of the distribution lies (see p. 59 in Ref. 110).

Measures of central tendency
Measures of central tendency include the following:
- Mean, or arithmetic average, the sum of all values divided by the number of individual values; mean $= \bar{x} = \sum \frac{x}{n}$, where x represents each value of the variable, n represents the number of observations, and $\sum$ means "the sum of."
  (i) Except for a dichotomous variable, don't compute the mean for a nominal or ordinal variable. As mentioned, if you code a dichotomous variable as $0/1$, then computing the mean gives the proportion of observations with value $= 1$.

(ii) Because it includes every value in the distribution, the mean can be strongly influenced by extreme but uncommon values. Sometimes such values are erroneous; other times they accurately describe an unusual observation. Although your main intent may be to summarize the group, "outliers" may have disproportionate influence on the group mean.

- Median, the 50th percentile value. Rank order all the values and find the value such that half the values are $\leq$ the median and half the values are $\geq$ the median. For an even number of observations, take the average of the two values in the middle of the ranking.

(i) May be used for ordinal, discrete, and continuous variables.

(ii) *The median is a robust estimator of central tendency, relatively stable to perturbations. If a distribution is not symmetrical, particularly if it contains extreme outliers, the median will be less affected than the mean.*

(iii) For a symmetric distribution as is the normal distribution, the mean and the median are the same.

- Mode, the most commonly occurring value(s).

(i) May be used for any type of variable.

(ii) For a symmetric distribution, the mean, median, and the mode are the same.

Figure 22.7 illustrates a bimodal distribution. Here, the mean and the median may lie between the two modes or peaks, marked by vertical lines, so neither the mean nor the median accurately summarize where the values tend to cluster. Reporting the two modes gives a more accurate summary.

When a distribution has more than one mode, consider that your data set may be over-aggregated, that is, you may be dealing with more than one distinct group.

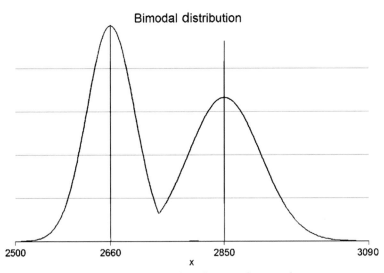

Figure 22.7 A bimodal distribution (produced using zdemo2.ado).

Measures of dispersion

Two distributions may have identical means, medians, and modes, yet represent very different data sets (Fig. 22.8). Clearly, we also need a way to summarize the spread of the values—close to the center or ranging far from it. This is what measures of dispersion do.

Measures of dispersion include the following:
- Range, the difference between the values at the extreme ends of a distribution.
  - (i) Very sensitive to extreme values, yet provides little information about where most of the values lie.
- Interquartile range, the values that lie between the 25th percentile and the 75th percentile.
  - (i) In combination with the range and by including the median, provides a better picture of the spread of values.

    Stata can draw a box and whiskers plot to represent all these measures (Fig. 22.9). The "whiskers" denote the range; the "box," the interquartile range; the horizontal line within the box, the median. The following command produced this figure (the variable is `birthweight`):

    ```
    graph box birthweight, ytitle ("Birth weight g") title("Birth
    weights of infants admitted to a NICU")
    ```
- Variance quantitates the extent to which the values deviate from the mean. The sum of the difference between the mean value ($\bar{x}$) and each value (x) above the mean and below the mean is not useful because it is always zero (reflect on the definition of the mean). We could, instead, square each such deviation $(x - \bar{x})^2$ before adding them all up so as to eliminate having the

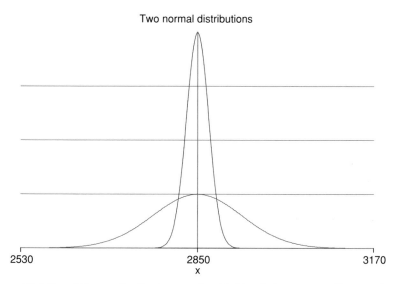

Figure 22.8 Two different distributions, each with identical means, medians, and modes (produced using zdemo2.ado).

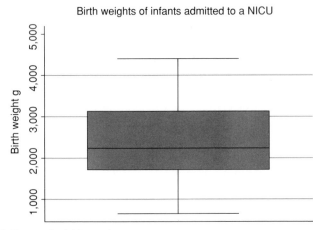

Figure 22.9 Box and whiskers plot.

negative and positive differences cancel each other out. Dividing the sum of those squares by the number of observations (n) minus 1, yields the variance:

$$s^2 = \sum \frac{(x - \bar{x})^2}{n - 1}.$$

(i) Why divide the sum of the squared deviations by ($n - 1$) and not n? The full explanation is beyond our scope, but the main idea is degrees of freedom (df), which happens to be ($n - 1$). Degrees of freedom measures information content in a data set (pp. 43 and 202 in Ref. 109). Only ($n - 1$) of the deviations are independent. Since the sum of the unsquared deviations $= 0$, the nth deviation can always be derived from the other ($n - 1$) deviations; the nth deviation contributes no additional information.

(ii) To square the deviations is also to square the variable's unit of measurement. People generally find it unintuitive to think about unit^2, for example, kg^2. Thus, to clarify this measure of dispersion we take the square root of s^2.

• Standard deviation (s): the square root of the variance. $s = \sqrt{s^2}$.

(i) A relatively small standard deviation indicates a relatively homogeneous set of measurements. A relatively large standard deviation indicates a relatively heterogeneous set of measurements. In Fig. 22.8, the broad, low curve has a larger standard deviation than the tall, narrow curve.

(ii) As mentioned, both s^2 and s include the unit of measurement for the variable they characterize. Therefore, it is only meaningful to compare the dispersion of variables when units of measurement are the same. In the case of one group of patient weights in kilograms (kg) and another group in pounds (lb), you could not compare the standard deviations of the weights in kg and in lb. To compare dispersions, first convert one unit of measurement to the other.

- Coefficient of variation (CV) relates s to $\bar{x}$, by expressing s as a percentage of $\bar{x}$.. $CV = (s/\bar{x}) \times 100\%$.
  (i) Thus, CV measures dispersion relative to central tendency.
  (ii) Because measurement units appear in both the numerator and the denominator, these can be deleted. Thus, a unit-free, CV provides a way to compare any two variables. However, Pagano and Gauvreau advise that CV is falling into disfavor and discourage its use.[109]

Summary measures for binomially distributed data

Aspects of summary measures for a binomially distributed variable differ from the overview given above. A value some call the mean, but I think is less confusingly termed the expected value (see Section 7.4 in Ref. 111), is computed by $n \times p$, where n is the number of observations and p is the probability of a success for the dichotomous outcome. The expected value of a probability distribution is the most likely number of successes, on average, when a set of trials is repeated many times. In the scenario illustrated by Figs. 22.3 and 22.4, the expected number of women who had prenatal care would be $7 \times 0.71 = 4.97$, or about 5 women out of 7 would be expected to have had prenatal care. It's easy to see this in Fig. 22.3. The standard deviation of a binomially distributed variable is computed as

$$s = \sqrt{np(1-p)}.$$

Normal distribution: greater depth

The formula for the theoretical normal probability distribution describes the parameters upon which it depends:

$$y = \frac{1}{\sqrt{2\pi\sigma^2}} e^{-1/2\left(\frac{x-\mu}{\sigma}\right)^2}$$

where $y =$ the height of the curve on the y axis (some authors instead denote this by $f(x)$); $x =$ a value on the x axis (a value of the random variable); $\pi =$ the constant approximated by 3.14159; $\sigma = s$, the standard deviation; $\mu = \bar{x}$, the mean; and $e =$ the base number of natural logarithms, approximated by 2.71828. The number e also appears in statistical functions we examine later. (See Ref. 112 for an enjoyable historical and mathematical overview of e.)

The main idea is that two parameters completely determine the normal distribution: $\mu = \bar{x}$, the mean; and $\sigma = s$, the standard deviation.

From knowledge of the normal probability distribution, we can estimate characteristics of the many normally distributed random variables in patient data sets. For example, in a population where birth weight is normally distributed, how unusual is it for an infant chosen at random to have a birth weight greater than 4.1 kg? We know that the total area beneath the curve, the sum of the probabilities of all possible outcomes, is 1. If we know $\mu = \bar{x}$, the mean; and $\sigma = s$, the standard deviation for this birth weight variable, then we also know the shape of the curve and we can estimate the probability of interest. We compute the proportion of the area of the curve that lies to the right of 4.1 kg. Theoretically, there are an infinite number of normal distributions, so each unique curve would call for a specific computation to estimate the probability of interest.

The standard normal distribution

Thankfully, each possible normal distribution may be related to a special one, with $\mu = 0$ and $\sigma = 1$. This special normal distribution is called the standard normal distribution. We relate the normal distribution of interest to the standard normal distribution, as follows:

$$SND = z = \frac{x - \mu}{\sigma}$$

where SND denotes the term standard normal deviate, alternately referred to as the z score.

We use the z score to estimate the probability of interest: the proportion of the population that has a value above or below a specified cutpoint. We need to merely know the areas contained in arbitrarily small sections of the standard normal curve. Knowing this, the z score allows us to compute the area under the curve bounded by the cutpoint value we have chosen for *any* normal distribution. Textbooks of statistics typically include in their appendices a table relating a particular z score to the proportion of the area of the standard normal distribution that is above or below that point.

Using Stata, you can easily compute the desired area under the curve. You also might enjoy exploring concepts we cover here using Stata add-in programs available on the UCLA instructional Stata web site (http://www.ats.ucla.edu/stat/stata; accessed June 22, 2004). Download them within Stata by running the following command while connected to the Internet: `findit [tdemo | ztable | zdemo | ztail | zcalc | zdemo2]` that is, `findit ztable`; or `findit zdemo`; etc. Following installation, from **Help** on the Stata main menu, select **Stata Command...**, type the name of the add-in, and then click **OK**. Philip B. Ender wrote these programs and kindly consented to my using them in this book (ender@ucla.edu, UCLA Department of Education, UCLA Academic Technology Services).

After you install the `ztable` add-in, run the command `ztable` to produce a table of the areas between 0 & z of the standard normal distribution (see below). For each z score you wish to evaluate, the leftmost column specifies the digit to the left of the decimal point and the first digit to the right of the decimal point; the top row below the title provides the second digit to the right of the decimal point. To find the area between 0 and a z score of 1.96, look down the first column to the 20th row: `1.90`. Follow that row out to the right until at the column headed by .06, the 4th column from the right. The value at that location is 0.4750: the area of the standard normal distribution that lies between 0 and 1.96.

. ztable

Areas between 0 & Z of the Standard Normal Distribution

	.00	.01	.02	.03	.04		.05	**.06**	.07	.08	.09
0.00	0.0000	0.0040	0.0080	0.0120	0.0160	|	0.0199	0.0239	0.0279	0.0319	0.0359
0.10	0.0398	0.0438	0.0478	0.0517	0.0557	|	0.0596	0.0636	0.0675	0.0714	0.0753
0.20	0.0793	0.0832	0.0871	0.0910	0.0948	|	0.0987	0.1026	0.1064	0.1103	0.1141
0.30	0.1179	0.1217	0.1255	0.1293	0.1331	|	0.1368	0.1406	0.1443	0.1480	0.1517
0.40	0.1554	0.1591	0.1628	0.1664	0.1700	|	0.1736	0.1772	0.1808	0.1844	0.1879
0.50	0.1915	0.1950	0.1985	0.2019	0.2054	|	0.2088	0.2123	0.2157	0.2190	0.2224
0.60	0.2257	0.2291	0.2324	0.2357	0.2389	|	0.2422	0.2454	0.2486	0.2517	0.2549
0.70	0.2580	0.2611	0.2642	0.2673	0.2704	|	0.2734	0.2764	0.2794	0.2823	0.2852
0.80	0.2881	0.2910	0.2939	0.2967	0.2995	|	0.3023	0.3051	0.3078	0.3106	0.3133
0.90	0.3159	0.3186	0.3212	0.3238	0.3264	|	0.3289	0.3315	0.3340	0.3365	0.3389
1.00	0.3413	0.3438	0.3461	0.3485	0.3508	|	0.3531	0.3554	0.3577	0.3599	0.3621
1.10	0.3643	0.3665	0.3686	0.3708	0.3729	|	0.3749	0.3770	0.3790	0.3810	0.3830
1.20	0.3849	0.3869	0.3888	0.3907	0.3925	|	0.3944	0.3962	0.3980	0.3997	0.4015
1.30	0.4032	0.4049	0.4066	0.4082	0.4099	|	0.4115	0.4131	0.4147	0.4162	0.4177
1.40	0.4192	0.4207	0.4222	0.4236	0.4251	|	0.4265	0.4279	0.4292	0.4306	0.4319
1.50	0.4332	0.4345	0.4357	0.4370	0.4382	|	0.4394	0.4406	0.4418	0.4429	0.4441
1.60	0.4452	0.4463	0.4474	0.4484	0.4495	|	0.4505	0.4515	0.4525	0.4535	0.4545
1.70	0.4554	0.4564	0.4573	0.4582	0.4591	|	0.4599	0.4608	0.4616	0.4625	0.4633
1.80	0.4641	0.4649	0.4656	0.4664	0.4671	|	0.4678	0.4686	0.4693	0.4699	0.4706
1.90	0.4713	0.4719	0.4726	0.4732	0.4738	|	0.4744	**0.4750**	0.4756	0.4761	0.4767
2.00	0.4772	0.4778	0.4783	0.4788	0.4793	|	0.4798	0.4803	0.4808	0.4812	0.4817
2.10	0.4821	0.4826	0.4830	0.4834	0.4838	|	0.4842	0.4846	0.4850	0.4854	0.4857
2.20	0.4861	0.4864	0.4868	0.4871	0.4875	|	0.4878	0.4881	0.4884	0.4887	0.4890
2.30	0.4893	0.4896	0.4898	0.4901	0.4904	|	0.4906	0.4909	0.4911	0.4913	0.4916
2.40	0.4918	0.4920	0.4922	0.4925	0.4927	|	0.4929	0.4931	0.4932	0.4934	0.4936
2.50	0.4938	0.4940	0.4941	0.4943	0.4945	|	0.4946	0.4948	0.4949	0.4951	0.4952
2.60	0.4953	0.4955	0.4956	0.4957	0.4959	|	0.4960	0.4961	0.4962	0.4963	0.4964
2.70	0.4965	0.4966	0.4967	0.4968	0.4969	|	0.4970	0.4971	0.4972	0.4973	0.4974
2.80	0.4974	0.4975	0.4976	0.4977	0.4977	|	0.4978	0.4979	0.4979	0.4980	0.4981
2.90	0.4981	0.4982	0.4982	0.4983	0.4984	|	0.4984	0.4985	0.4985	0.4986	0.4986
3.00	0.4987	0.4987	0.4987	0.4988	0.4988	|	0.4989	0.4989	0.4989	0.4990	0.4990
3.10	0.4990	0.4991	0.4991	0.4991	0.4992	|	0.4992	0.4992	0.4992	0.4993	0.4993
3.20	0.4993	0.4993	0.4994	0.4994	0.4994	|	0.4994	0.4994	0.4995	0.4995	0.4995
3.30	0.4995	0.4995	0.4995	0.4996	0.4996	|	0.4996	0.4996	0.4996	0.4996	0.4997
3.40	0.4997	0.4997	0.4997	0.4997	0.4997	|	0.4997	0.4997	0.4997	0.4997	0.4998
3.50	0.4998	0.4998	0.4998	0.4998	0.4998	|	0.4998	0.4998	0.4998	0.4998	0.4998

The z score indicates how many standard deviations a specific value of the normally distributed variable lies from the mean (Fig. 22.10). Thus, a z score = 1 means that the value lies 1 standard deviation above the mean; a z score = -1 means the value lies 1 standard deviation below the mean. Using the table of areas (see above) to compute the area between the two vertical lines in Fig. 22.11, we find that the area between 0 and $z = 1.00$ of the standard normal

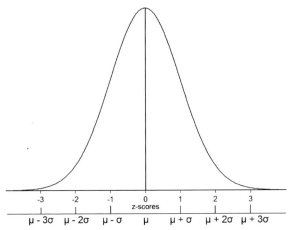

Figure 22.10 The z score indicates how many standard deviations a specific value of the normally distributed variable lies from the mean (produced using zdemo.ado; after Kirkwood and Sterne[113])

distribution is 0.3413. The area between 0 and $z = -1.00$ of the standard normal distribution is also 0.3413. Although z is -1.00, the area between 0 and -1 is still a positive value, and because the normal distribution is symmetric, that area must be the same as the area between 0 and 1.00. So we add 0.3413 + 0.3413 = 0.6826, the shaded area in Fig. 22.11.

Applying the same method as above, we find the area between -1.96 and $+1.96 = 0.95$ (0.4750 + 0.4750 = 0.95). Therefore, the remaining 0.05 of the total area of 1 is equally distributed in the two tails beyond -1.96 and

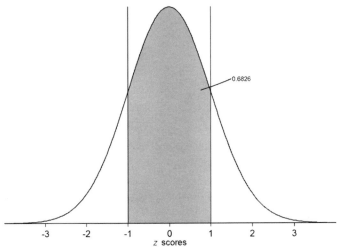

Figure 22.11 The area between $z = -1.00$ and $z = +1.00$ (produced using zdemo.ado).

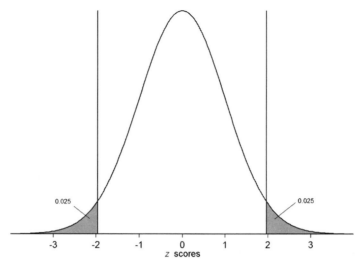

Figure 22.12 1 minus the area between $z = -1.96$ and $z = +1.96$ (produced using zdemo.ado).

+1.96, as shown in Fig. 22.12. You already know that about two thirds of normally distributed values occur within 1 standard deviation from the mean, and about 95% of the values occur within 2 standard deviations from the mean. Now you understand why.

Let's work with these ideas

On the accompanying CD, find the file called practice_dataset.txt. This is a tab-delimited data set saved as a text file (an option in Microsoft® Excel). The observations were made between 1996 and 2000. The patient data has been "de-identified" to conform with the United States Federal Government "Safe Harbor" standard (see Section 164.514 in Ref. 114; for other requirements relating to uses and disclosures of protected health information, see pp. 29–30 of Ref. 114). And it is to comply with the "Safe Harbor" standard that some of the Stata output in the following chapters may reference a variable that does not appear in the provided data set. I do provide derived variables when it is not possible for you to reconstruct the censored observations that produced them.

To work with our practice data set, we must bring it into Stata. Later, before saving it, we shall convert it to a Stata data file. Subsequently, you need only double-click on the Stata data file icon to open Stata and immediately load the data.

```
. insheet using "C:\BMJ Books\ Managing and Learning from Perinatal
and Pediatric Data\Manuscript\Datasets\practice_dataset.txt",clear
(40 vars, 4321 obs)
```

Stata found a text file containing 40 variables and 4321 observations. Let's examine the birth weight variable.

. summarize birthweight,det **det is an acceptable abbreviation for the option "detail"**

```
                              birthweight
--------------------------------------------------------------
no observations
```

oh,oh... what went wrong?

. describe birthweight

```
              storage    display    value
variable name  type      format     label      variable label
--------------------------------------------------------------
birthweight    str9      %9s
```

Look at the data in the Stata browser window. Many of the values resemble: "1,250.00." When created, the birthweight variable format was not specified as numeric. The database interpreted the presence of a comma in many of the observations to indicate that this was string data. This problem could have been prevented by specifying in the source database that the data are numeric and setting a field input mask. Anyway, this is great for us because we have *dirty data* to clean! The Stata function called "real" converts string data to numeric.

. gen BW = real(birthweight)   **gen is an acceptable abbreviation for "generate," a command that creates a new (derived) variable.**

(4022 missing values generated)

Now what happened? There are 4321 total observations in the original data set, so this maneuver worked for *some* of the observations. Check the browser to find that all observations contain patient data up to observation number 3076. Observations 3077 to 4321 are entirely missing. The source data set was originally created by merging patient data with census data, by zip code. The empty observations had no corresponding patient zip code with which to merge. But that accounts only for some of the missing observations. Let's examine our new variable:

. sum BW,det

```
                                BW
--------------------------------------------------------------
Percentiles          Smallest
  1%       3.31        2.88
  5%       400         3
 10%       480         3.31      Obs              299
 25%       580         34        Sum of Wgt.      299

 50%       720                   Mean         706.6394
```

		Largest	Std. Dev.	190.4812
75%	865	985		
90%	940	985	Variance	36283.1
95%	970	990	Skewness	-.762941
99%	985	995	Kurtosis	3.947862

It seems Stata knew what to do with values <1,000.00 but not with values >1000.00. Stata was foiled by the comma. Let's try again; we'll get rid of the variable we just created but don't want.

. drop BW

Often in Stata various strategies can solve your data management problems. Here's a simple and clean approach I discovered by searching Stata documentation.

. destring birthweight, generate(BW) ignore(,)
birthweight: characters, removed; BW generated as double
(1256 missing values generated)   **1244 of the missing values are accounted for by observations containing only missing values; the remainder are incomplete observations that are missing values in the birthweight variable. We can also check this out by running the codebook command for the birthweight variable (distinguish from BW).**

. codebook birthweight

```
-------------------------------------------------------------------
-----------------------------------------------------------
```

birthweight
(unlabeled)

```
-------------------------------------------------------------------
-----------------------------------------------------------
```

```
                    type: string (str9)

           unique values: 1138                    missing "": 1256/4321

                examples: ""
                          "1,600.00"
                          "2,420.00"
                          "3,440.00"
```

Notice that here too there are 1256 missing values. Now let's examine the new BW variable we created.

. sum BW, det

```
                              BW
-------------------------------------------------------------------
      Percentiles      Smallest
 1%        480           2.88
 5%        730            3
```

10%	1005		3.31	Obs	3065
25%	1600		34	Sum of Wgt.	3065
50%	2325			Mean	2413.55
		Largest		Std. Dev.	1320.854
75%	3241	5422			
90%	3802	5500		Variance	1744654
95%	4090	5557		Skewness	12.60113
99%	4600	47000		Kurtosis	424.759

Success!

**Be sure to save work you plan to use again: select <u>F</u>ile, Save <u>A</u>s
..., and choose a location and type in a file name. Make sure to
save the file as a Stata data file (.dta), for example,**

. save "C:\BMJ Books\Datasets\practice_10aug_2004.dta "

**Did you notice that although we successfully converted the
variable, the data still appear dirty? The four smallest BW values
range from 2.88 to 34 [grams]; three of the four largest values
are plausible, but I know of no infant with a birth weight of 47,000
[grams]. We may have to make informed but uncertain judgments. For
example, if we're reasonably sure that no infant ever was admitted
to our NICU who weighed <400 g or >12,000 g, we might drop
observations outside these boundaries. Whenever possible, better to
review each infant's patient record containing an apparent outlier
value and correct it as indicated by other data in that record. So
that I may write this book instead of dig through archives, I choose
to amputate outlier data.**

. drop if BW<400 | BW>12000
(1271 observations deleted)

**Don't worry that 1271 observations were dropped. Remember that
there were 1256 missing observations for birth weight in the
original data set. Stata codes missing values as a period (.), and
orders missing values as higher than any particular number. Stata
considers a missing value as a number certainly higher than our
criterion of BW > 12000 and therefore dropped such observations.
The remaining observations have reasonable values:**

. sum BW,det

BW

	Percentiles	Smallest		
1%	515	400		
5%	755	400		
10%	1025	420	Obs	3050
25%	1610	425	Sum of Wgt.	3050
50%	2330		Mean	2408.937
		Largest	Std. Dev.	1038.892

75%	3250	5380		
90%	3803.5	5422	Variance	1079296
95%	4090	5500	Skewness	.1510304
99%	4593	5557	Kurtosis	2.211746

**Let's further explore the BW variable. (Don't forget to save the
cleaned data set with a new name; I chose practice_10aug_2004_clean
.dta)**

. histogram BW, normal fraction
(bin=34, start=400, width=151.67647)
See Fig. 22.13; consider the distribution approximately normal.

**Some readers may have trouble accepting the distribution in Fig.
22.13 as "approximately" normal. Sometimes, we may transform
a variable to better resemble the theoretical distribution by
performing a mathematical operation to all the values. The details
are beyond our scope, but you should appreciate that transforms
may result in more than your desired aims.[115] Stata has a command
called** gladder **that helps you explore whether performing some
mathematical operations improves the fit of the variable to the
theoretical normal distribution. Figure 22.14a illustrates the
result of running** gladder **on the BW variable. Another command,**
qladder **(the letter q, rather than the letter g precedes "ladder"),
displays the quantiles of each transformation against the quantiles
of a normal distribution; this display may help you decide among
possibilities that look too close to call on** gladder **(Figure
22.14b). I'm not persuaded that these transforms improve the fit;
the data may, in fact, be bimodal.**

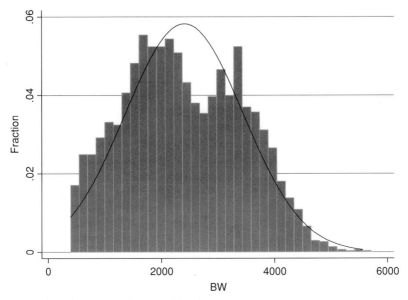

Figure 22.13 Histogram BW, normal fraction.

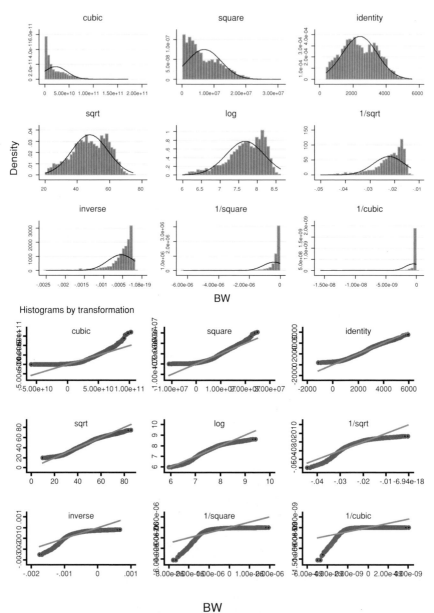

Figure 22.14 (a) `gladder` and (b) `qladder`. Some axis labels appear compressed at the scale of reproduction, but it doesn't matter.

We know from the tabular summary of BW, above, that μ = 2409 (rounded off) and σ = 1039. Suppose we want to find the proportion of infants in our population who have a birth weight >4000 g. We solve for the standard normal deviate, the z score.
. disp norm(1.5312801)

.93714991   **disp is an acceptable abbreviation for display, a command that puts Stata in calculator mode. norm(z) returns the cumulative standard normal distribution: the proportion of the area to the left of z. To answer our question, we subtract this quantity from 1.**

. disp 1-.93714991
.06285009   **Thus, if the population values are normally distributed, 6.3% of our population has a birth weight >4000 g.**

Tails

Evaluative decisions about data distributions are commonly either "one-tailed" or "two-tailed." The tail of a statistical distribution is the smaller portion of the curve divided by a vertical line placed at a chosen x value. When we determined that approximately 6.3% of our population had a birth weight >4000 g, our group of interest is represented in one tail, at the right side of the distribution. If we have no way to know in advance that an observed value may turn out to be higher *or* lower than the expected value for the distribution, then we include the area of the tail that lies at the other end of the distribution along with the area of the tail that the current observation has directed us.

To understand how to compute the shaded area between -1σ and $+1\sigma$ (Fig. 22.11), we had to keep track of specific portions of the area beneath the curve. We arrived at an approximate area of 0.68 by adding the areas to the left and to the right of $\mu = 0$. We extended this line of reasoning in computing the area of the two tails that lie to the left of -2σ and to the right of $+2\sigma$ (Fig. 22.12), by computing the area between these two cutpoints, subtracting that value from 1 to find the remaining area, and dividing that result by 2, since the curve is symmetric around $x = 0$ and we were interested in the area of each tail.

The methods of hypothesis testing to be presented in the forthcoming chapters each involve, in some way, computing the probability of obtaining a result equal to, or more extreme than, the one obtained.

Figures 22.15 and 22.16 both illustrate a shaded area = 0.05. In Fig. 22.15 the area is contained in one tail and in Fig. 22.16 the same area is contained in two tails. Compared with the situation illustrated in Fig. 22.15, a z score in Fig. 22.16 signifying a difference between groups must be farther from the mean, $\mu = 0$, to have an occurrence probability ≤ 0.05; $z = 1.645$ in Fig. 22.15 and $z = 1.96$ in Fig. 22.16. When you compute a two-tailed probability, to conclude that groups differ the value must be farther from $\mu = 0$ than when you

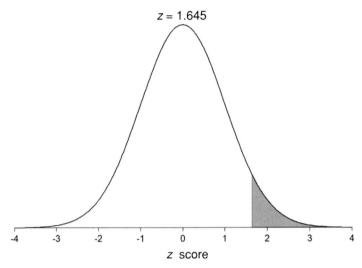

Figure 22.15 Shaded area = 0.05 in one tail (produced using ztail.ado).

compute a one-tailed probability. It's "easier" to find a significant difference when you compute a one-tailed probability.

Deciding whether to include one or two tails is a key step in testing a hypothesis. You probably are familiar with the convention of using a probability (P value) of 0.05 as a criterion to establish a statistically significant difference between groups. If the P value is ≤ 0.05 we conclude that the groups most likely are different, and if the P value is ≥ 0.05 we conclude the groups most

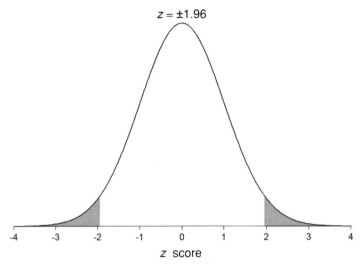

Figure 22.16 Shaded area = 0.05 in two tails (produced using ztail.ado).

likely are the same. But now you appreciate that the area determining the *P* value may be defined in more than one way.

Publication bias is a term acknowledging that studies are more likely to be published if they find a difference among the study groups than if they do not (Ch. 13 in Ref. 116). You now understand how the same data set may or may not show a difference among study groups depending on whether the *P* value represents a one- or two-tailed computation. So if you, or study authors, choose a one-tailed *P* value, make sure the rationale to do so was sound, beyond trying to improve the chance of publication. Most of the time, two-tailed computation is more appropriate. To paraphrase Rowntree[110], if you know so much about how groups differ that you can be confident about the direction in which they differ, by what criteria do you claim to be testing a hypothesis, whose key assumption is uncertainty about outcomes, rather than describing a predictable phenomenon?

CHAPTER 23

Data from all versus some: populations and samples

Estimating population parameters based on a sample

A data set may contain an observation on every subject of interest, that is, an entire defined population, or it may contain a sample of observations from that population. We are most interested to learn about defined populations of individuals, but practical considerations often force us to study samples from those populations. If your observations are but a sample from the population, you only may *estimate* population parameters like the mean (μ) and standard deviation (σ). To use data from a sample to draw conclusions about the population of origin is to make statistical inferences. For the inferences to be valid, your sample must accurately represent the population of origin. This is most likely when you have randomly selected the sample observations: every observation in the population had an equal probability to appear in the sample. The precision of your estimate of the population mean reflects how much the individual values in the sample vary.

The extent to which we may apply what we learn from data sampled from a population relates to the answers to two questions:
1 To what extent does the sample resemble the wider population?
2 Does our conclusion about the sample also apply to the wider population?

Parameters and statistics

Consider birth weight (BW) in the population represented by the data set we worked with in the last chapter. Assume this is a normally distributed random variable with mean $= \mu$ and standard deviation $= \sigma$. Suppose we randomly select a sample of n_i infants from this population of n_j infants. The mean of BW values $= \bar{x}_1$. If we randomly select another sample of n_i infants, the mean of their BW values will probably be not $\bar{x}_1$ (p. 180 in Ref. 109); let's call it $\bar{x}_2$. This variability is called sampling variation. Imagine we repeat this random sampling procedure many times to obtain a data set consisting of all the means of all the samples. The distribution of these sampling means is called a sampling distribution. To illustrate this idea, I had Stata draw four repeated random samples of 10% of the population (Table 23.1 and Fig. 23.1; compare with Fig. 22.13).

In statistical theory, the numerical values of the characteristics that describe a sample drawn from a population are called statistics; the numerical values of the same characteristics that describe the entire population are called

Table 23.1 Four random samples of 10% of a population

Sample no.	x, Sample mean	s, Sample SD
1	2380	1041
2	2539	1054
3	2449	1055
4	2527	1048

parameters (pp. 82–83 in Ref. 110). The convention is to use Roman letters to represent statistics and Greek letters to represent parameters (I used this convention in the previous paragraph). We may now define statistical inference as the process of using statistics to estimate parameters,[110] or perhaps more soberly, as the process of using data, subject to random variation, to determine a system characteristic.[117]

Central limit theorem

While introducing the idea of a sampling distribution I asked you to imagine a process of repeated sampling. We usually don't engage in such a process, but you should know about some of the properties of the theoretical distribution of sampling means. These properties, upon minimal assumptions, tell us quite a bit about what can be inferred from a sample to the population. These properties are described by the central limit theorem: for "large enough" sample sizes,

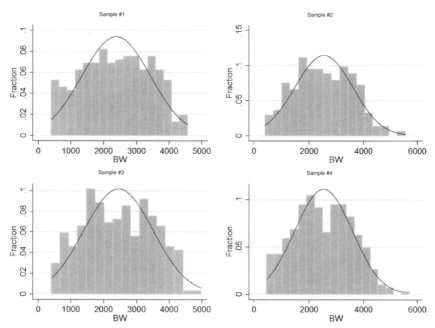

Figure 23.1 Four random samples of 10% of a population.

Table 23.2 Four random samples of 50% of a population

Sample no.	x, Sample mean	s, Sample SD
1	2405	1034
2	2390	1033
3	2408	1032
4	2430	1044

n ($n \geq 15$, usually[113]), *the distribution of the sample means is approximately normal even when the individual observations are not normally distributed.* [If the population of origin is itself normally distributed, n need only equal 1. The farther from normality the population distribution, the larger the n must be.] The central limit theorem underpins statistical analysis. Authors tend to gush as they write about the theorem: "remarkable," "very powerful," "startling," "amazing," and "beautiful."[109,111,113] I shall try to help you appreciate the basis for this passion.

Theoretically, the mean of a sampling distribution is the same as the mean for the population itself. It's intuitively reasonable that sample means would tend to fall around the population mean. The mean for the population from which the samples in Table 23.1 were drawn is 2409 (see Stata output in Chapter 22); the mean of the four samples is 2473.75, not spot on because of sampling variation and a relatively small n.

Each random sample from a population varies somewhat in its estimate of the population mean. The larger the sample, the narrower the variability, but for any sample smaller than the whole population, sampling variability remains. Table 23.2 and Fig. 23.2 illustrate 50% samples drawn from the same

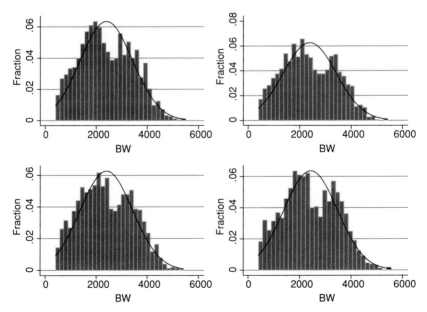

Figure 23.2 Four random samples of 50% of a population (arranged in same sample order as Fig. 23.1).

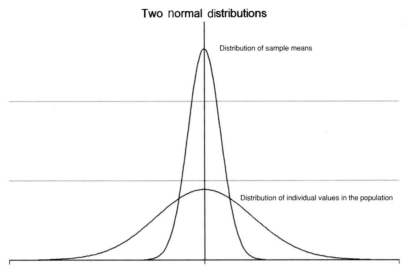

Two normal distributions

Distribution of sample means

Distribution of individual values in the population

Figure 23.3 Distribution of individual values in a population and of sample means drawn from the same population (produced using zdemo2.ado).

population as the 10% samples in Table 23.1 and Fig. 23.1 ($\bar{x}$ for sample 3 happened to round off to 2408, but actually isn't exactly the same as μ, which is 2408.937).

But where does that leave us for a data set obtained from only *one* sample? Well, we *are* likely to make an error estimating the population mean from one sample mean, as illustrated in Tables 23.1 and 23.2, because that one sample mean is unlikely to fall exactly at the center of the sampling distribution. However, by the nature of the normal distribution, the size of the error is likely to be relatively small. Most values in a normal distribution cluster around the center. For a sampling distribution, that's the location of both the sampling mean and the population mean. *So most of the time, an individual sample mean will be relatively close to the population mean*, and only infrequently will an individual sample mean lie out in one of the tails; that is, only infrequently will an individual sample mean reflect a relatively large error in estimating the population mean.

It gets better yet. The standard deviation of the distribution of the sampling means is called the standard error of the mean: $SE = \frac{\sigma}{\sqrt{n}}$. (see Ref. 111 for a derivation of the theorem and the SE, aimed at nonmathematicians.) This means that the dispersion of the distribution of sampling means is *narrower* than the dispersion of the population distribution (σ) itself, because σ is divided by the square root of the sample size, n. The sample means do more than tend to cluster around the population mean, they cluster *rather closely* around the population mean (Fig. 23.3)!

CHAPTER 24

Estimating population parameters: confidence intervals

To careful readers, the importance and beauty of the central limit theorem might not yet be compelling. The utility of the central limit theorem is framed in terms of population parameters. If you work only with a sample, what use is it to know how to compute the standard error, $SE = \frac{\sigma}{\sqrt{n}}$, when the formula requires the value for σ? Nor do we know μ; so what use is it to know how to compute the z score? That is what we next explore.

We are at a crucial place in the story, the very core of statistical theory. Even if we had the funding to try, still we could not collect the data we desire for some populations. For example, suppose we study the effect of intervention I on all individuals in a defined population of patients who were born between 1996 and 2000. Our study indicates that I provides a large protective effect; we decide henceforth to use it in routine clinical practice. In deciding henceforth to apply what we learned, we drew inference to an even *wider* target population: similarly defined people not yet born. Carefully reflect on the notion of inference because it largely constitutes our warrant to collect and analyze health care data. The point is that if we apply what we learn from a population-based study, we return to the principles governing a sample drawn from a larger population.

Point and interval estimates

Each sample mean is a *point estimate* of the population mean, a single number estimating the mean. Though the point estimate varies with each sample, a single estimate cannot indicate that variability. Therefore, we commonly also make an *interval estimate*, called a confidence interval (CI). The confidence interval estimates the population mean in terms of a range of values that probably contains the actual value, taking into account the amount of variability in the sample estimate. To compute a confidence interval we draw on knowledge of the normal distribution and the central limit theorem. We usually don't know σ, so we substitute s, the sample standard deviation, as our estimate of σ.[109,113] However, as we saw, s varies from sample to sample, and this alters the shape of the theoretical sampling distribution that we use to infer our population parameters. [The extent the distribution is altered depends inversely on sample size.] This relationship is described by the t distribution, also a symmetrical bell-shaped curve.

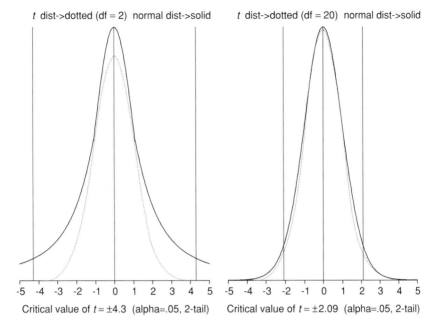

Figure 24.1 *t* distribution at low and high df, related to the normal distribution (produced using tdemo.ado).

The *t* distribution

The *t* distribution, like the normal distribution, has an area under the curve equal to 1. But compared to the normal distribution the *t* distribution is flatter, more spread out and with somewhat more area contained in the tails. Its particular shape is a function of the number of degrees of freedom (df) in the sample: df = $(n - 1)$ (see the discussion of variance in Chapter 22). Every value of df produces a different *t* distribution, so textbooks of statistics usually present abridged tables of the area under the curve. Stata can compute the exact area you specify. As df → ∞, the *t* distribution approaches the normal distribution (Fig. 24.1). The *t* score is computed analogously to the *z* score and is converted to an area or probability by referring to the corresponding *t* distribution. We expand these ideas in Chapter 25, when we compare means from two different samples.

Confidence Interval

Repeating, the confidence interval estimates the population mean in terms of a range of values that probably contains the actual value. "Probably" has a specific meaning in this context. A 95% confidence interval (CI_{95}) has a 95% probability of containing the actual, but unknown, population mean. Imagine selecting 100 random samples from a population and computing a

CI for the mean of each sample. If your method was designed to arrive at the CI$_{95}$, then on average, 95 of the 100 CIs would include the value of the population mean (μ). The 95% cutpoint is common, but other cutpoints, as suitable to the context, could be chosen. The cutpoint value affects the width of the resulting interval: a 99% CI will be wider than a corresponding 95% CI. For a given percentile cutpoint, a more precise estimate will be narrower than one less precise. The precision of an estimate reflects the variability of individual values in the sample.

The formula to compute a two-sided confidence interval derives from the standard normal deviate for a sampling distribution of means:

$$z = \frac{\bar{x} - \mu}{\sigma / \sqrt{n}}.$$

The central limit theorem states that z is normally distributed; therefore, as illustrated by Fig. 22.16, 95% of the observations lie between a z score of -1.96 and $+1.96$. If we knew σ, the 95% CI would be bounded by the interval $\left(\bar{x} - 1.96\frac{\sigma}{\sqrt{n}}, \bar{x} + 1.96\frac{\sigma}{\sqrt{n}}\right)$.

In Chapter 22, we examined the variable BW for a population of 3050 infants. The value of σ was 1038.892. Table 23.1 presented statistics for four 10% samples ($n = 305$) drawn from this population. $\bar{x}$ for sample 1 was 2380 g. The 95% CI for this sample is therefore $\left(2380 - 1.96\frac{1038.892}{\sqrt{305}}, 2380 + 1.96\frac{1038.892}{\sqrt{305}}\right) = (2263.4059, 2496.5941)$, which contains the actual population mean, $\mu = 2408.937$.

Similarly, to compute a 95% CI *when we don't know* σ, which is often the case, we estimate it by s, and replace the value of -1.96 and $+1.96$ with $\pm$ the appropriate t statistic (t score) for the df in the sample. As a rule of thumb, when df >30, substituting the normal distribution for the t distribution produces less than a 5% error in the interval estimate (Fig. 24.1). Although it is important to understand how CIs are computed, Stata takes care of the computational details for you.

The Stata command cii requires n, $\bar{x}$, and s. To compute CI$_{95}$ for the mean of sample 1 in Table 23.1:

```
. cii· 305 2380 1041

    Variable |   Obs     Mean    Std.Err.    [95% Conf.    Interval]
-------------+---------------------------------------------------------
             |   305     2380    59.60749    2262.705      2497.295
```

Because n is relatively large, the confidence limits are almost identical to those when σ was given: 2263.4059, 2496.5941. To compute the confidence limits for a data set containing individual observations, run the command ci *var-name*.

The central limit theorem is not a universal warrant

Sometimes you'll work with methods that assume a normally distributed variable yet the central limit theorem won't be applicable. The sample size may be extremely small or the population distribution may drastically deviate from normal. In Chapter 22, I discussed transforming the measurement scale of the variable as a way to get a closer approximation to normal (gladder and qladder commands). Another approach is to use nonparametric methods, the subject of Chapter 31. In general, check the distribution before proceeding with further analysis.

CHAPTER 25

Comparing two sample means and testing a hypothesis

Overview

Often, we have data that we suspect come from more than one distinct group. One way to explore the possibility is to compare the mean outcomes in these groups. The simplest comparison involves two groups, considered to be independent. Later we shall extend the approach and examine how to compare means from more than two groups. A special case of two sample comparisons (which is beyond our scope) involves paired data; examples include collecting data on the same individuals before and after some treatment, or matching cases and controls in an epidemiologic study. You should know that special methods are required to analyze such data.[109,113]

H_0 and H_A

For health care data, the typical distinction among two groups you suspect are different rests in one group having received some exposure, or treatment, while the other did not. Be careful about calling these controls (see the discussion on case-control studies in Chapter 18). We may evaluate the differences between groups by considering the width and extent of overlap of their confidence intervals. We also may explicitly test the hypothesis that the mean outcome of the exposed group is equal to the mean outcome of the unexposed group. This does not mean that the two means must literally be equal, only that the difference we observe between the means can be explained by sampling variation. This formulation articulates the null hypothesis, H_0. The alternate hypothesis, H_A, posits that the mean outcome of the exposed group is not equal to the mean outcome of the unexposed group; the observed difference between the means is unlikely to be explained by sampling variation. So formulated, one of these hypotheses always must be true.

Testing a null hypothesis

The actual hypothesis test depends on the probability, *assuming the null hypothesis were true,* of obtaining a difference between the group means as extreme or more extreme than that observed. When the probability is sufficiently low, we conclude that there is a difference between the groups. The value of this computed probability is known as a *P* value. The *P* value, as we have seen, is determined by a specified area of a relevant theoretical probability distribution. For hypothesis testing, this distribution displays all possible values of a measure derived from the differences between the groups' outcome measures, for example, means. This measure is called a test statistic. The area of the distribution that determines the P value is that portion containing values of the test statistic that are as extreme, or more extreme, than the one observed between the groups.

This may seem more complicated than it is. Look again Figs. 22.15 and 22.16 and imagine that the curves are of a t distribution instead of a z distribution, because our present focus is on samples rather than populations, and that the distributions describe all possible values of the relevant test statistic. The boundaries of the shaded areas, then, represent the values as extreme or more extreme than the cutpoint value (the actual value of the test statistic).

If the P value is sufficiently low, that is, *if we presume H_0 were true* and find that the probability of obtaining a difference between the group means as extreme or more extreme than that observed is lower than some small specified value, then we are compelled to reject H_0 and accept H_A. Many investigators set the specified value, which is called the level of statistical significance and denoted by α, for a P value at ≤ 0.05. When the z score, or the t score, or some other test statistic, falls far enough out in the tails of the distribution so that the delimited area is ≤ 0.05 (5% of the area under the curve), we say the difference between the group means – or other appropriate summary outcome statistics – is *statistically significant*. Understand that $\alpha = 0.05$ means that if H_0 were true, the probability of obtaining a difference between the group summary measures as extreme or more extreme than that observed is 5%. Accordingly, if we perform many hypothesis tests, then on average, 5 times in 100 we will incorrectly reject H_0. When you desire a smaller probability of making such an error you should select a lower α. With $\alpha = 0.01$, you risk rejecting H_0 1% of the time when in fact you should not.

If the probability of obtaining a difference between the group summary measures as extreme or more extreme than that observed is $>\alpha$, then although we cannot reject H_0, we also do not have firm grounds to accept it. For example, if $P = 0.07$ we would not reject H_0; but must understand that *assuming H_0 were true,* the probability of obtaining a difference between sample group summary measures as extreme or more extreme than we have observed still is only 7%. The value may not satisfy conventional criteria of statistical significance, but this is still a relatively unlikely finding. We return to this issue in Chapter 26, where we examine the types of errors we may make when testing hypotheses and strategies to minimize these errors.

Test statistics and testing a hypothesis

Consider what a hypothesis test represents: in the main, we seek to establish whether the two or more sample distributions came from different populations or the same population. Our task is illustrated in Fig. 25.1. Your intuition,

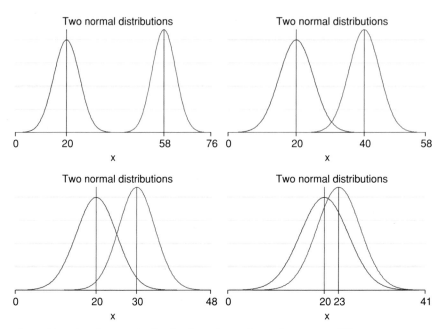

Figure 25.1 Are the sample distributions drawn from the same or different populations? (Produced using zdemo2.ado and the Stata `graph combine` command.)

informed by what you've learned so far about distributions, may lead you to guess that the two graphs at the top probably represent samples drawn from different populations; harder to evaluate is the graph at the lower left, and at the lower right, indicating that probably two samples were drawn from one population. The notion of a significant difference rests upon the distributions of the group outcomes. The test statistic describes precisely how different are those distributions. Methods to compute test statistics differ according to the nature of the data. Although you need not know the relevant formulas, you should always understand the essential ideas underpinning the test statistics you ask statistical software to compute.

A test statistic describes the signal-to-noise ratio in the data you wish to compare (see p. 96 in Ref. 118). Consider the signal as the difference in effect observed among the groups. This difference in effect is expressed by some measure of the difference in the central tendency. Consider the noise as the inherent variation in the values of the random variable you measure for each group. This variation is expressed by the variance in our estimate of the central tendency. Thus, a test statistic is

$$\frac{\text{some measure of difference in central tendency}}{\text{some measure of variance in the estimate of the central tendency}} = \frac{\text{signal}}{\text{noise}}.$$

Recall, the central limit theorem says that for "large enough" sample sizes[113] (n usually $\geq$15), the distribution of the sample means is approximately normal even when the individual observations are not normally distributed. Therefore, the distribution of the differences in central tendency among groups also is approximately normal. In other words, the distribution of the values of the test statistic, as broadly defined above, is approximately normal. Essentially, what we have learned about other theoretical distributions applies to the sampling distribution of the test statistic.

The *t* test

Imagine we select two independent samples of size n from population A and population B. We denote the mean value of some random variable, X, in the sample from each respective population by $\bar{X}_A$ and $\bar{X}_B$. The exact method by which we compare these samples depends on the variance of the underlying populations. If we know the population variances or can reasonably assume they are equal, then we compare the samples using the two-sample t test. When we cannot assume equal variances in the two populations then we compare the samples using a special modification of the two-sample t test.

In Fig. 25.2, the plotted z score of ± 2.878 reflects a two-tailed hypothesis test of the mean for group A and the mean for group B. Assume n in each group is large; also, I made up the particular z-score value. Values on the x-axis to the right of 0 reflect MeanA $-$ MeanB > 0; values to the left of 0 reflect MeanA $-$ MeanB < 0. I show a z distribution because the t distribution approaches the

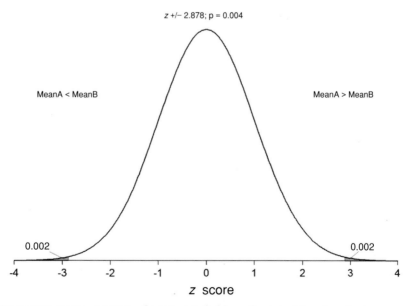

Figure 25.2 z score ± 2.878 reflects two-tailed hypothesis test (produced using ztail.ado).

normal distribution as df $\rightarrow \infty$ and we assume large samples here. The test is two tailed because in this hypothetical situation we do not know before collecting the data in which direction the difference, if any, would lie. In each tail, the z score of ± 2.878 cuts off an area $= 0.002$. Thus, *assuming H_0 were true*, the probability of obtaining a difference between sample group means as extreme or more extreme than we have observed is 0.004.

Explore some of these ideas using Stata

Open the Stata data file (.dta) you saved from the exercise in Chapter 22. One of the variables in this data set is called ante. This variable records whether each infant's mother received antenatal care. Let's summarize the observations:

```
. sum ante,det
```

	ante
no observations	

Can you guess what's going on? You can explore the values of this variable in the Stata browser, but it's a good habit to use the codebook command to get an overview.

```
. codebook ante
ante
(unlabeled)
```

type:	string (str1)

unique values: 2	missing "": 31/3050

```
   tabulation: Freq.   Value
                 31    " "
               1875    "N"
               1144    "Y"
```

ante is formatted as a string variable. Data values were entered as Y = yes and N = no. For 31 of the 3050 observations, no data were entered for this variable. Once again we have "dirty" data; to analyze ante as a categorical variable we must convert to numeric format. Stata initially reported there were no observations because "summarize" is a so-called analytic command. As such, it expects observation values to be numbers. When they are not, it treats the data as missing values. To solve the problem, generate a new numeric variable, antecare:

```
. encode ante, generate(antecare)
```

Let's see what we've accomplished.

```
. codebook antecare
```

```
antecare
(unlabeled)
```

type:	numeric (long)				
label:	antecare				
range:	[1,2]		units:	1	
unique values:	2		missing .:	31/3050	

tabulation:	Freq.	Numeric	Label
	1875	1	N
	1144	2	Y
	31	.	

```
. sum antecare,det
```

                                antecare

	Percentiles	Smallest		
1%	1	1		
5%	1	1		
10%	1	1	Obs	3019
25%	1	1	Sum of Wgt.	3019
50%	1		Mean	1.378933
		Largest	Std. Dev.	.4852019
75%	2	2		
90%	2	2	Variance	.2354209
95%	2	2	Skewness	.4991186
99%	2	2	Kurtosis	1.249119

I'm satisfied, so I'll save my work. By the way, note that the mean value is approximately 1.38. Based on coding no antenatal care, N, as a 1 (see codebook output), it can be said that 38% of this population did not receive antenatal care, an unusually large proportion for many regions.

I suspect BW may be associated with a mother receiving antenatal care, so I look at BW for the group with, and the group without, antenatal care exposure.

```
. sum BW if antecare=1,det
invalid syntax
r(198);
```

Based on the coding scheme in the codebook antecare **output, you might think the previous command asked Stata to summarize the BW variable for infants whose mothers did not receive antenatal care. However, Stata has two ways to indicate "equals." Use a single "=" with a mathematical expression, but use "=="if you are specifying a value for a variable.**

```
. sum BW if antecare==1,det
```

	BW			
	Percentiles	Smallest		
1%	600	400		
5%	1330	400		
10%	1720	420	Obs	1875
25%	2325	425	Sum of Wgt.	1875
50%	3000		Mean	2920.901
		Largest	Std. Dev.	905.5782
75%	3565	5380		
90%	4005	5422	Variance	820071.9
95%	4300	5500	Skewness	-.341056
99%	4755	5557	Kurtosis	2.888539

sum BW if antecare==2,det

	BW			
	Percentiles	Smallest		
1%	490	445		
5%	615	450		
10%	750	450	Obs	1144
25%	1110	460	Sum of Wgt.	1144
50%	1580		Mean	1576.126
		Largest	Std. Dev.	607.3113
75%	1990	3572		
90%	2320	3725	Variance	368827.1
95%	2570	4080	Skewness	.3642829
99%	3200	4082	Kurtosis	3.182301

**Surprised? Mean BW of infants whose mothers did not receive
antenatal care is substantially higher than the mean BW of infants
whose mothers did receive antenatal care. You might have expected
that the higher low birth weight rate generally known to occur
among mothers who do not receive prenatal care would be reflected
in the data. My primary aim here is to illustrate hypothesis
testing, but I must digress: I suspect we're exploring a confounded
relationship. Possible confounders include maternal residence
and access to care. For example, a greater proportion of mothers
who receive antenatal care may live relatively far from this
hospital, so their infants tend come to this hospital only if
they're born prematurely. Mothers living near this hospital,
presumably for socio/cultural/economic reasons, may be less
likely to receive prenatal care but it is more likely that all
these infants come to this hospital, rather than only those who are
premature (that is, the distribution of gestational ages may be
approximately normal).**

**Anyway, let's do some hypothesis testing. Let's test the null
hypothesis that the mean BW of infants whose mothers did not
receive antenatal care equals the mean BW of infants whose mothers
did receive antenatal care.**

. ttest BW,by(antecare)

Two-sample t test with equal variances

Group	Obs	Mean	Std. Err.	Std. Dev.	[95% Conf.	Interval]
N	1875	2920.901	20.91343	905.5782	2879.885	2961.917
Y	1144	1576.126	17.95554	607.3113	1540.896	1611.355
combined	3019	2411.321	18.86689	1036.649	2374.328	2448.314
diff		1344.775	30.2259		1285.51	1404.041

Degrees of freedom: 3017

Ho: mean(N) - mean(Y) = diff = 0

Ha: diff <0	Ha: diff != 0	Ha: diff > 0
t = 44.4908	t = 44.4908	t = 44.4908
P < t = 1.0000	P > |t| = 0.0000	P > t = 0.0000

Stata has given us lots of output. It has performed a two-sample t test after computing the group means, standard deviations, and 95% confidence intervals. Similar data appear for the combined group. Why are there 3017 degrees of freedom when there are 3019 total observations and df = n - 1? df = n - 1 for *each group*. For the group without antenatal care (N), n = 1875, so df = n - 1 = 1874; and for the group with antenatal care (Y), n = 1144, so df = n - 1 = 1143. 1874 + 1143 = 3017.

Below the count of df, Stata articulates the null hypothesis, Ho: mean(N) - mean(Y) = diff = 0. **And below that, the three analytical options, two of which I've sort of discouraged your using because they're one-tailed.** Ha: diff < 0 **describes the one-tailed possibility that the difference in means is <0;** Ha: diff > 0 **describes the one-tailed possibility that the difference in means is >0; and the one in the center,** Ha: diff != 0 **describes the two-tailed possibility that the difference in means is not = 0 (in Stata, ! or ~ symbolize "not").**

Below each Ha: **statement is the associated** t **statistic (an exceedingly high value, in this case), and below that, the** P **value. For the two-tailed test,** P > \|t\| = 0.0000 **means that** *assuming H_0 were true,* the probability of obtaining an absolute value (two-tailed test looks at -t and + t) of a t statistic for the difference in sample group means as extreme or more extreme than 44.4908 is <0.00005. (Stata displays 0.0000 to denote a value <0.00005.)

Astute readers noticed that the summaries of the BW variable showed rather different variance according to antenatal care. Recall that I said we must use a special modification of the two-sample t test when we can't assume the variances of the two populations are equal. It's easy in Stata:

. ttest BW,by(antecare) unequal

Two-sample t test with unequal variances

```
--------------------------------------------------------------------
  Group|   Obs      Mean    Std. Err.   Std. Dev. [95% Conf. Interval]
---------+----------------------------------------------------------
      N|  1875   2920.901   20.91343   905.5782 2879.885   2961.917
      Y|  1144   1576.126   17.95554   607.3113 1540.896   1611.355
--------------------------------------------------------------------
combined|  3019   2411.321   18.86689  1036.649  2374.328   2448.314
--------------------------------------------------------------------
    diff|           1344.775   27.56398            1290.729   1398.822
--------------------------------------------------------------------
Satterthwaite's degrees of freedom: 2990.71
```

$$. \ Ho: \ mean(N) \ - \ mean(Y) \ = \ diff \ = \ 0$$

Ha: diff <0	Ha: diff != 0	Ha: diff > 0
t = 48.7874	t = 48.7874	t = 48.7874
P < t = 1.0000	P > |t| = 0.0000	P > t = 0.0000

In our example, results are about the same for the CI for the difference, the *t* statistic, and the inference that may be drawn.

Confidence intervals aid evaluating group differences and statistical significance

Earlier, I said that we may evaluate differences between groups by considering the width and extent of overlap of their CIs or by testing the null hypothesis. Although derived from the same statistics as the P value, the CI for the mean of the differences between groups communicates substantially more evaluative information. By definition, if the CI_{95} for the mean of the differences between groups includes 0 – more generally, if it includes the null value, i.e., the value denoting no difference – then the P value >0.05. If you examine the CI_{95} for each group and find the ranges overlap, the P value will usually be >0.05. Sometimes, however, confidence intervals overlap by as much as 25% yet may still be compatible with statistical significance.[115] If the ranges do not overlap, then the P value <0.05.

Confidence intervals tell you things that a P value by itself does not: the magnitude of the difference between groups (the effect size) and the precision of the estimate. Test statistics are a function of sample size, n. For very large n, relatively small differences between groups can achieve high levels of statistical significance. Thus, you want to know more than just a P value. Imagine I select a sample of 10,000,000 infants from some government registry that recorded birth weight (BW) and maternal favorite color. I wish to test the hypothesis that mothers whose favorite color is red ($n = 5,500,000$) have infants of different birth weight than mothers whose favorite color is blue ($n = 4,500,000$). I find that mean BW of infants whose mothers prefer red is 3260 g, with a standard deviation of 247 g, and the mean BW for those whose mothers prefer blue is 3262 g with a standard deviation of 249 g. Not much of a difference, is there? From my perspective as a neonatologist, a difference in 2 g is of no clinical significance whatever. Let's run the hypothesis test:

```
. ttesti 5500000 3260 247 4500000 3262 249

Two-sample t test with equal variances
                  Obs     Mean   Std. Err.  Std. Dev. [95% Conf. Interval]
---------+-----------------------------------------------------------------
       x | 5500000     3260   .1053212        247   3259.794    3260.206
       y | 4500000     3262   .1173797        249    3261.77     3262.23
---------+-----------------------------------------------------------------
combined | 10000000 3260.9   .0783941    247.904   3260.746    3261.054
---------+-----------------------------------------------------------------
    diff |                -2   .1575769              -2.308845   -1.691155

Degrees of freedom: 9999998

                  Ho: mean(x)  - mean(y)  = diff = 0

    Ha: diff < 0              Ha: diff != 0              Ha: diff > 0
      t = -12.6922              t = -12.6922               t = -12.6922
  P < t =   0.0000         P > |t|  =  0.0000         P > t =   1.0000
```

Assuming H_0 were true, the probability of obtaining an absolute value of a t statistic for the difference in sample group means as extreme or more extreme than 12.6922 is <0.00005. As I warned, when n is very large, small differences in effect size (of a magnitude often *clinically insignificant*) may be highly *statistically significant*.

To help you interpret this maternal color preference data you would want to know about the effect size and the precision of the estimate. You get that from the CI_{95} for the difference between the groups. From the Stata output above, that interval is (-2.308845, -1.691155). In other words, the probability that the population mean is somewhere between 1.69 and 2.31 g is 95%. The magnitude of the effect seems very small, perhaps less than the measurement accuracy itself. However, the interval is rather narrow and so I conclude that the estimate of effect is rather precise. I know the P value is highly significant because the interval bounding the mean difference did not contain 0 and was relatively far from 0. This illustration is intended to make one point only, so I merely point out the possibility that confounding may be involved.

We should also consider how to interpret a CI that on one side just barely includes 0, but ranges quite far in the other direction. Such a CI_{95} denotes a $P > 0.05$ and also relatively low precision in estimating the effect size. Should you think differently about those underlying data than about a data set that also yields a CI_{95} just barely including 0, but with a narrow range? The tight interval means the precision of this second estimate of effect size is much better. By the convention of setting α at 0.05, we'd not reject H_0 in either case. However, we're more likely to be wrong not rejecting H_0 in the first case than in the second. The explanation is in the next chapter.

CHAPTER 26

Type I and type II error in a hypothesis test, power, and sample size

Careful reasoning only prevents some mistaken conclusions

Drawing a mistaken conclusion is built-in to testing a hypothesis. Some mistaken conclusions result from faulty logic. Others predictably occur even when logic is correct. The predictable errors are of two types: type I and type II. Before exploring the predictable errors, let's look at one important example of faulty logic.

In Chapter 25, I emphasized an important aspect of hypothesis testing logic by italicizing some words. I described the P value as the probability, *assuming the null hypothesis were true*, of obtaining a difference between the group means as extreme or more extreme than that observed. This is commonly, but wrongly, thought to mean the P value is the probability that the null hypothesis is true. Be sure you understand why this statement is wrong.

The P value is an outcome of a *conditional* probability scenario. The P value is the answer to the question: "What is the probability of getting these data, *given* H_0"? If the P value were the probability that H_0 is true, it would be the answer to a different question: "What is the probability that H_0 is true, given these data"? The difference between these two questions resembles the difference between the following: (a) "What is the probability of getting this diagnostic test result, *given that the patient does not have disease D*"? (b) "What is the probability that the patient does not have disease D, *given this diagnostic test result*"? (For more discussion and references, see Ch. 3 in Ref. 119).

Type I error

If we set the significance level, α, at 0.05 to reject H_0 and we perform many hypothesis tests, then on average 5 times in 100 we will incorrectly reject H_0. Figure 26.1 illustrates the relevant portions of the z distribution. The point is that unlikely outcomes nonetheless occur simply by chance, a matter of sampling variation. If we reject H_0 because $P \leq \alpha$ when the observed difference was due only to sampling variation, and not because the samples really came from different populations, we make a type I error. In making a type I error, we conclude from the hypothesis test that the samples originate from different

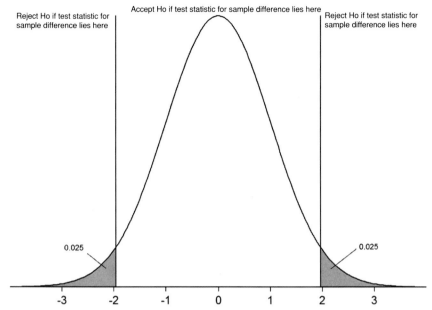

Figure 26.1 Type I error (produced using ztail.ado).

source populations when they actually do not. In conditional probability notation, $\alpha = P$ (reject $H_0 \mid H_0$ true), that is, the probability of rejecting H_0, given that H_0 is true.

Type II error

If we do not reject H_0 because $P > \alpha$ when the observed difference was not due to sampling variation – the samples really do come from different source populations – we make a type II error. We make a type II error when we conclude from the hypothesis test that the samples come from the same source (i.e., they are not different), when they actually come from different sources (i.e., they are different).

Type II errors arise when we are mistaken about the applicable sampling distribution describing the data under consideration. In Fig. 26.2, the curve on the left is the one we *think* represents the sampling distribution given the values we have observed. For a two-tailed hypothesis test with $\alpha \leq 0.05$, to achieve significance the sample mean of interest must lie on either of the parts of the horizontal axis beneath the shaded portion with area = 0.025. Sample means in the remaining area are judged consistent with sampling variation and we do not reject H_0. However, the *actual* sampling distribution lies to the right of the distribution that we mistakenly think is the correct one. Some of the values in the *actual* distribution overlap with the distribution upon which we based our hypothesis test. Those overlapping values that happen

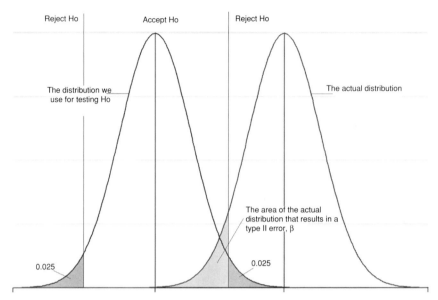

Figure 26.2 Type II error (produced using zdemo2.ado).

to lie to the left of the part of the horizontal axis beneath the shaded portion with area $= 0.025$, in our mistaken idea of the distribution, will be considered compatible with sampling variation when, in fact, they are out in the tail of the actual distribution. These are the values that produce a type II error and are so indicated in the figure. The probability of a type II error is denoted by β and equals the identified shaded area under the curve. In conditional probability notation, $\beta = P\,(\text{do not reject } H_0 \mid H_0 \text{ false})$, that is, the probability of not rejecting H_0, given that H_0 is false.

As you can see from Fig. 26.2, the value of β will vary with the location of the actual distribution and the cutpoint value under consideration. Essentially, β depends on the size of the difference you don't want to miss.

Power

The power of a hypothesis test is defined as $1 - \beta$. In other words, power is the probability that you *won't* commit a type II error. In conditional probability notation, power $= P$ (reject $H_0 \mid H_0$ false).

Power is about the probability of not missing an important difference. The power of a study is often set arbitrarily at 0.80.[116] Suppose a therapeutic trial reports no effect for a new treatment. Before you accept the treatment as ineffective, determine the study's power to identify an effect of a magnitude you consider important. Power computations derive from the formula for the relevant test statistic. Therefore, power depends on the actual values of the measure of central tendency for each group.

Sample size

Since power computations derive from the relevant test statistic, which tend to be a function of sample size, n, the size of the samples for a hypothesis test must not be determined arbitrarily. The sample size should reflect
- values of α and β appropriate to the question. You seek to identify
    - **(a)** a small effect (difference) when
        - **(i)** the exposure (intervention) is low cost and low risk.
        - **(ii)** the outcome is important and clearly measurable.
    - **(b)** only a large effect (difference) when
        - **(i)** the exposure (intervention) is high risk and high cost.
        - **(ii)** the outcome is not so important and hard to measure accurately or directly.
- the size of a difference you don't want to miss.

The formula to compute the sample size, n, needed to obtain a specified power for a hypothesis test is obtained by algebraically rearranging the terms in the expression for the appropriate test statistic. By specifying the desired level for α and β, and plugging in the corresponding value of the appropriate test statistic and the values of the sample measures of central tendency, we obtain the minimum sample size. See Ref. 113 for more details.

Computing sample size and power using Stata

`sampsi` computes power or sample size. Similar to the `ttesti` command, which we used in Chapter 25, `sampsi` is an immediate command. All of its arguments are numbers, usually *derived* from a data set, that you must enter directly in the command line, in distinction to the commands (such as `ttest`) that work on the observations in a data set loaded in memory. The syntax follows: `sampsi #1 #2 [, alpha(#) power(#) n1(#) n2(#) ratio(#) pre(#) post(#) sd1(#) sd2(#) method(post|change|ancova|all) r0(#) r1(#) r01(#) onesample onesided ]`.
- `#1` and `#2` refer to the postulated or actual means of the samples.
- `alpha(#)` specifies the significance level of the test; the default is `alpha(.05)`.
- `power(#)` is power of the test; the default is `power(.90)`.
- `n1(#)` specifies the size of the first sample.
- `n2(#)` specifies the size of the second sample.

If you specify n then `sampsi` reports the power calculation. If you don't specify n, then `sampsi` computes sample size. The options `sd1(#)` and `sd2(#)` denote the standard deviations for comparing means. If you don't specify these, Stata assumes its dealing with proportions. Here is a sample computation where `n1 = n2`. Of course, one must estimate as best one can the means and standard deviations.

```
. sampsi 132.86 127.44, p(0.8) sd1(15.34) sd2(18.23)

Estimated sample size for two-sample comparison of means
```

```
Test Ho: m1 = m2, where m1 is the mean in population 1
                       and m2 is the mean in population 2
Assumptions:

          alpha = 0.0500 (two-sided)
          power = 0.8000
             m1 = 132.86
             m2 = 127.44
            sd1 =  15.34
            sd2 =  18.23
          n2/n1 =   1.00

Estimated required sample sizes:

              n1 = 152
              n2 = 152


. sampsi 5.6 6.1, n1(100) sd1(1.5) a(0.01)

Estimated power for two-sample comparison of means

Test Ho: m1 = m2, where m1 is the mean in population 1
                       and m2 is the mean in population 2
Assumptions:

          alpha = 0.0100 (two-sided)
             m1 =    5.6
             m2 =    6.1
            sd1 =    1.5
            sd2 =    1.5
 sample size n1 =    100
             n2 =    100
          n2/n1 =   1.00

Estimated power:
          power = 0.4134
```

Strategies to minimize error

To minimize a type I error
- set α to a lower level.
- decrease the standard error by increasing the size of n.
  To minimize a type II error
- set α to a higher level. In Fig. 26.2, where the curves overlap, setting α to a higher level would move the line demarcating values that support rejecting H_0 to the left. This would simultaneously decrease the area for β.
- look for a larger main effect: a larger effect size, that is, difference in measures of central tendency. In Fig. 26.2, this would amount to moving the curves farther apart, decreasing the amount of overlap, ultimately to where there is no overlap.
- decrease the standard error by increasing the size of n.

Table 26.1 Outcomes of interpreting a hypothesis test

What we do as a result of the hypothesis test	What's actually the case	
	H_0 true (no difference, effect size = null)	H_0 false (groups are different, effect size matters)
Reject H_0	Type I error: $P = \alpha$	Correct conclusion: $P = \text{power} = 1 - \beta$
Do not reject H_0	Correct conclusion: $P = 1 - \alpha$	Type II error: $P = \beta$

These strategies entail tradeoffs between improvements in α and β. The exception is when you reduce the overlap of the curves. This may occur either by looking for a larger main effect or by increasing n, which will narrow the sampling distribution.

Summary

Table 26.1 sums up the outcomes of interpreting a hypothesis test.

$\alpha = p$ (reject $H_0 \mid H_0$ true)
$\beta = p$ (do not reject $H_0 \mid H_0$ false)
$\text{power} = p$ (reject $H_0 \mid H_0$ false)

CHAPTER 27

Comparing proportions: introduction to rates and odds

To compare outcomes expressed as proportions is to evaluate count data: the number of events that pertain to one of two alternative conditions. The alternative conditions might be yes/no, female/male, disease/no disease, etc. Thus, the type of outcome variable for comparing proportions is categorical, more specifically, dichotomous, or binary. Such variables are often *coded* by 0's or 1's. [In Chapter 25, Stata used 1's or 2's when it converted the `ante` variable to `antecare`.] Although the methods entail counts, the conceptual focus is on the proportion of the total that experienced the outcome and the proportion that didn't.

Fractions: ratios, proportions, and rates

A proportion is a specific type of fraction. The most generic type of fraction is a ratio (what you get when you divide one quantity by another).[120] No matter which quantity goes in the numerator and which in the denominator, it's still a ratio. A proportion is a particular kind of ratio: it describes the relation of a part to the whole. What goes in the numerator also must be included in the denominator, because the denominator counts all events. If our dichotomous outcome variable records survival as lived (L) or died (D), then the proportion of the sample who died is defined as D/N, where $N = (L) + (D)$.

A rate is an even more specific type of ratio: the numerator still counts events and the denominator includes a term for time. For example, an infection rate might be reported as (# individuals with positive blood culture reports)/month, or (# individuals with positive blood culture reports)/100 patient days. Technically, [(# individuals with positive blood culture reports)/ # patients] is not a rate, it's a proportion. Even in the medical literature, authors vary in how they use the term rate, so check for explicitly defined measures and methods of computation. I am reminded of an article I once reviewed about a process improvement effort aimed at decreasing an undefined "pneumothorax rate" in an NICU. Did the numerator count each occurrence of intrapleural air in any pleural space, or individuals with one or more pneumothoraces, or something else yet? The article also did not provide a time unit for the denominator. The "rate" was actually an implicit proportion.

244

Assumption of independent events

The statistical methods we examine in this book rest on the assumption that each individual outcome event is independent of the outcome of any other individual. For example, the occurrence of each death in no way influences the occurrence of any other death. However, within an institution, might some deaths be related to understaffing, or extraordinarily high work load, or an inexperienced group of trainees? When considering deaths from different facilities, might risk of death be associated with where an infant receives care? When the independence of individual observations may be questioned, special analytical techniques are necessary. Details involve making statistical adjustment for clustering of outcomes, and are beyond our scope. Another assumption about independence concerns independence among the variables in a predictive model. We return to this point when we examine multivariate regression.

Sampling distribution of a proportion

The binomial, or Bernoulli, distribution, (see Chapter 22) describes the possible outcomes of a dichotomous random variable. Thus, the sampling distribution of a proportion is the binomial distribution. The distribution is a function of the probability of the event occurring, p, and the number of observations, n(denoted as N in Chapter 22, to conform to factorial notation); the mean number of successes $= np$; the variance $= np(1 - p)$.

As n becomes increasingly large, the distribution of a binomial variable increasingly resembles the normal distribution. When np and $np(1 - p)$ both exceed 5, we may use the corresponding normal distribution with the same mean and variance of the corresponding binomial distribution.[109,113] However, for values of np and $np(1 - p)$ between 5 and 10 the numerator of the formula for the standard normal deviate, z, needs to be fudged just a little — we are, after all, approximating a discrete distribution by a continuous one (see Fig. 22.1). Therefore, statisticians add a continuity correction factor.[113] Adding 0.5 to the terms in the numerator of the standard normal deviate brings the resulting P values much closer to what they would be if we used the binomial formula with all its factorial terms. The main idea is that we can use the approximation to the normal distribution to test hypotheses and estimate required sample sizes.

Using Stata: prepare to compare proportions

In the next section, we shall consider the relationship between an infant requiring mechanical ventilation while in the NICU and the outcome of being discharged from the hospital with a home monitor. The data set that we worked with in previous chapters contains a variable called `homemonitor`.

```
. sum homemonitor,det
```

```
                              homemonitor
-----------------------------------------------------------------
no observations
```

By this point you know that this is probably dirty data.

```
. codebook homemonitor
```

```
---------------------------------------------------------------------
-----------------------------------------------------------------
homemonitor
 (unlabeled)
---------------------------------------------------------------------
-----------------------------------------------------------------

                  type:   string (str1)

         unique values:   2                            miss-
ing "":  0/3050

            tabulation:   Freq.   Value
                          2891    "N"
                           159    "Y"
```

It's a string variable. We must convert it to numeric.

```
. encode homemonitor, gen(HM)
```

```
. codebook HM
```

```
----------------------------------------------------------------------
-----------------------------------------------------------------
HM
(unlabeled)
----------------------------------------------------------------------
-----------------------------------------------------------------

                  type:   numeric (long)
                 label:   HM

                 range:   [1,2]                    units:   1
         unique values:   2                        miss-
ing .:  0/3050

            tabulation:   Freq.   Numeric  Label
                          2891          1  N
                           159          2  Y
```

**I've created a new variable, HM, that's numeric. I prefer to code
a "no" as a 0 and a "yes" as a 1.**

```
. recode HM (1=0) (2=1)
```

```
(HM: 3050 changes made)

. codebook HM

----------------------------------------------------------------
------------------------------------------------------
HM
(unlabeled)
----------------------------------------------------------------
------------------------------------------------------

                  type:  numeric (long)
                 label:  HM, but 1 value is not labeled

                 range:  [0,1]                         units:  1
         unique values:  2                          miss-
ing .:  0/3050

             tabulation:  Freq.   Numeric  Label
                          2891          0
                           159          1  N
```

**Stata transferred the label mapping that was automatically done
when I encoded the new variable, but can't figure out the new
assignment scheme;therefore, it kept 1 = N, but assigned no label
to 0. We'll drop the current labeling scheme and start over.**

```
. label drop HM

. label define HM 0 No 1 Yes

. codebook HM

----------------------------------------------------------------
------------------------------------------------------
HM
(unlabeled)
----------------------------------------------------------------
------------------------------------------------------

                  type:  numeric (long)
                 label:  HM

                 range:  [0,1]                         units:  1
         unique values:  2                          miss-
ing .:  0/3050

             tabulation:  Freq.   Numeric  Label
                          2891          0  No
                           159          1  Yes
```

**We've achieved the desired result. Notice that the codebook output
indicated that the variable name, HM, itself is unlabeled. To help**

someone unfamiliar with the data set, or if we ourselves forget
what **HM** represents, let's label the variable.

. label var HM "Went home with a monitor"

. codebook HM

```
-------------------------------------------------------------------
-----------------------------------------------------------
HM
Went home with a monitor
-------------------------------------------------------------------
-----------------------------------------------------------
```

                    [remainder of output same as previously shown]

HM is ready to go. Now let's explore our exposure variable.

. codebook mechvent

```
-------------------------------------------------------------------
-----------------------------------------------------------
mechvent
(unlabeled)
-------------------------------------------------------------------
-----------------------------------------------------------

                  type:  string (str1)

       unique values:  2                      missing "":  121/3050

          tabulation:  Freq.  Value
                        121   ""
                       2415   "N"
                        514   "Y"
```

**This is another string variable that must be converted. Also, we
don't know the value of mechvent for 121 of the observations;
they're missing. Note that missing values for string variables
are empty quotes.**

. encode mechvent, gen(MV)

. codebook MV

```
-------------------------------------------------------------------
-----------------------------------------------------------
MV
(unlabeled)
-------------------------------------------------------------------
-----------------------------------------------------------

                  type:  numeric (long)
```

```
                   label:  MV

                   range:  [1,2]                          units:  1
           unique values:  2                         miss-
ing .:  121/3050

              tabulation:  Freq.   Numeric  Label
                            2415         1  N
                             514         2  Y
                             121         .
```

Next, we recode MV and label it in the same way as we've just done for HM.

```
. recode MV (1=0) (2=1)
(MV: 2929 changes made)

. codebook MV

----------------------------------------------------------------------
----------------------------------------------------------
MV
(unlabeled)
----------------------------------------------------------------------
----------------------------------------------------------

                    type:  numeric (long)
                   label:  MV, but 1 value is not labeled

                   range:  [0,1]                          units:  1
           unique values:  2                         miss-
ing .:  121/3050

              tabulation:  Freq.   Numeric  Label
                            2415         0
                             514         1  N
                             121         .

. label drop MV

. label define MV 0 No 1 Yes

. codebook MV

----------------------------------------------------------------------
----------------------------------------------------------
MV
(unlabeled)
----------------------------------------------------------------------
----------------------------------------------------------

                    type:  numeric (long)
                   label:  MV

                   range:  [0,1]                          units:  1
```

```
          unique values:   2                              miss-
ing .:    121/3050

              tabulation:   Freq.    Numeric   Label
                            2415           0   No
                             514           1   Yes
                             121           .

. label var MV "required mechanical ventilation"
```

Don't forget: **always save your data set after you've created new variables, changed labels, or changed data.**

Chi-square (χ^2) test

The typical framework for comparing proportions is a contingency table. To compare two proportions, use a 2 × 2 table; more generally, use an $r \times c$ table, where r = # rows and c = # columns. Depending on the author, exposure may be represented in either the rows or the columns, so check this for each table you review.

You could test a hypothesis about a pair of independent proportions using the normal approximation to the binomial distribution, but a more general way exists to achieve the same thing: the chi-square (χ^2) test. For a 2 × 2 table, the χ^2 and z test for the difference between two proportions yield the same results. To see how χ^2 works, we first cross tabulate the data from the HM and MV variables recently created. Relate the following Stata output to the general formulation that follows in Table 27.1.

Table 27.1 A 2 × 2 outcome matrix

| | Exposure variable | | |
Outcome variable	Yes	No	Total
Yes	a	b	$a + b$
No	c	d	$c + d$
Total	$a + c$	$b + d$	n

```
. tab HM MV,cell

+------------------+
| Key              |
|------------------|
|     frequency    |
| cell percentage  |
+------------------+
```

```
+-----------------+
Went home | required mechanical
   with a |       ventilation
  monitor |      No        Yes |      Total
----------+----------------------+----------
      No |    2,347       428 |      2,775
         |    80.13      14.61 |      94.74
----------+----------------------+----------
     Yes |       68        86 |        154
         |     2.32      2.94 |       5.26
----------+----------------------+----------
   Total |    2,415       514 |      2,929
         |    82.45      17.55 |     100.00
```

Table 27.1 is a general representation of a 2 × 2 table of observed frequencies for a sample of size n. We may express H_0, no association between exposure and outcome, as follows: the proportion of individuals who experience the outcome among all those who receive the exposure is equal to the proportion of individuals who experience the outcome among those who do not receive the exposure. The alternate hypothesis, H_A, may be expressed thus as follows: the proportion of individuals who experience the outcome is not the same in the two exposure groups.

Under H_0 and if the numbers in each cell in Table 27.1 are held constant, we may represent expected frequencies as in Table 27.2. The formula in each cell describes the following relationship:

$$\text{Expected value of a cell} = \frac{(\text{Row total}) \ (\text{Column total})}{\text{Grand total}}$$

Table 27.2 Computing expected outcomes[109]

Outcome variable	Exposure variable		Total
	Yes	**No**	**Total**
Yes	$(a + b)(a + c)/n$	$(a + b)(b + d)/n$	$a + b$
No	$(c + d)(a + c)/n$	$(c + d)(b + d)/n$	$c + d$
Total	$a + c$	$b + d$	n

Thus, we may express H_0 in terms of the HM and MV variables: the proportion of infants who go home with a monitor (HM) among all those who receive mechanical ventilation (MV = 1) is equal to the proportion of infants who go home with a monitor (HM) among those who do not receive mechanical ventilation (MV = 0). Similarly we may express H_A: the proportion of infants who go home with a monitor (HM) is not the same in the two exposure groups (MV = 0; MV = 1).

The χ^2 test compares the observed (O) and expected (E) frequencies in each cell of the $r \times c$ table:

$$\chi^2 = \sum_{i=1}^{rc} \frac{(O_i - E_i)^2}{E_i} \quad \text{(see p. 314 in Ref. 109)}$$

In words, take the sum of the squares of all differences between observed and expected values for each cell in a table of r rows and c columns, divide by the expected value in that cell, and then start the summation at cell number one and continue through cell number ($r \times c$) (for a 2 $\times$ 2 table, through cell number 4). The χ^2 test statistic approximates a theoretical probability distribution also called χ^2. The shape of the distribution varies with the degrees of freedom (df) in the relationship you are investigating. The notion of df here resembles what we considered for the t distribution in Chapter 25, but for an $r \times c$ table, df $= (r - 1)\,(c - 1)$. Thus, a 2 $\times$ 2 table has 1 df. Consider a 2 $\times$ 2 table with the marginal totals filled in. You would only have to know the value of one of the four cells to be able to deduce the values of the other three.

I mentioned that the χ^2 test statistic approximates the χ^2 theoretical probability distribution. The approximation is close enough to compute your p value unless

- the *expected* count in each cell of a 2 $\times$ 2 table is <5; more generally, Pagano and Gauvreau[109] suggest that no more than one in five cells have an expected count <5.
- any cell has an expected count <1.

When either exclusion applies, you must compute the actual binomial probability. This method is called Fisher's exact test. If manually computed, Fisher's exact test is very time-consuming; but using Stata, it's a piece of cake.

Also, in discussing the method to compare means I mentioned that different methods are needed when the samples are not independent but paired. In the case of proportions, the appropriate test is McNemar's test, which is beyond our scope.

Comparing proportions using Stata

Stata has a useful collection of tabulation commands grouped under the title "epitab," tables for epidemiologists. The cc command creates a 2 $\times$ 2 table for a case-control study. Recall, such studies are based on outcomes and do not incorporate exposure times. We can't compute an incidence rate because rates include the time dimension. Note that case-control studies employ a random sample of controls, representing some fraction of the population. However, we don't know just what that fraction is. Therefore, we can't accurately estimate the risk of occurrence of the outcome of interest. Remember, risk means probability of occurrence, probability means proportion, and a proportion describes the relation of a part to the *whole*. We can, however, for a case-control study compute and compare odds. Let's analyze the HM and MV variables as if they came from a case-control study; in fact, our data set represents a cohort and we shall analyze the variables that way later in this chapter.

```
. cc HM MV
                                                       Proportion
                 |  Exposed   Unexposed  |    Total     Exposed
-----------------+----------------------+----------------------
         Cases   |    86          68    |     154       0.5584
      Controls   |   428        2347    |    2775       0.1542
-----------------+----------------------+----------------------
         Total   |   514        2415    |    2929       0.1755
                 |                      |
                 |   Point estimate     |  [95% Conf. Interval]
                 |----------------------+----------------------
    Odds ratio   |      6.935198        |  4.896184    9.835117  (exact)
 Attr. frac. ex. |       .855808        |  .7957593    .8983235  (exact)
 Attr. frac. pop |      .4779188        |
                 +----------------------------------------------
                      chi2(1) =  164.75  Pr>chi2 = 0.0000
```

If we had small samples, we'd have run Fisher's exact test. Remember, I said it was easy with Stata; just add it as an option.

```
. cc HM MV, exact
                                                       Proportion
                 |  Exposed   Unexposed  |    Total     Exposed
-----------------+----------------------+----------------------
         Cases   |    86          68    |     154       0.5584
      Controls   |   428        2347    |    2775       0.1542
-----------------+----------------------+----------------------
         Total   |   514        2415    |    2929       0.1755
                 |                      |
                 |   Point estimate     |  [95% Conf. Interval]
                 |----------------------+----------------------
    Odds ratio   |      6.935198        |  4.896184    9.835117  (exact)
 Attr. frac. ex. |       .855808        |  .7957593    .8983235  (exact)
 Attr. frac. pop |      .4779188        |
                 +----------------------------------------------
                      1-sided Fisher's exact P = 0.0000
                      2-sided Fisher's exact P = 0.0000
```

Since our samples are large, the output is the same with either χ^2 or Fisher's exact test. The concept of odds ratio is introduced shortly.

Probability and odds

The probability of an event occurring, by the frequentist definition, is equal to the proportion of times it occurs on many repeated trials. Thus, by our definition of a proportion, the probability of an event ranges in value between 0 and 1. Probability values may also be expressed as a percentage, in which case values range between 0 and 100%. A probability value that describes the proportional occurrence of an unwanted outcome has a special name, risk.

In health care we often speak of ~odds instead of probability. I find the notion of odds much less intuitive than the notion of probability. However, methods for analyzing dichotomous outcomes often report odds and odds ratios, so we should examine the notion. Returning to our dichotomous survival variable, the odds of dying are defined by

$$\text{Odds}(D) = \frac{P(D)}{P(\text{not}\,D)} = \frac{P(D)}{P(L)} = \frac{P(D)}{1 - P(D)}.$$

Rearranging terms allows us to express probability in terms of odds:

$$P(D) = \frac{\text{Odds}\,(D)}{1 + \text{Odds}\,(D)}.$$

Thus, to say the odds of dying are 2 to 1 means that the probability of dying is 2 times greater than the probability of not dying. Expressed as a probability value, 2 to 1 odds means $2/(1 + 2) = 2/3 = .67 = 67\%$.

The relationship between P and odds is such that when $P \leq 0.1$, odds and P values are about equal. From that point on, they increasingly differ: when $P = 1$, odds $= \infty$. Think about what odds $= 1$ means. For our survival variable, odds $= 1$ for dying means that the probability of dying is onefold greater than the probability of not dying; $P(D) = 1/(1 + 1) = 1/2 = .5 = 50\%$. We now consider the meaning of an odds ratio.

Odds ratio

The Stata output earlier in the section "Comparing proportions using Stata" gave us a P value of <0.00005 for H_0, suggesting that there is probably an association between exposure to MV and the outcome of HM $= 1$. Although the P value by itself doesn't tell us about the *strength* of the association, the Stata output does, via the odds ratio. The odds ratio (OR) describes the odds of the outcome occurring among exposed individuals divided by the odds of the outcome occurring among unexposed individuals. When OR $= 1$, exposure does not matter.

From the notion of odds defined earlier in this chapter:

$$\text{Odds (outcome|exposure)} = \frac{P(\text{outcome|exposure})}{P(\sim\text{outcome|exposure})}$$

$$= \frac{P(\text{outcome|exposure})}{1 - P(\text{outcome|exposure})}$$

the OR may be expressed as

$$\text{OR} = \left(\frac{P(\text{outcome|exposure})}{1 - P(\text{outcome|exposure})} \right) \text{divided by} \left(\frac{P(\text{outcome|no exposure})}{1 - P(\text{outcome|no exposure})} \right)$$

In terms of Table 27.1 (remember, probability = proportion): $P(\text{outcome}|\text{exposure}) = a/a + c$ and $P(\text{outcome}|\text{no exposure}) = b/b + d$. So sparing you the algebraic derivation, we may estimate the OR ($\hat{\text{OR}}$: the $\wedge$ above the term denotes an estimated quantity and we pronounce the term "OR-hat") by

$$\hat{\text{OR}} = \frac{ad}{bc}$$

The Stata output in the previous section tells us the point estimate of the odds ratio for going home with a monitor is about 6.9. The 95% CI for that estimate is 4.896184, 9.835117. Recall that sometimes a variable is better analyzed after transforming the measurement units by some mathematical operation. The CI for OR is computed analogously to the CI for a mean, and therefore assumes normally distributed values. However, the probability distribution of OR is skewed: a natural log transform results in a better approximation to normal. You need not trouble yourself about this when Stata runs the computation. I just thought you might want to know a little about what goes on behind the scenes. (For further details see Ch. 16 in Ref. 113.) For this reason, use a log scale when graphically displaying the CI for OR: you'll get a symmetric interval (pp. 91–94 in Ref. 121).

Relative risk or risk ratio

The relative risk, or risk ratio, is expressed as

$$\hat{\text{RR}} = \frac{P(\text{outcome} \mid \text{exposure})}{P(\text{outcome} \mid \text{no exposure})} = \frac{a/(a+c)}{b/(b+d)} = \frac{a/(b+d)}{b/(a+c)} = \frac{ab+ad}{ba+bc}$$

To compute relative risk, divide the probability of the outcome among exposed individuals by the probability of the outcome among unexposed individuals. The relative risk may be a more intuitively clear way to describe the strength of the association between exposure and outcome. When H_0 applies, RR = 1. Values of RR >1 indicate increased risk above null; values of RR <1 indicate decreased risk, a protective effect of the exposure.

Stata uses RR to report cohort study results. Cohort studies entail following groups over time, from onset of exposure through occurrence of outcome, if it occurs. Comparisons rest on accounting for exposure time. If you know that exposure time is the same for those who did and did not experience the outcome of interest, then you can use Stata's cs command, which produces a similar 2 × 2 table to that produced by the cc command but provides RR instead of OR. Here's the result for the HM and MV variables we examined previously.

```
. cs HM MV

                | required mechanical   |
                | ventilation           |
                |  Exposed    Unexposed |     Total
----------------+-----------------------+----------
```

```
          Cases |      86           68  |       154
       Noncases |     428         2347  |      2775
      ----------------+-------------------------+----------
          Total |     514         2415  |      2929
                |                        |
           Risk | .1673152     .0281573  | .0525777
                |                        |
                |      Point estimate    | [95% Conf. Interval]
                |------------------------+----------------------
 Risk difference |          .1391578     |  .1062221    .1720936
      Risk ratio |         5.942149      |  4.386791    8.048968
   Attr. frac. ex. |        .8317107     |  .7720429    .8757605
   Attr. frac. pop |        .4644618     |
                +------------------------------------------------
                      chi2(1) =    164.75  Pr>chi2 = 0.0000
```

**The cs command computes CI. In this output we see the risk of HM
for the exposed (0.1673152) and unexposed (0.0281573) group, the
risk difference, and the RR (5.942149). The risk of going home with
a monitor is about 5.9-fold greater for infants exposed to
mechanical ventilation than those not exposed. (Once again, I call
your attention to the possibility of confounding of the
relationship, but do not explore it here.)**

Odds ratios and relative risk

Be careful that you not generally interpret an OR as if it were a RR. As already
mentioned, when $P \leq 0.1$, odds and P values are about equal; when $P \geq 0.1$,
they diverge so that when $P = 1$, odds $= \infty$. Thus, only when the outcome
occurs *very* infrequently will OR and RR be approximately equal. Recall

$$\hat{RR} = \frac{P(\text{outcome}|\text{exposure})}{P(\text{outcome}|\text{no exposure})} = \frac{a/(a+c)}{b/(b+d)} = \frac{a/(b+d)}{b/(a+c)} = \frac{ab+ad}{ba+bc}$$

In this context, to speak of very infrequently occurring outcomes means the
values for a and b are small enough that their product is almost zero. When
that is the case,

$$\frac{ab+ad}{ba+bc} \approx \frac{ad}{bc} \quad \text{and} \quad \hat{OR} = \frac{ad}{bc}.$$

For our analyses of the association between MV and HM, the OR was about
6.9 and the RR was about 5.9. Not the same, but the magnitudes of effect size
are similar. The risk of the outcome in the unexposed group is rather small,
0.028. Above a risk of about 0.1 in the unexposed group, OR and RR will
quickly diverge.

Although it is an intuitive measure to some people, the OR is a more robust
measure of effect, especially for analyses involving more than one exposure
variable. And as mentioned, the OR is the appropriate effect measure for

case-control studies. Therefore, though perhaps an unintuitive measure, the OR is the more commonly used measure of exposure effect on an outcome.

What about $r \times c$ tables?

Stata has commands for working with $r \times c$ tables where $r > 2$. See Stata help for `tab`, `tab2`, `tabi`. We explore techniques for more than two levels of exposure in Chapter 28. The most generalized method to analyze the exposure outcome relationship uses logistic regression, the subject of Chapter 34.

Stratifying the analysis of dichotomous outcomes: confounders and effect modifiers; the Mantel–Haenszel method

Overview

The purpose of stratifying is to identify and measure the effect of known confounders on an outcome of interest. When we think that an outcome is affected by yet another variable besides the exposure entered in a single 2 × 2 table, we can examine the primary exposure–outcome relationship by decomposing it on the basis of the different levels, or strata, of that third variable. Of course, the stratification variable must be categorical. In general, if we find that the association between exposure and outcome is not substantially different across the strata, then we may describe the association using one summary odds ratio. However, if we discover that the association differs across the strata, then the association between exposure and outcome is more accurately reported as a stratified analysis. We shall consider a more general way to control for confounding when we examine regression techniques.

Simpson's paradox

Simpson's paradox describes an intuitively unexpected change in either the magnitude or direction of the relationship between an exposure and an outcome, when subgroups are pooled. The change is due to the influence of a third factor. To illustrate, let's study the relationship between some exposure and the outcome of dying within the study interval. We create a 2 × 2 table for the entire group of study subjects; let's say 2000. We use the Stata `csi` command to produce the tables. I chose the numbers in each cell to make the necessary points.

```
. csi 150 75 850 925        All 2000 subjects

                 | Exposed   Unexposed |     Total
-----------------+---------------------+----------
         Cases   |    150          75  |       225
      Noncases   |    850         925  |      1775
-----------------+---------------------+----------
         Total   |   1000        1000  |      2000
```

```
               |                    |
          Risk |     .15      .075  |     .1125
               |                    |
               | Point estimate     | [95% Conf. Interval]
               |--------------------+---------------------
Risk difference |        .075       |  .0474993    .1025007
    Risk ratio |           2        |  1.53755     2.601541
Attr. frac. ex. |          .5        |  .3496148    .6156124
Attr. frac. pop |    .3333333       |
               +-------------------------------------------
                    chi2(1) =      28.17  Pr>chi2 = 0.0000
```

This table reports the exposure outcome relationship for all subjects pooled together. We think that gender affects the relationship, so we stratify the analysis, creating similar tables for males and females.

. csi 50 25 450 475   **This table presents the data for males.**

```
               | Exposed  Unexposed |    Total
---------------+--------------------+----------
       Cases   |    50        25    |     75
    Noncases   |   450       475    |    925
---------------+--------------------+----------
       Total   |   500       500    |    1000
               |                    |
        Risk   |    .1       .05    |    .075
               |                    |
               | Point estimate     | [95% Conf. Interval]
               |--------------------+---------------------
Risk difference |         .05       |  .0174977    .0825023
    Risk ratio |           2        |  1.257763    3.180248
Attr. frac. ex. |          .5        |  .2049379    .6855592
Attr. frac. pop |    .3333333       |
               +-------------------------------------------
                    chi2(1) =       9.01  Pr>chi2 = 0.0027
```

. csi 100 50 400 450   **This table presents the data for females.**

```
               | Exposed  Unexposed |    Total
---------------+--------------------+----------
       Cases   |   100        50    |    150
    Noncases   |   400       450    |    850
---------------+--------------------+----------
       Total   |   500       500    |    1000
               |                    |
        Risk   |    .2        .1    |    .15
               |                    |
               | Point estimate     | [95% Conf. Interval]
               |--------------------+---------------------
Risk difference |          .1       |  .0561739    .1438261
    Risk ratio |           2        |  1.458068    2.743356
Attr. frac. ex. |          .5        |  .3141611    .6354829
```

```
Attr. frac. pop |         .3333333        |
                +-------------------------------------------
                        chi2(1) =        19.61  Pr>chi2 = 0.0000
```

Whether we consider all subjects together or stratify by gender, the risk ratio (RR) remains 2. We may conclude that gender does not confound the relationship between the exposure and outcome variables.

Consider the next series of tables, based on different data.

```
. csi 45 30 455 470        All subjects; here the total is 1000

                 | Exposed   Unexposed |     Total
-----------------+---------------------+----------
         Cases |    45          30 |       75
      Noncases |   455         470 |      925
-----------------+---------------------+----------
         Total |   500         500 |     1000
               |                     |
          Risk |   .09         .06 |     .075
               |                     |
               | Point estimate    | [95% Conf. Interval]
               |---------------------+----------------------
Risk difference |         .03        | -.0025967     .0625967
     Risk ratio |         1.5        |  .961211      2.340797
 Attr. frac. ex. |       .3333333    | -.0403543     .5727951
 Attr. frac. pop |         .2        |
               +-------------------------------------------
                        chi2(1) =       3.24   Pr>chi2 = 0.0717
```

```
. csi 5 20 95 380 This table presents the data for males.

                 | Exposed   Unexposed |     Total
-----------------+---------------------+----------
         Cases |     5          20 |       25
      Noncases |    95         380 |      475
-----------------+---------------------+----------
         Total |   100         400 |      500
               |                     |
          Risk |   .05         .05 |      .05
               |                     |
               | Point estimate    | [95% Conf. Interval]
               |---------------------+----------------------
Risk difference |          0        | -.0477584     .0477584
     Risk ratio |          1        |  .3847474     2.599108
 Attr. frac. ex. |          0        | -1.599108     .6152526
 Attr. frac. pop |          0        |
               +-------------------------------------------
                        chi2(1) =       0.00   Pr>chi2 = 1.0000
```

```
. csi 40 10 360 90 This table presents the data for females.

                 | Exposed   Unexposed |     Total
-----------------+---------------------+----------
```

```
          Cases |      40        10 |      50
       Noncases |     360        90 |     450
-----------------+-------------------+----------
          Total |     400       100 |     500
                |                   |
           Risk |      .1        .1 |      .1
                |                   |
                | Point estimate    | [95% Conf. Interval]
                |-------------------+----------------------
Risk difference |              0    | -.0657392     .0657392
     Risk ratio |              1    |  .5182011    1.929753
  Attr. frac. ex.|             0    | -.9297528     .4817989
 Attr. frac. pop |             0    |
                +------------------------------------------
                    chi2(1) =     0.00   Pr>chi2 = 1.0000
```

The RR for the entire group is 1.5 but the RR for males is 1 (no effect) and the RR for females is 1 (no effect). These three tables illustrate Simpson's paradox. How can a strong exposure effect disappear when we stratify by gender? The effect disappears when gender is associated with the exposure variable and with the outcome. In the first table in this series, describing the pooled data, there appears to be a relationship between being exposed and getting the outcome, with a RR of 1.5; that is, those exposed have a 50% increased risk of becoming a case. That the relationship between exposure and outcome disappears with stratification by gender indicates that

- there is no real association between the exposure and the outcome; rather, the association is between gender and outcome.
- the distribution of males and females among exposed and unexposed groups is unequal.

Another way to think about Simpson's paradox is to make explicit the question to which each table is the answer.

- The first table, displaying the pooled data, is the answer to "Among the entire study group, what is the association between exposure and outcome?".
- The second table is the answer to "Among the males in the study group, what is the association between exposure and outcome?".
- The third table is the answer to "Among the females in the study group, what is the association between exposure and outcome?".

That is, each table answers the same basic question about the exposure–outcome association, but for a different group.

Effect modification

To affect an exposure–outcome relationship, a third factor need not be a confounder. If the exposure–outcome effect size is a function of the value of the third factor, then the third factor is an effect modifier. Note that a confounder distorts the association between exposure and outcome. Instead of distorting the association, an effect modifier *modifies* the size or direction of the effect produced by the exposure. The exposure–outcome association is real, the magnitude or direction of the effect is influenced by the value taken on by the third factor (i.e. the effect modifier). Another term for effect modification is interaction. For example,

```
. csi 100 60 900 940 All 2000 subjects
                    |   Exposed    Unexposed   |       Total
--------------------+------------------------+-----------
           Cases |       100            60   |         160
        Noncases |       900           940   |        1840
--------------------+------------------------+-----------
           Total |      1000          1000   |        2000
                    |                            |
            Risk |        .1           .06   |         .08
                    |                            |
                    |   Point estimate         |   [95% Conf. Interval]
                    |------------------------+--------------------
 Risk difference |               .04        |   .0162852    .0637148
      Risk ratio |          1.666667        |   1.225074    2.267437
  Attr. frac. ex. |                .4        |   .1837226    .5589735
 Attr. frac. pop |               .25        |
                    |------------------------------------------
                              chi2(1) =    10.87    Pr>chi2 = 0.0010


. csi 26 24 474 476 This table presents the data for males.

                    |   Exposed    Unexposed   |       Total
                    |------------------------+-----------
           Cases |        26            24   |          50
        Noncases |       474           476   |         950
--------------------+------------------------+-----------
           Total |       500           500   |        1000
                    |                            |
            Risk |      .052          .048   |         .05
                    |                            |
                    |   Point estimate         |   [95% Conf. Interval]
                    |------------------------+--------------------
 Risk difference |              .004        |  -.0230151    .0310151
      Risk ratio |          1.083333        |   .6308182    1.860459
  Attr. frac. ex. |         .0769231        |  -.5852429    .4624981
 Attr. frac. pop |               .04        |
                    |------------------------------------------
                              chi2(1) =     0.08    Pr>chi2 = 0.7717


. csi 75 35 425 465 This table presents the data for females.

                    |   Exposed    Unexposed   |       Total
--------------------+------------------------+-----------
           Cases |        75            35   |         110
        Noncases |       425           465   |         890
```

```
-----------------+---------------------+----------
          Total |      500        500 |    1000
                |                     |
           Risk |      .15        .07 |     .11
                |                     |
                |   Point estimate    |  [95% Conf. Interval]
                |---------------------+---------------------
Risk difference |              .08    |  .0415327    .1184673
     Risk ratio |          2.142857   |  1.463092    3.138448
 Attr. frac. ex.|          .5333333   |  .3165159    .6813711
 Attr. frac. pop|          .3636364   |
                |---------------------+---------------------
                      chi2(1) =    16.34  Pr>chi2 = 0.0001
```

The preceding three tables illustrate quantitative effect modification. The *magnitude* of the effect size is influenced by the value of the third factor, gender. The RR in the whole group is 1.67. Among males, the RR is 1.08; in this case, not significantly different from 1, but for the point of discussion, the direction of the risk is still increased with exposure, albeit only 8%. Among females, the RR is 2.14.

A qualitative interaction or effect modification produces a change in the direction of the effect according to the value of the effect modifier. For example,

```
. csi 75 75 925 925 All 2000 subjects

                |  Exposed   Unexposed |    Total
----------------+---------------------+----------
          Cases |       75          75 |     150
       Noncases |      925         925 |    1850
----------------+---------------------+----------
          Total |     1000        1000 |    2000
                |                     |
           Risk |     .075        .075 |    .075
                |                     |
                |   Point estimate    |  [95% Conf. Interval]
                |---------------------+---------------------
Risk difference |              0      |  -.0230868    .0230868
     Risk ratio |              1      |  .7350442    1.360462
 Attr. frac. ex.|              0      |  -.3604623    .2649558
 Attr. frac. pop|              0      |
                |---------------------+---------------------
                      chi2(1) =     0.00  Pr>chi2 = 1.0000
```

```
. csi 50 25 450 475 This table presents the data for males.

                |  Exposed   Unexposed |    Total
----------------+---------------------+----------
          Cases |       50          25 |      75
       Noncases |      450         475 |     925
----------------+---------------------+----------
```

```
         Total |       500          500   |       1000
               |                          |
          Risk |        .1          .05   |       .075
               |                          |
               |   Point estimate         |   [95% Conf. Interval]
               |-------------------------+-----------------------
Risk difference |                 .05     |    .0174977   .0825023
    Risk ratio |                   2     |    1.257763   3.180248
Attr. frac. ex. |                .5     |    .2049379   .6855592
Attr. frac. pop |           .3333333    |
               |-------------------------+-----------------------
                        chi2(1) =     9.01    Pr>chi2 = 0.0027
```

. csi 25 50 475 450 **This table presents the data for females.**

```
               | Exposed   Unexposed |    Total
---------------+---------------------+----------
        Cases |    25          50    |     75
     Noncases |   475         450    |    925
---------------+---------------------+----------
        Total |   500         500    |   1000
              |                      |
         Risk |   .05          .1    |    .075
              |                      |
              |   Point estimate     |   [95% Conf. Interval]
              |---------------------+-----------------------
Risk difference |             -.05     |   -.0825023   -.0174977
    Risk ratio |               .5     |    .3144408    .7950621
Prev. frac. ex. |             .5     |    .2049379    .6855592
Prev. frac. pop |            .25     |
              |---------------------+-----------------------
                       chi2(1) =     9.01    Pr>chi2 = 0.0027
```

The *direction* of the effect size is influenced by the value of the third factor, gender. RR in the whole group = 1. Among males, RR = 2. Among females, RR = 0.5. In other words, gender, the effect modifier, acts on the exposure–outcome relationship to produce a twofold increased outcome risk among males, but a 50% decreased outcome risk among females. Male gender interacts with exposure to make exposure a risk factor, while female gender interacts with exposure to make exposure a protective factor.

Mantel–Haenszel method

When we considered the results of the stratified analyses in the two previous sections we used no formal evaluative method to interpret the results. How much of a difference ought there to be between the strata to conclude we're dealing with a confounder or effect modifier? To answer this question, we may use the Mantel–Haenszel method. The Mantel–Haenszel method

- assesses homogeneity, that is, is the variation in the magnitude of the exposure–outcome association across the tables probably due to sampling variation?
  - **(a)** If the test of homogeneity yields a P value >0.05, typically we accept H_0: the ORs among the tables are the same. We have a reasonable basis to combine the stratified data and report a summary OR. If $P \leq 0.05$, typically we reject H_0. In that case, we cannot combine the data; we report the stratified analysis.
  - **(b)** The test for homogeneity involves computing weighted averages for the strata, to reflect those strata that contain greater numbers of observations. (For methodological details, see Refs. 109 and 113.)
  - **(c)** The test statistic has the χ^2 distribution.
- tests a second H_0: the summary OR $= 1$.

Kirkwood and Sterne caution that the Mantel–Haenszel method has low power to detect effect modification.[113] This point comes up in the following illustration.

```
. use "C:\wherever_you_stored_the_data\practice_dataset.dta", clear

. encode sex, gen(gender)   the sex variable is a string variable

. codebook gender
----------------------------------------------------------------------
----------------------------------------------------------------
gender
(unlabeled)
----------------------------------------------------------------------
----------------------------------------------------------------

                   type:  numeric (long)
                  label:  gender

                  range:  [1,3]                          units:  1
          unique values:  3                           missing .:  8/3050

             tabulation:  Freq.   Numeric  Label
                           1379         1  F
                              1         2  I
                           1662         3  M
                              8         .

. recode gender (3=0)
(gender: 1662 changes made)

. label drop gender

. label define gender 0 male 1 female 2 indeterminate

. codebook gender

----------------------------------------------------------------------
----------------------------------------------------------------
```

```
gender
(unlabeled)
-------------------------------------------------------------------
----------------------------------------------------

               type:  numeric (long)
               label:  gender

               range:  [0,2]                          units:  1
       unique values:  3                            missing .:  8/3050

          tabulation:  Freq.   Numeric  Label
                       1662          0  male
                       1379          1  female
                          1          2  indeterminate
                          8          .

. codebook disposition

-------------------------------------------------------------------
----------------------------------------------------
disposition
(unlabeled)
-------------------------------------------------------------------
----------------------------------------------------

               type:  numeric (byte)

               range:  [1,5]                          units:  1
       unique values:  4                            missing .:  18/3050

          tabulation:  Freq.   Value
                       2464    1
                        402    2
                        165    3
                          1    5
                         18    .
```

Infants who died were coded as "3."   Create a new variable called survived.

```
. gen survived = 1 if disposition~=3
(165 missing values generated)

. replace survived = 0 if disposition ==3
(165 real changes made)

. replace survived = . if disposition>5
(18 real changes made, 18 to missing)

. codebook survived

-------------------------------------------------------------------
----------------------------------------------------
```

```
survived
(unlabeled)
------------------------------------------------------------------
--------------------------------------------------
```

```
                    type:  numeric (float)

                   range:  [0,1]                     units:  1
           unique values:  2               missing .:  18/3050

              tabulation:  Freq.  Value
                            165   0
                           2867   1
                             18   .
```

. label var survived "0 if died, 1 if lived"

. gen veryprem = 1 if gestage <=28
(2682 missing values generated)

. replace veryprem = 0 if gestage >28 & gestage <=44
(2671 real changes made)

. label var veryprem "0 if gestage >28 & <44, 1 if gestage <=28"

. codebook veryprem

```
------------------------------------------------------------------
--------------------------------------------------
veryprem
0 if gestage >28 & <44, 1 if gestage <=28
------------------------------------------------------------------
--------------------------------------------------
```

```
                    type:  numeric (float)

                   range:  [0,1]                     units:  1
           unique values:  2               missing .:  11/3050

              tabulation:  Freq.  Value
                           2671   0
                            368   1
                             11   .
```

Remember to save the new dataset.

**Let's examine the association between exposure to mechanical
ventilation (MV) and survival (survived: 0 = died, 1 = lived) among
very premature infants (veryprem: 0 if gestage >28 & <44, 1 if
gestage $\leq$ 28), stratified by gender. Stata uses the Mantel-Haenszel
method for a stratified cc analysis.**

. cc survived MV if veryprem==1, by(gender)

```
  gender |       OR     [95% Conf. Interval]   M-H Weight
---------+------------------------------------------------
    male |   1.128205   .3994124   2.905571    4.482759 (exact)
  female |   2.459627   .9311001   6.212438    2.96319 (exact)
---------+------------------------------------------------
   Crude |   1.643082   .8389843   3.124654             (exact)
M-H combined | 1.658058 .9011271   3.050798
------------------------------------------------------------
Test of homogeneity (M-H)      chi2(1) =    1.53   Pr>chi2 = 0.2156

                    Test that combined OR = 1:
                          Mantel-Haenszel chi2(1) =      2.68
                                       Pr>chi2 =      0.1018
```

The *P* value for the test of homogeneity (in earlier versions of
Stata, the test was called the test for heterogeneity) is 0.2156,
so we do not reject H_0. But remember the caution about low power to
detect a difference if it exists. The point estimate of OR for
survival among females seems substantially higher than the OR for
males (2.46 vs. 1.13), but the CIs are wide. Gender may be an
effect modifier, but we may not have enough observations to detect
the effect at α = 0.05. Nor can we reject the hypothesis that the
combined OR = 1. This is based on comparing observed and expected
counts in each cell in each stratum.

Note also that the crude OR and M-H combined ORs are essentially
identical. This suggests no confounding by gender.

CHAPTER 29

Ways to measure and compare the frequency of outcomes, and standardization to compare rates

In this chapter, we consider the two general ways to measure outcome frequency. In medicine and epidemiology, this often means disease frequency. Given that people experience some outcome – let us say some disease – how shall we count these occurrences? We may do so in different ways, thereby answering different questions.

Prevalence

Prevalence describes the number of individuals in a defined population who have the disease at the time of measurement. Prevalence is a proportion, defined for a particular point in time, and therefore, also referred to as point prevalence:

$$\text{Prevalence} = \frac{\#\text{cases}}{\#(\text{population})}$$

The proportion of individuals ill at some time estimates the probability that an individual in the defined population has the illness. Although you may sometimes see the term prevalence rate, prevalence does not include time in the denominator, so it isn't really a rate.

Incidence

New occurrences of a disease are measured in incidence terms. An incidence denominator includes only those individuals who could theoretically develop the disease, that is, those at risk. Existing cases therefore should not appear in the denominator. Nor, for example, were you measuring some pregnancy outcome would you count in the denominator women who had a hysterectomy. The point is, incidence aims to measure during some specified time period the new occurrences of the disease among those who *can actually get it*. Thus, the denominator also must include a specified time period. Incidence measures help illuminate disease etiology. In a study of etiology, using prevalent cases would introduce possible confounding by treatment.

One measure of incidence that may seem a bit confusing, because it's expressed as a proportion, is cumulative incidence:

$$\text{Cumulative incidence} = \frac{\text{\# new cases during the specified time interval}}{\text{\# in population at risk during the specified time interval}}$$

Cumulative incidence estimates the probability that an individual at risk will get the disease during the specified time interval. Note that this is a different probability estimate than that provided by point prevalence. The specified time interval is crucial. A cumulative incidence of 1 out of 100, or 1%, during a 1-*month* interval indicates a very different process from a cumulative incidence of 1% during a 1-*year* interval. Clearly, a cumulative incidence without an associated time interval is not meaningful.

Computing cumulative incidence rests on an important assumption that in the real world often is hard to satisfy. It assumes everyone was followed for the same amount of time, that is, the specified time interval. We used cumulative incidence, the `cs and csi` commands, in some of the Stata computation for Chapters 27 and 28, on the basis of an oversimplified set of assumptions about risk of exposure and outcome in our cohort. In fact, exposure times varied among the neonates. Sometimes, if the individual exposure times vary but they nonetheless all occur within a relatively short total observation interval, those exposure times may practically be rounded off to approximate that relatively short time interval. If we restricted the time interval of observation to some shorter period during which all individuals indeed provide exposure–outcome information, we'd better satisfy the computational assumptions at the price of eliminating data from which we otherwise might be able to learn.

To use all the data available and get a more precise estimate of the rate of disease occurrence, we compute incidence rate, also called incidence density (ID):

$$\text{ID} = \frac{\text{\# new (incident) cases during the specified time interval}}{\text{total person-time}}$$

Total person-time describes the sum of the time that each individual was observed. If patient A was observed for 10 days, patient B for 5 days, and patient C for 14 days, then total person-time = 29 patient days.

Let's compute the ID for the MV–HM relationship. We assume exposure time equals length of stay (LOS) in the hospital. We compute LOS as the difference between the values of the variables describing date of disposition, or discharge of some kind, and date of admission. To protect patient confidentiality, these variables are not provided in your data set. I include the following output nonetheless, because it illustrates new analytical methods you'll find helpful.

```
. codebook dateofdisposition
```

```
--------------------------------------------------------------------
--------------------------------------------------
dateofdisposition
(unlabeled)
--------------------------------------------------------------------
--------------------------------------------------

              type:   string (str8)

      unique values:   1359                    missing "":   22/3050

           examples:   "11/16/98"
                       "2/27/97"
                       "5/2/00"
                       "7/3/99"
```

```
. codebook admdate
```

```
--------------------------------------------------------------------
--------------------------------------------------
admdate
(unlabeled)
--------------------------------------------------------------------
--------------------------------------------------

              type:   string (str8)

      unique values:   1352                    missing "":   0/3050

           examples:   "11/22/98"
                       "2/6/98"
                       "5/25/97"
                       "7/31/98"
```

Stata won't compute differences on string variables. We must
convert these variables to numeric with date formatting. We also
must tell Stata whether to append the digits 19 or 20 in front of
two-digit years like 98 or 00. Searching Stata Help for dates
leads you to information about the Stata date function, illustrated
below.

```
. gen admitd = date(admdate, "mdy", 2002)
```

```
. gen dischd = date(dateofdisposition, "mdy", 2002)
(22 missing values generated)
```

To save space, unless there's a special point to make, I don't show
some of the data-checking output. In your work, you should
routinely scrutinize such output. From left to right, the items
specified for the date function are the name of the variable
containing the string data you want Stata to consider as dates; the
format - from the codebook output above - you see that the string

data was entered as month, day, year, so we specify "mdy"; 2002
is the cutpoint for whether year values get a 19 or a 20 prefix.
That is, 2-digit years are considered to represent the maximum year
that does not exceed YYYY. So if we specify YYYY = 2002, then
98 would mean 1998 but 00 would mean 2000. The split point would
be years 02 and 03; 02 would mean 2002 but 03 would mean 1903.

Next, we create the LOS variable.

```
. gen LOS = dischd - admitd
(22 missing values generated)

. sum LOS,det
```

```
                                    LOS
-----------------------------------------------------------------
          Percentiles        Smallest
   1%           0             -24397
   5%           1              -356
  10%           2              -354        Obs              3028
  25%           4              -353        Sum of Wgt.      3028

  50%          10                          Mean          21.24868
                             Largest       Std. Dev.     745.2959
  75%          23              312
  90%          49              319         Variance        555466
  95%          70             1107         Skewness      16.76623
  99%         108            32907         Kurtosis      1633.482
```

Evidently, some of the patients in the NICU have traveled back
in time. More likely, we still have dirty data. Let's look more
closely to see if values make sense within an observation.

```
. list LOS if LOS<0

          +--------+
          |   LOS  |
          |--------|
   339. |    -30  |
   366. |   -271  |
   510. |    -20  |
   518. |   -353  |
   894. |     -8  |
          |--------|
   979. |     -4  |
  1280. |    -39  |
  1641. |   -354  |
  1664. |    -81  |
  1671. | -24397  |
          |--------|
  1876. |   -356  |
  2619. |    -13  |
          +--------+
```

Observation no. 1671 has an interesting LOS: -24397 days. Looking at this individual's data in the browser window, the admission date is in 1999 and the disposition date is 3/10/33. In your actual work, you'd want to check the records and correct the obvious error. This infant's birth weight was 1995 g and discharge weight was 3595 g, so I suspect the actual disposition date was in the year 1999 or 2000. For simplicity here, I'll just exclude observations with LOS values below 0 or above 365. Of course, having created new variables, I should save the data set. Now, we're ready to start the analysis.

```
. ir HM MV LOS if LOS > 0 & LOS <=365
```

	required mechanical ventilation		
	Exposed	Unexposed	Total
Went home with a Monitor	86	67	153
LOS	22094	33190	55284

	Point estimate	[95% Conf. Interval]	
Incidence Rate	.0038925 .0020187	.0027675	
Inc. rate diff.	.0018738	.0009196 .0028279	
Inc. rate ratio	1.92822	1.384768 2.694769	(exact)
Attr. frac. ex.	.4813869	.2778573 .6289107	(exact)
Attr. frac. pop	.2705835		

```
              (midp)   Pr(k>=86) =                      0.0000  (exact)
              (midp) 2*Pr(k>=86) =                      0.0001  (exact)
```

My aim is simply to illustrate how to compute an incidence rate. As a study design, there are problems; to mention just one: LOS is undoubtedly confounded by MV along with other unmeasured exposures.

We have a total of 55284 days of patient observation. Among those infants exposed to MV the incidence of HM was about 4 per 1000 days in the NICU, while among those not exposed to MV the incidence of HM was about 2 per 1000 days in the NICU. The incidence rate ratio is 1.93. We don't go into the methods here (see Ch. 23 in Ref. 113), but the 2-tailed P value for the incidence rate ratio is 0.0001. That is, we have reason to reject H_0 (RR = 1).

Note also that this rate ratio is quite different from the risk ratio of 5.942149 we obtained when we computed CI for HM and MV using the cs command. This suggests that follow-up periods varied for the individual observations and therefore the cumulative incidence is not an accurate measure of outcome frequency.

Some specific measures of outcome frequency

Table 29.1 summarizes some common outcome measures. Clinicians often speak of a birth defect "rate," but technically, this is a prevalence measure, and therefore a proportion. The population at risk for birth defects is all products of conception, but information about congenital anomalies often is not available for aborted pregnancies and stillbirths.

Table 29.1 Common outcome measures

Measure	Category	What goes in the numerator	What goes in the denominator	Example
Morbidity rate	Incidence	New cases	Population at risk during a specified time interval	Retinopathy of prematurity rate
Mortality rate	Incidence	# Deaths	Population at risk during a specified time interval	Neonatal mortality rate
Birth defect "rate"	Prevalence	# Births with a congenital anomaly	# (Live) births	Structural congenital heart defect "rate"

Comparing rates: standardization

To make a fair rate comparison among two or more groups, it often is necessary to account for one or more confounders that may distort the relationship between exposure and outcome. We shall examine two processes of adjusting rates so they may be fairly compared: indirect and direct standardization.

Let's examine infant mortality rates in two states in the United States: New Hampshire and New York (data source: linked birth/infant death for 1997 through 1998, obtained at http://wonder.cdc.gov/lbdJ.html (accessed July 8, 2004); data descriptions at: http://wonder.cdc.gov/wonder/help/lbd.html (accessed July 8, 2004)). Table 29.2 shows the unadjusted data.

On the basis of the crude infant mortality rates (unadjusted for known confounders), it seems an infant born in New York is more likely to die in the first year than an infant born in New Hampshire. Race is a well-known

Table 29.2 Unadjusted infant mortality rates: New York and New Hampshire, 1997–1998

State	Births	Deaths	Rate/1000 births
New Hampshire	28,419	124	4.36
New York	515,394	3332	6.46

Table 29.3 The data of Table 29.2, stratified by race

	New Hampshire		New York	
Race	Births	% of all births	Births	% of all births
Black	238	0.8	109,677	21.3
White	28,073	98.8	370,864	71.9
Other	108	0.4	34,853	6.8
Total	28,419	100	515,394	100

confounder of this relationship, so we should explore the racial distribution in these two populations. Table 29.3 indicates a substantial difference in racial distribution between the states. Almost all births (98.8%) in New Hampshire were to white mothers compared to about 72% of births in New York. Is the difference in crude infant mortality rates due to location or due to maternal race? The association between maternal race and infant mortality may be confounded as well, but that is beyond our scope.

Table 29.4 Unadjusted infant mortality rates: United States, 1997–1998

Race	Births	Deaths	Rate/1000 births
Black	1,209,815	16,628	13.74
White	6,191,367	37,153	6.00
Other	421,265	2,512	5.96
Total	7,822,447	56,293	7.20

When comparing rates among groups, two methods are used to adjust for differences in the distribution of a confounding factor. The direct method of standardization applies the stratum-specific rates from study data to a standard population. The indirect method of standardization applies stratum-specific rates from a standard population to study data. Standardized mortality ratios (SMRs) are computed using indirect standardization (see Table 29.7).[113] With either method, the first step is to examine comparable data for the standard population. For the illustration in this section, we shall use the data for all births in the United States from 1997 to 1998 (Table 29.4).

In Table 29.4, the infant mortality rate that appears in the row describing the totals reflects a weighted average of the stratum-specific rates. Race seems to be associated with infant mortality. We saw in Table 29.3 that race also seemed to be associated with location, that is, state of residence. Therefore, race confounds the association between location and infant mortality. We therefore may question whether New York State's higher infant mortality rate (Table 29.2) simply reflects a higher proportion of black mothers giving birth in that state. Stratifying by race for each state reveals the data necessary

Table 29.5 Infant mortality rates: New York and New Hampshire, stratified by race

Race	New Hampshire			New York		
	Births	Deaths	Rate/1,000 Births	Births	Deaths	Rate/1,000 Births
Black	238	2	8.40	109,677	1291	11.77
White	28,073	120	4.27	370,864	1903	5.13
Other	108	2	18.52	34,853	138	3.96
Total	28,419	124	4.36	515,394	3332	6.46

to draw a conclusion, but it's still difficult to determine what the conclusion is just by visual inspection of Table 29.5.

Direct standardization

To directly standardize the data for each state, we compute the expected number of infant deaths in each race category. We assume that each state has the racial distribution of the United States as a whole and apply each state's stratum-specific infant mortality rate (Table 29.6). The direct-adjusted infant mortality rates of 5.68/1000 births for New Hampshire and 6.09/1000 births for New York are what we would expect in each of those states if they had the racial distribution seen in the United States overall, and if each state's race-specific mortality rate applied to the respective stratum. The direct-adjusted infant mortality rate is computed by dividing the total expected number of deaths by the total births in the standard population, the United States. New Hampshire's adjusted rate rises, while New York's falls a little.

Table 29.6 Direct standardized infant mortality rates

Race	United States (births)	New Hampshire			New York		
		Rate/ 1000 births	Expected # deaths	Direct adjusted infant mortality rate/1000 births	Rate/ 1000 births	Expected # deaths	Direct adjusted infant mortality rate/1000 births
Black	1,209,815	8.40	10,162.45		11.77	14,239.52	
White	6,191,367	4.27	26,437.14		5.13	31,761.71	
Other	421,265	18.52	7,801.83		3.96	1,668.21	
Total	7,822,447		44,401.42	5.68		47,669.44	6.09

Indirect standardization

To indirectly standardize the data for each state, we again compute the expected number of infant deaths in each race category. Now we assume that each state has the stratum-specific infant mortality rate of the United States

Table 29.7 Indirect standardized infant mortality rates

| | United States (rate/1000 births) | New Hampshire | | | New York | | |
		Births	Expected # deaths	Indirect-adjusted rate/1,000 births*	Births	Expected # deaths	Indirect-adjusted rate/1,000 births†
Race							
Black	13.74	238	3.27		109,677	1,506.96	
White	6.00	28,073	168.44		370,864	2,225.18	
Other	5.96	108	0.64		34,853	207.73	
Total	7.20	28,419	172.35	5.18	515,394	3,939.86	6.12

*SMR crude rate for US; SMR = O/E = 124/172.35 = 0.72.
†SMR crude rate for US; SMR = O/E = 3332/3939.86 = 0.85.

as a whole and apply those rates to each stratum of observed births (Table 29.7). By this method, New Hampshire's rate is a little lower than with that from direct standardization, while New York's stays about the same. Indirect adjustment may be preferable when stratum rate numerators are small, as is the case for the New Hampshire data (review the number of deaths among infants of black or other race in Table 29.3). In such a case, sampling variation can have a large effect on the stratum-specific rate, causing direct standardization to yield a less reliable estimate. Indirect standardization, by using the stratum-specific rate from the standard population, addresses this problem. With either method, however, bear in mind that the rates reflect a set of hypothetical circumstances aimed at controlling for a confounder.

Stata computes standardized rates

I used data totals to illustrate the main points of this chapter. When you have a complete set of individual observations for which you wish to compute and compare rates, Stata can help. The commands are `dstdize` and `istdize`, for direct and indirect standardization, respectively. You must specify the stratifying variable(s), of course. See Stata Help for details.

CHAPTER 30

Comparing the means of more than two samples

The problems embedded in multiple comparisons

We shall expand the analysis begun in Chapter 25, where we compared mean birth weight (BW) for infants born to mothers who did or did not receive antenatal care. Now, imagine we wish know whether BW differs according to five possible race/ethnicity values. How do we make the comparisons? Do we perform a series of two-sample t tests for each of the possible pairs of samples? For example, compare BW for whites and for blacks, for whites and for Asians, for whites and ...; for blacks and for Asians, for blacks and ..., etc. What if we wish to know whether BW differs by maternal race/ethnicity *and* by three age categories? Although lightning-fast statistical programs mitigate the job of performing the many repetitive calculations needed, there remains an important reason to look for a different way to make multiple comparisons.

If α is set at 0.05 and we do 20 such comparisons, then *by chance alone* one of those comparisons will show a significant difference. If extremely high or low values occur uncommonly, then the more tests we do, the more likely it is we will find such a value. If we compare the means of seven different groups, sampling variation leads to an almost 50% chance of finding a "significant" difference (α set at 0.05) even though the populations have the same mean.[122] Thus, we must account for this phenomenon when we make multiple comparisons.

To compare the mean outcomes from each stratum of an exposure variable with multiple categories we use a technique called analysis of variance (ANOVA). ANOVA may be used with an exposure variable having as few as two categories. ANOVA generalizes the approach we used to compare two sample means; when comparing two-sample means the two-sample t test yield the same results. ANOVA is a special case of multiple regression, which we explore in Chapter 33. This chapter provides a brief overview of the theory behind the method and introduces you to using Stata to execute the computations.

Analysis of variance

One-way ANOVA tests the null hypothesis that the population means of the groups being compared are *all* identical. Although several groups are compared, it is called one-way because the focus is on one variable. For example, we use one-way ANOVA to compare the mean BWs of infants among categories of gestational age. To compare group means by more than one classification scheme we use multiway ANOVA. For example, we use multiway ANOVA to compare the mean BWs of infants by gestational age category, by gender, and by maternal race. Our scope here is limited to one-way ANOVA. Either method assumes equal variances among the groups and that the outcomes do not severely depart from the normal distribution.[113,122]

As the name of the method indicates, ANOVA focuses on variance. In particular, the methods assess "within-groups" and "between-groups" variability. Within-groups variability estimates the extent that individual observations vary around their respective group's population means. Between-groups variability estimates the extent that population means vary around their so-called grand mean, computed by pooling all the sample observations across groups.

One-way ANOVA replaces multiple t tests with a single test that accounts for multiple comparisons. The test statistic for this single test is called the F statistic. The distribution of values for the F statistic differs from those we have considered so far, and also varies with the degrees of freedom in the comparison.

$$F \text{ statistic} = \frac{\text{between-groups variability}}{\text{within-groups variability}}$$

Illustrative analysis and interpretation of results follows shortly.

Which groups differ?

Sometimes we desire more information than a test of the null hypothesis in one-way ANOVA provides: the population means of the groups being compared are *all* identical. Multiple comparison techniques allow us to test the pairwise differences among group means. When the number of comparisons is relatively small, one suitable technique is that of Bonferroni. It fixes the frame of reference for statistical significance, α, on the complete set of comparisons instead of an individual pairwise comparison. A method more suited for comparing many different groups is that of Scheffé. Both these tests have relatively low power to detect a difference. On the other hand, Scheffé's method is tolerant of "data dredging" (comparisons not planned before the data were collected).

One-way ANOVA using Stata

We return to the data set we used in earlier chapters, and begin by exploring the data.

```
. sum BW,det

                              BW
-------------------------------------------------------------
          Percentiles       Smallest
   1%           515             400
```

```
   5%            755            400
  10%           1025            420         Obs                 3050
  25%           1610            425         Sum of Wgt.         3050

  50%           2330                        Mean            2408.937
                             Largest        Std. Dev.       1038.892
  75%           3250           5380
  90%         3803.5           5422         Variance         1079296
  95%           4090           5500         Skewness        .1510304
  99%           4593           5557         Kurtosis        2.211746
```

Mean and median are fairly close.

. histogram BW if gestcat ==1, bin(50) fraction normal
**gestcat is a derived variable: see GAcat in Chapter 20 for method,
and gestcat variable label or one-way tabular output below for
categories**
(bin=50, start=400, width=58)   **Output appears in Fig. 30.1.**

. list BW if BW >3000 & gestcat==1

```
        +------+
        |  BW  |
        |------|
  2735. | 3300 |
        +------+
```

. browse **gestage was entered as "4"; I suspect the correct value
was "40," for our purpose, we'll just drop this observation**

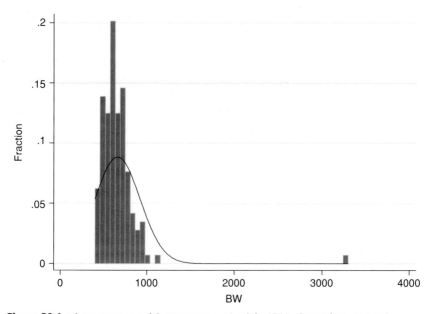

Figure 30.1 Histogram BW if gestcat ==1, bin(50) fraction normal.

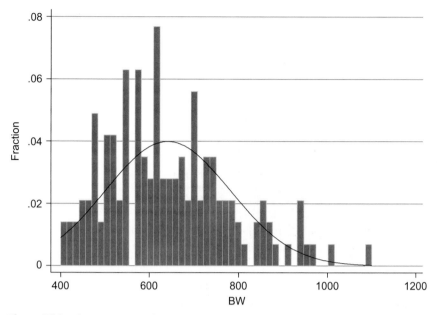

Figure 30.2 Histogram BW if gestcat ==1, bin(50) fraction normal **(obs.2735 dropped).**

```
. drop in 2735
(1 observation deleted)

. histogram BW if gestcat ==1, bin(50) fraction normal
(bin=50, start=400, width=14)         Output appears in Fig. 30.2.
```

The distribution is now closer to normal.

```
. histogram BW if gestcat ==2, bin(50) fraction normal
(bin=50, start=485, width=30)         Output appears in Fig. 30.3.

. list BW if BW >1500 & gestcat==2

        +------+
        |  BW  |
        |------|
 338.   | 1985 |
        +------+

. browse
```
Looking at the values across variables for this one record, it's hard to tell whether this is an erroneous value or an outlier. I'll keep it in the data set.

```
. histogram BW if gestcat ==3, bin(50) fraction normal
(bin=50, start=550, width=57)         Output appears in Fig. 30.4.
```

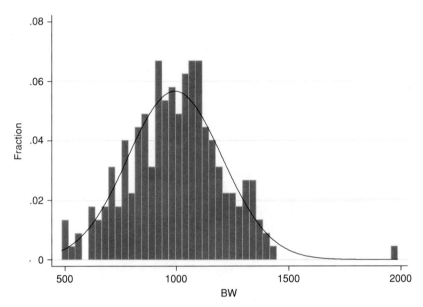

Figure 30.3 Histogram BW if gestcat ==2, bin(50) fraction normal.

. histogram BW if gestcat ==4, bin(50) fraction normal
(bin=50, start=990, width=74.5)   **Output appears in Fig. 30.5.**

. histogram BW if gestcat ==5, bin(50) fraction normal
(bin=50, start=635, width=98.44)   **Output appears in Fig. 30.6.**

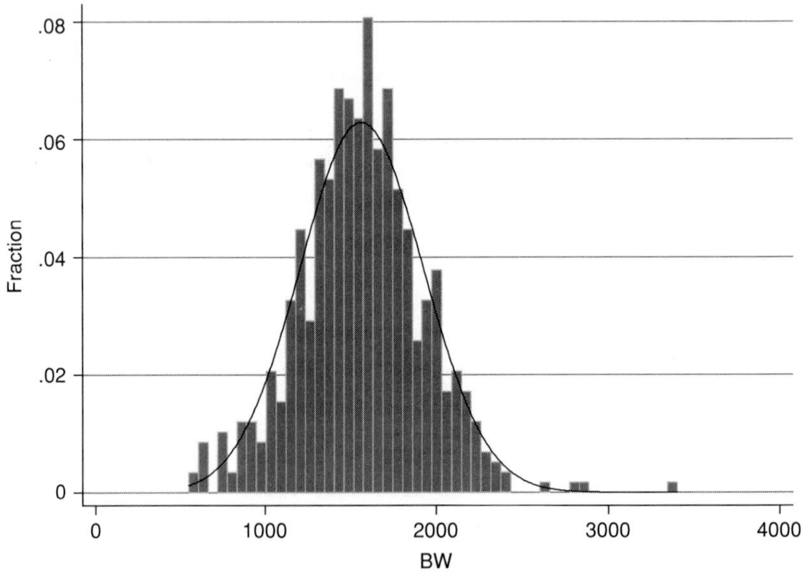

Figure 30.4 Histogram BW if gestcat ==3, bin(50) fraction normal.

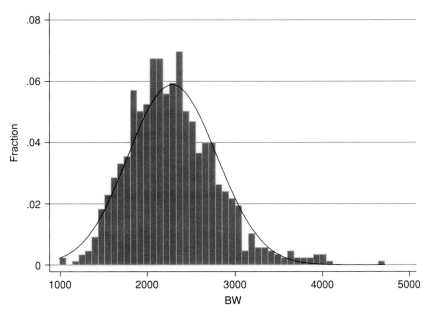

Figure 30.5 Histogram BW if gestcat ==4, bin(50) fraction normal.

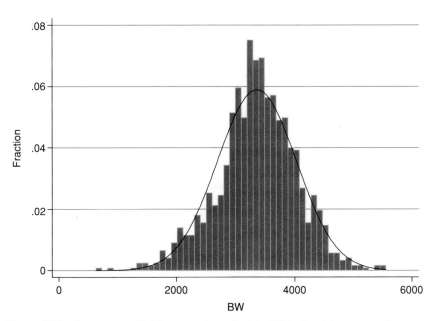

Figure 30.6 Histogram BW if gestcat ==5, bin(50) fraction normal.

Let's explore some of the values in the left tail of Fig. 30.6.

. list BW if BW <1500 & gestcat==5

```
        +------+
        |  BW  |
        |------|
 337.   | 1361 |
 785.   | 1385 |
 850.   |  910 |
1110.   | 1400 |
1675.   | 1446 |
        |------|
1860.   | 1270 |
2924.   |  635 |
        +------+
```

**The most extreme value, observation #2924, had a missing value
for gestage. By the rules by which gestcat was generated, missing
values were categorized as a 5. Here's one way to work around this
issue:**

. list BW if BW <1500 & gestcat==5 & gestage <=42

```
        +------+
        |  BW  |
        |------|
 337.   | 1361 |
 785.   | 1385 |
 850.   |  910 |
1110.   | 1400 |
1675.   | 1446 |
        |------|
1860.   | 1270 |
        +------+
```

We'll keep the other observations and consider them outliers.

. drop in 2924
(1 observation deleted)

**I must mention, as we start our ANOVA, that in general you should
not use ANOVA when you know in advance that the means among the
groups are different. For didactic purposes, we shall compare the
mean BW for the various values of gestcat as if we did not know
that they are different. The resulting Stata output clearly
illustrates this chapter's main ideas.**

. oneway BW gestcat,scheffe tabulate

```
1<=25wks      |
2>25&<=28wks  |
```

```
3>28 &<=32wks|
4>32 &<=36wks|
5>36wks      |              Summary of BW
             |       Mean     Std. Dev.        Freq.
-------------+-------------------------------------
           1 |    641.53846   139.91938          143
           2 |    993.70982   211.10387          224
           3 |    1564.3368   361.54353          582
           4 |    2288.282    504.80944          876
           5 |    3363.8692   662.71347         1223
-------------+-------------------------------------
       Total |    2409.2264   1038.6099         3048
```

```
                    Analysis of Variance
    Source            SS        df       MS           F     Prob > F
-------------------------------------------------------------------
Between groups    2.4385e+09     4     609625249   2186.75   0.0000
 Within groups    848330264    3043   278780.895
-------------------------------------------------------------------
     Total        3.2868e+09   3047   1078710.62
```

Bartlett's test for equal variances: chi2(4) = 748.3442 Prob>chi2 =
0.000

```
                       Comparison of BW
    by 1 <=25wks 2 >25 & <=28wks 3 >28 & <=32wks 4 >32 & <=36wks
       5  >36wks                                     (Scheffe)
```

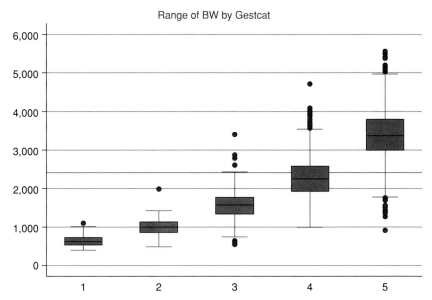

Figure 30.7 Graph box BW, over(gestcat) yline(2409.23) ylabel(#6)
title ("Range of BW by Gestcat").

```
Row Mean-|
Col Mean |           1             2             3             4
---------+-------------------------------------------------------
       2 |      352.171
         |        0.000
         |
       3 |      922.798       570.627
         |        0.000         0.000
         |
       4 |      1646.74       1294.57       723.945
         |        0.000         0.000         0.000
         |
       5 |      2722.33       2370.16       1799.53       1075.59
         |        0.000         0.000         0.000         0.000
```

**The *P* value for the *F* statistic of the test of the null hypothesis
that the group means are identical is <0.00005.   The Scheffé
pairwise comparisons all have P values <0.0005.   We use a box plot
to display the ANOVA results, as follows:**

```
. graph box BW, over(gestcat) yline(2409.23) ylabel(#6) title
("Range of BW by Gestcat")
```
Output appears in Fig. 30.7.

CHAPTER 31

Assuming little about the data: nonparametric methods of hypothesis testing

Sometimes data don't conform to analytical assumptions

Most of the analytical methods covered in this book are based on information about how the data are distributed. For example, when we compared sample means we assumed a normal distribution. Methods based on such information are called parametric methods. Recall from Chapter 23, the numerical values of the characteristics that describe a sample drawn from a population are called statistics; the numerical values of the same characteristics that describe the entire population are called parameters. To analyze a data set, good analytical practice proceeds, after data checking, by examining the distribution of the values of the variables. In past chapters, we've produced such frequency distribution histograms and explored whether transforming measurement units achieved a better approximation to the normal distribution.

Despite transformation, however, sometimes the data just don't conform to the assumptions of parametric analysis methods. Sometimes the difficulty hinges on a very small sample size. The central limit theorem tells us that the sampling distribution of means approximates the normal distribution even if the underlying distribution is not normal. But we also know that the degree to which the sampling distribution approximates a normal distribution is a function of sample size. Difficulty with assumptions of parametric methods also arises when dealing with ordinal variables. In general, when you can't make distributional assumptions about the data, use nonparametric methods to analyze them.

This chapter introduces you to nonparametric methods – methods that rely on fewer distributional assumptions than do parametric methods. Parametric methods use the actual values of the observations. The nonparametric methods we consider here are based not on values, but on the *ranks* of the individual values of a variable after sorting them in ascending order. Although we shall not consider analysis of paired data, you should know that appropriate nonparametric tests are available.

Wilcoxon rank sum test

The Wilcoxon rank sum test is the nonparametric counterpart of the two-sample *t* test. The assumption here is that each of the distributions has a similar shape. The method tests the following null hypothesis, H_0: the *medians* of the two populations are the same. Here is an overview of the method:

1 List the values from the two samples together, in ascending order.
2 Assign the rank "1" to the lowest value, incrementing by 1 as you proceed up the list. In the event of tie values, average the rank assignments and give that average rank to each tied observation value.
3 Arrange the rank designations to correspond to the original samples. Create two groups of rank assignments, where each group is made up only of the members of each of the original samples.
4 Compute the test statistic from the difference of the sums of the smaller group and the expected value of the sum of the ranks, if the ranks were evenly distributed among the groups, divided by the variance of the ranks for the smaller group. For details see Ref. 109.

The Stata command for the Wilcoxon rank sum test is `ranksum`. See Stata **Help** for details.

Spearman's rank correlation

Spearman's rank correlation is the nonparametric counterpart of the correlation coefficient, also known as Pearson's correlation coefficient. (I apologize for introducing the term correlation before the chapter devoted to it. I shall refer back to this when we later arrive at that topic. My aim is to discuss nonparametric methods as a group, in one chapter.) Here is an overview of the method:

1 Sort the values of each variable in ascending order.
2 For each variable, assign the rank "1" to the lowest value and increment by 1 as you proceed up the list.
3 Compute Pearson's correlation coefficient (interestingly, this entails a parametric method) for the ranks instead of the actual observation values.[113]

We shall use Stata to compute Spearman's rank correlation in Chapter 32.

Kruskal–Wallis test

A nonparametric way to perform a one-way ANOVA is the Kruskal–Wallis test. Here's a nonparametric way to make the same comparison we examined in Chapter 30.

```
. kwallis BW, by(gestcat)

Test: Equality of populations (Kruskal-Wallis test)
```

```
+---------------------------+
| gestcat |  Obs  | Rank Sum |
|---------+------+-----------|
|       1 |  143 |  13849.00 |
|       2 |  224 |  66078.00 |
|       3 |  582 | 436758.00 |
|       4 |  876 |  1.27e+06 |
|       5 | 1223 |  2.86e+06 |
+---------------------------+
```

```
chi-squared  =   2323.337 with 4 d.f.
probability  =      0.0001

chi-squared with ties =  2323.344 with 4 d.f.
probability  =      0.0001
```

If nonparametric methods make fewer assumptions, why not use them always

Nonparametric methods are less sensitive to errors in measurement because they rely on ranks and not the actual measurement values. These methods are also suited to working with ordinal data. Recall from Chapter 21, ordinal data represent categories for which order matters, for example, mild = 0, moderate = 1, and severe = 2. But the interval magnitude is undefined. Further, the categories could have been inversely coded, and the coding scheme does not necessarily imply any relative scale of gradation, that is, severe does not necessarily mean twice as bad as moderate and mild does not necessarily mean negligible just because it's coded by a zero. Because to consider a mean or standard deviation for data like this would make no sense, we can't use parametric methods to compare groups.

If nonparametric methods are broadly applicable and relatively insensitive to measurement error, why not use them always? When distributional assumptions are met, nonparametric methods have disadvantages that make them less attractive than parametric methods:

- By its very definition, the null hypothesis for a nonparametric test is anchored by less specific information than the null hypothesis for the parametric counterpart.
- Confidence intervals using nonparametric techniques often require a special method called bootstrapping (well beyond our scope).
- Perhaps most important, nonparametric techniques have less power than their parametric counterparts.

  If H_0 is false, a larger n is needed to reject it by nonparametric methods than by parametric methods. Applying the Wilcoxon rank sum test when the two-sample t test is apt gives only 95% of the power a t test would have to detect a significant difference.

CHAPTER 32

Correlation: measuring the relationship between two continuous variables

Pearson's correlation coefficient

Thus far, we have considered ways to measure the relationship between categorical exposure variables and either categorical or continuous outcome variables. Now we consider measuring the relationship between a continuous exposure variable and a continuous outcome variable. Examples of continuous exposure variables include pCO2 and serum triglyceride level. The method is called correlation analysis. It assumes a linear relationship between the exposure and outcome variables.

The mathematical function that estimates the magnitude of the linear correlation is Pearson's correlation coefficient, r. It reflects the product of the standard normal deviates for the two variables, X and Y, which are being assessed.

$$r = \frac{1}{(n-1)} \sum_{i=1}^{n} \left(\frac{x_i - \overline{x}}{s_x} \right) \left(\frac{y_i - \overline{y}}{s_y} \right)$$

where s_x and s_y are the respective sample standard deviations (p. 365 in Ref. 109). The correlation coefficient r is a number with no unit of measurement. Possible values span -1 to $+1$. $r < 0$ indicates a negative correlation: as the value of the independent variable increases, the value of the dependent variable decreases. $r > 0$ indicates a positive correlation: as the value of the independent variable increases, the value of the dependent variable also increases. The two extreme values indicate a perfect linear relationship between the variables (don't expect that for health care data). Figures 32.1a–32.1d summarize the range of relationships that r may describe. Note that $r = 0$ may, but need not, correspond to a shapeless and directionless cloud of plotted points. $r = 0$ simply means there is *no straight line* correlation. Figure 33.4 shows the scatter of observations where $r = 0.53$.

To comply with the methodological assumption of a linear relationship between the exposure and outcome variables, before computing a correlation coefficient we must examine a two-way scatter plot of the data. Let's look at two variables in our practice data set.

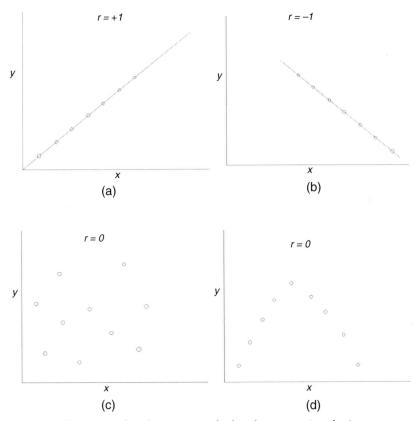

Figure 32.1 The relationships between *x* and *y* for *r* between −1 and +1.

. twoway scatter BW gestage   **The first listed variable is the**
dependent variable. Therefore, here I explore a hunch that
gestational age is associated with birth weight. Output appears
in Fig. 32.2.

The scatter plot suggests the data broadly satisfy the linearity
assumption. Let's measure the degree of correlation.

. correlate BW gestage
(obs=3038)

```
            |      BW   gestage
------------+------------------
         BW |  1.0000
    gestage |  0.8768   1.0000
```

The correlation coefficient is +0.8768. This indicates a strong
positive correlation - no surprise to clinicians working with
neonates.

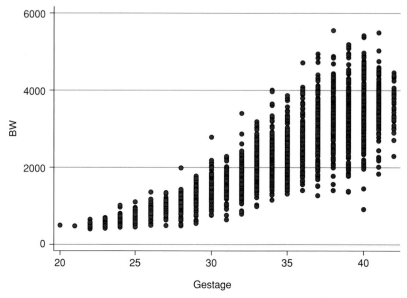

Figure 32.2 `twoway scatter BW gestage`.

We may determine if the magnitude of a correlation is statistically significant by computing the probability of obtaining a value for r as extreme or more extreme than what we observed, assuming the null hypothesis. The population correlation coefficient is denoted by ρ. The null hypothesis maintains that at the population level the variables are uncorrelated, $\rho = 0$. The test statistic to evaluate the null hypothesis is $\frac{r-0}{\text{SE}(r)}$. For randomly obtained observations from two variables with a normal distribution, this test statistic has a t distribution with $n - 2$ df.[109]

The Stata `correlate` command does not evaluate this test statistic for a test of H_0. To do that we use `pwcorr`, this computes pairwise correlations. In our example, we consider only one pair of variables. The `sig` option displays the significance level of each correlation coefficient and the `obs` option, the number of observations.

```
. pwcorr BW gestage, obs sig

             |       BW  gestage
-------------+------------------
         BW  |   1.0000
             |
             |     3048
             |
    gestage  |   0.8768   1.0000
             |   0.0000
             |     3038     3038
             |
```

This tabulation displays the Pearson correlation coefficient, the number of observations (3038), and the *P* value for the test of H_0 (<0.00005).

Nonparametric correlation analysis

Recall that we when we looked at BW distributions stratified by gestcat, we encountered some outlier values. Parametric methods are sensitive to outliers, so let's evaluate the correlation of BW and gestage using the nonparametric Spearman's rank correlation coefficient, introduced in Chapter 31.

```
. spearman BW gestage

 Number of obs =      3038
Spearman's rho =       0.8883

Test of Ho: BW and gestage are independent
    Prob >  |t| =      0.0000
```

Pretty similar results compared to the parametric method.

Two important caveats

It's so easy to run a correlation analysis that you may be tempted to skip exploring the two-way scatter plots first. *Beware*: none of the correlation commands in Stata tells you about linearity of the data. If the relationship between the variables is not indeed linear (see Fig. 32.1d), then the correlation coefficient will be misleading. *Always* look at the two-way plot before computing the correlation coefficient.

It can also be very tempting to extrapolate a relationship displayed in a two-way scatter plot beyond the range bounded by the actual observations. The same goes for regression relationships (see the next chapter). However, the plotted points contain no information about points not plotted. We simply have no way to know what the relationship is between the variables at values we have not actually observed.

CHAPTER 33

Predicting continuous outcomes: univariate and multivariate linear regression

Overview of linear regression

Correlation analysis measures the *strength* of the linear association. Regression techniques explore how the value of an outcome variable may change in response to changes in one or more independent variables. In this context, the outcome, or dependent variable, may be called the response variable; the independent, or predictor variable(s) may be called the explanatory variable. Correlation analysis is a symmetrical computation method, and regression is asymmetrical. If we flip the position of the variables in the relationship we obtain a different result. In this chapter, we explore linear regression. These methods apply when the relationship is essentially linear: a straight line fit to the scatter plot of the variables reasonably summarizes the relationship.

Linear regression estimates, from the equation of the straight line that best describes the relationship between explanatory and response variables, the slope and y-axis intercept. From the equation of this straight line, we can plug in a given value of the explanatory variable(s) and estimate the value the response variable would take. However, usually the observed and predicted values are not exactly the same. We denote an observed value for the response variable by y, and the predicted value for the response variable by placing a "hat" above y to denote the response value based on the fitted straight line: $\hat{y}$. To measure the strength of the association the method also computes the estimated value of the linear correlation coefficient.

When only one explanatory variable is involved, the technique is called simple linear regression. When multiple explanatory variables are involved, the technique is called multiple regression.

Simple linear regression

Using the practice data set, we shall focus on infants with gestational age ≤ 38 weeks. We explore the relationship between birth weight (BW) as an explanatory variable and lowest measured systolic blood pressure (lowestsystolicbp) as the response variable. Linear regression assumes the variables are normally distributed, so we begin by checking their distributions.

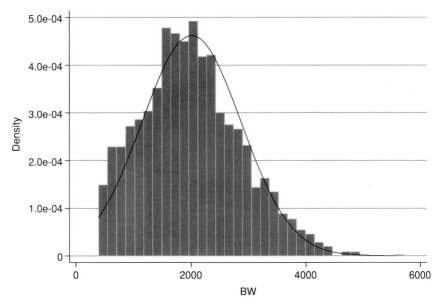

Figure 33.1 Histogram BW if gestage<=38, normal.

```
. histogram BW if gestage<=38, normal
(bin=33, start=400, width=156.27273) Output appears in Fig. 33.1.
```

This distribution is right-skewed a bit. Let's explore the effect of some transforms.
```
. gladder BW if gestage<=38          Output appears in Fig. 33.2.
```

Transforming BW to the square root (sqrt) of birth weight yields a closer approximation to normal. Let's create the transformed variable.

```
. gen BWsqrt = sqrt(BW)
```

Now we examine the original and new variables in more detail. We compare the number of observations as a check on the process that generated the new variable, and examine the mean and median values to evaluate the transform's mitigating the skew.

```
. sum BW if gestage<=38, det

                              BW
-------------------------------------------------------------
        Percentiles      Smallest
 1%          490            400
 5%          675            400
10%          890            420      Obs              2235
25%         1400            425      Sum of Wgt.      2235

50%         1950                     Mean          2013.857
                          Largest    Std. Dev.     863.6213
75%         2565           4845
```

```
90%          3200             4880      Variance      745841.7
95%          3555             4945      Skewness       .4306448
99%          4210             5557      Kurtosis      2.900643


. sum BWsqrt if gestage<=38, det

                                 BWsqrt
-------------------------------------------------------------
        Percentiles      Smallest
  1%      22.13594            20
  5%      25.98076            20
 10%      29.83287       20.4939      Obs                2235
 25%      37.41657      20.61553      Sum of Wgt.        2235

 50%      44.15881                    Mean           43.77288
                        Largest       Std. Dev.      9.891208
 75%      50.64583      69.60603
 90%      56.56854      69.85699      Variance         97.836
 95%      59.62382      70.32069      Skewness       -.1141802
 99%      64.88451      74.54529      Kurtosis        2.60368
```

Next, let's explore lowestsystolicbp.

```
. histogram lowestsystolicbp if gestage<=38, normal
(bin=32, start=0, width=3.4375)        Output appears in Fig. 33.3.
```

Pretty good. We won't quibble with the measurement values of "0." For an actual investigation we'd want to determine if those values might in fact denote "missing."

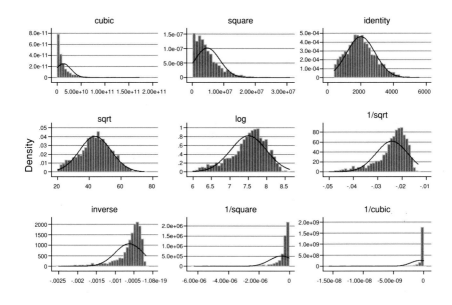

Histograms by transformation

BW

Figure 33.2 gladder BW if gestage<=38.

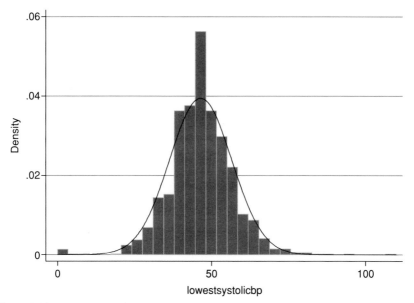

Figure 33.3 histogram lowestsystolicbp if gestage<=38, normal.

. sum lowestsystolicbp if gestage<=38,det

                        lowestsystolicbp

          Percentiles   Smallest
   1%   23   0
   5%   30   0
  10%   34   0   Obs   1699
  25%   41   0   Sum of Wgt.   1699

  50%   46   Mean   46.42319
                           Largest   Std. Dev.   10.10559
  75%   52   83
  90%   58   88   Variance   102.1229
  95%   63   96   Skewness   -.0813266
  99%   73   110   Kurtosis   6.353585

Now, the two-way scattergram:

. twoway scatter BWsqrt lowestsystolicbp if gestage<=38   **Output appears**
in Fig. 33.4.

There appears to be a linear trend toward higher lowestsystolicbp values as
BWsqrt increases.
Next, we evaluate the correlation:

pwcorr lowestsystolicbp BWsqrt,sig

              | lowest~p   BWsqrt
--------------+------------------

```
lowestsyst~p |   1.0000
             |
             |
      BWsqrt |   0.5349   1.0000
             |   0.0000
             |
```

Now, let's try a regression analysis:

```
. regress  lowestsystolicbp BWsqrt if gestage<=38

      Source |       SS       df       MS              Number of obs =    1699
-------------+------------------------------           F(  1,  1697) =  714.14
       Model |  51359.514      1   51359.514           Prob > F      =  0.0000
    Residual |  122045.212   1697  71.9182159          R-squared     =  0.2962
-------------+------------------------------           Adj R-squared =  0.2958
       Total |  173404.726   1698  102.122925          Root MSE      =  8.4805

------------------------------------------------------------------------------
lowestsyst~p |    Coef.   Std. Err.      t    P>|t|     [95% Conf. Interval]
-------------+----------------------------------------------------------------
      BWsqrt |  .6008278   .0224832    26.72   0.000     .55673    .6449256
       _cons |  21.14796   .9679294    21.85   0.000     19.2495   23.04642
------------------------------------------------------------------------------
```

**We shall focus on a few details of this simple linear regression output. There
are 1699 observations, corresponding to the number of observations in the
response variable (the explanatory variable contains 2235 observations). The
coefficient (Coef.) = .6008278 and the intercept (_cons) = 21.14796. The
coefficient and the intercept describe the fitted line for the observations:**
$\hat{y}$ **= 21.14796 + .6008278 x**
Next, we fit the best straight line.

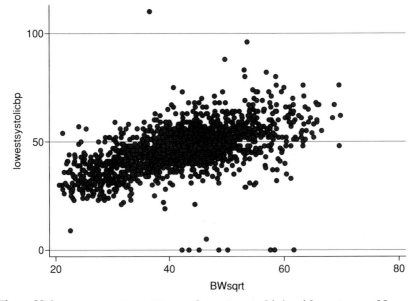

Figure 33.4 twoway scatter BWsqrt lowestsystolicbp if gestage<=38.

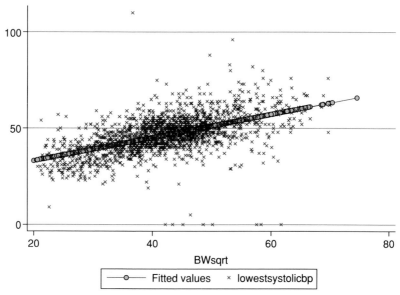

Figure 33.5 `twoway scatter psystbp lowestsystolicbp BWsqrt if gestage<=38, connect(l) msymbol(O x) mlcolor(gs5) mfcolor(gs14).`

```
. predict psystbp
(option xb assumed; fitted values)
```
This command is based on the antecedent regression computation. psystbp is the name I assigned to the variable describing predicted response values

```
. twoway scatter psystbp lowestsystolicbp BWsqrt if gestage<=38, connect(l)
msymbol(O x) mlcolor(gs5) mfcolor(gs14)          Output appears in Fig. 33.5.
```

Notice the options included with this scatterplot command. Check Stata regress and graph Help for details.

Slope describes the increase in the value of the response variable, *y*, for every unit increase in the value of the explanatory variable, *x*. Intercept is the point where the fitted straight line would cross the *x*-axis. The fitted straight line in Fig. 33.5 has a particular slope, 0.6008278, and a particular intercept at the *y*-axis, 21.14796. Although no infant would actually have a value for $\sqrt{BW} = 0$, sometimes we nonetheless must extrapolate the fitted line to obtain this theoretical value for *y* when *x* = 0. Recognize, however, that this process entails estimating the outcome value associated with predictor variable values not actually observed. Relationships that appear well explained over the range of observations may behave differently outside that range.

Centering an explanatory variable
One way to make meaningful an extrapolated value such as the *y*-axis intercept where $\sqrt{BW} = 0$ is to work with a "centered" explanatory variable.

A centered variable has mean $= 0$. (In Chapter 35, I explain how this idea facilitates interpreting a predictive model against a baseline hazard.) To generate this variable we subtract the mean value from each observation in the original variable. The y-intercept of the simple linear regression for this centered explanatory variable thus represents the mean value. As you know, other than for line-fitting or creating a centered variable, we ought not extrapolate a relationship beyond the range of observation values.[109]

The regression equation

We may describe the fitted regression line by an equation of the form: $\hat{y} = \beta_0 + \beta_1 x$. The β symbols denote the parameters of the regression line. β_0 describes the y-intercept and β_1 the slope. A positive β_1 indicates y increases as x increases; a negative β_1 indicates y decreases as x increases. Figure 33.5 illustrates natural variation among observed infants: most "×" markers on the plot do not lie along the fitted regression line. Therefore, in using a regression equation to describe our observations we include a term, ε, to account for the individual scatter of points. The model is thus more accurately described by

$$\hat{y} = \beta_0 + \beta_1 x + \varepsilon,$$

where ε is called the error term of the equation, and describes the positive or negative distance of any outcome y from the fitted line. The value of ε for each value of y is called the residual. Thus in Fig. 33.5, the fitted line illustrates the amount of information in the observations that the model can explain; the residuals indicate the information in the observations that the model could not explain.[123]

Assumptions underlying linear regression

Stata executes a regression command whether or not the data satisfy the assumptions underlying linear regression. Therefore, first verify that

1 for each value of x, the distribution of y values is normal.
2 the relationship between x and y can be summarized as a plotted straight line.[123]
3 all y are independent: the outcome for one individual in no way affects another.
4 for any value of x, the associated values for y have constant variance. This is called homoscedasticity. How to verify this is described shortly.

Regression methodology and Stata output

For any given set of observations, an infinite number of linear models could theoretically be generated. The method to determine the best fitting line is called least squares. We find the values for the parameters β_0 and β_1 such that the sum of the squared distances of each observed point from the fitted regression line is minimized, that is, we minimize the sum of the squares of the residuals. Note that the values of β_0 and β_1 *estimate* the population parameters and therefore β_0 and β_1 will vary with each sample. The standard errors and confidence intervals that appear in the Stata regression output describe the precision of the estimate.

For example, here is the lower half of the regression table from the Stata output presented between Figs. 33.4 and 33.5.

```
lowestsyst~p |    Coef.   Std. Err.      t     P>|t|     [95% Conf. Interval]
-------------+----------------------------------------------------------------
      BWsqrt |   .6008278   .0224832    26.72   0.000      .55673      .6449256
       _cons |   21.14796   .9679294    21.85   0.000     19.2495     23.04642
-------------------------------------------------------------------------------
```

The point estimate of β_1 is 0.6008278; the standard error is 0.0224832; the CI_{95} is (.55673, .6449256). Thus, each unit increase in BWsqrt (square root of BW) increases the value of lowestsystolicbp by 0.6 units, on average. The value of t and the P value relate to the test of H_0 that $\beta_1 = 0$ (df = sample size − # of regression coefficients). Statistical software packages uniformly report P values for the intercept even though this test of H_0 often is of no interest.[113] The Stata output shown here reports $P < 0.0005$ for the H_0 positing no association between $\sqrt{BW}$ and lowest measured systolic blood pressure in infants ≤ 38 weeks gestation. Therefore, we have grounds to reject H_0.

The upper half of the regression output reports an ANOVA table (introduced in Chapter 30 in the context of categorical data).

```
      Source |       SS       df       MS              Number of obs =    1699
-------------+------------------------------            F(  1,  1697) =  714.14
       Model |  51359.514       1   51359.514           Prob > F       =  0.0000
    Residual | 122045.212    1697   71.9182159          R-squared      =  0.2962
-------------+------------------------------            Adj R-squared =  0.2958
       Total | 173404.726    1698   102.122925          Root MSE       =  8.4805
```

The tabular entries denote "sum of squares" (SS), df, and "mean square" (MS) accounted for by the model and that left unexplained – residual. Summary statistics appear to the right of the ANOVA table. The F statistic for the ANOVA table tests that all coefficients except the intercept (_cons) have a value of 0. The probability of observing an F statistic that large or larger is listed as 0.0000: meaning in Stata, a number <0.00005. The R-squared value (R^2) is the coefficient of determination. R^2 measures how well the model, that is the fitted straight line, fits the data – the plotted observations. R^2 is the square of the Pearson correlation coefficient, r. It expresses the proportion of the variance in y that is explained by x. Therefore, $1 - R^2$ represents the unexplained variance. Our model explains about 30% of the variance. The adjusted R^2 is adjusted for the df. The Root MSE describes the square root of the mean square error of the residual, or unexplained part of the model – a measure of the variability around the regression line.

In thinking about how to increase the value of R^2, reflect on whether the model might require additional explanatory variables – a situation sometimes termed an underspecified model. Low model explanatory power also arises when the explanatory variable(s) measures something not as close to the true causal factor as you'd like. We explore these ideas further in Chapter 36.

Plotting residuals against fitted values; outliers

Another way to evaluate the fitted line and also the assumption of homoscedasticity is to plot the residuals against the predicted values. If the relationship between x and y is linear, then we expect to see a random scatter of these residuals rather than some trend or discernable pattern. The latter would imply that some systematic variation remains in the data, and a good model should account for nonrandom variation in the data. Further, for a well-fitting model, the cloud of dots should appear to have a slope of 0 and center around $y = 0$.[123] If the assumption of homoscedasticity is violated, then as $\hat{y}$ increases (the values on the horizontal axis of this plot) the range of values for the residuals plotted on the vertical axis may either increase or decrease so that the pattern of points is V-shaped. On this basis, Fig. 33.6 suggests that this assumption is satisfied. The Stata command, `rvfplot, yline(0)`, does all you may need; but it's not the only way to achieve this; see Stata **Help** on `regress` for details.

Plotting the residuals against the predicted values also calls attention to outlier values in the data set. For example, early in our illustrative regression analysis I noted that lowestsystolicbp contained several values $= 0$. We expect living infants have some value of systolic blood pressure >0. On the other end of the range, one infant had a value >100, also unusual. Some of the outliers appear in Fig. 33.6, as values that cluster around -50 and one value at about $+60$, on the residuals axis. The least squares method of fitting a

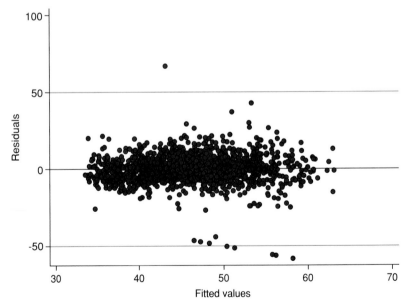

Figure 33.6 `rvfplot, yline(0).`

straight line is very sensitive to outlier values.[109] Discarding outlier values based on erroneous measurements can improve the explanatory power of the model, but don't be too hasty to drop these observations. Outliers may be real and may uniquely illuminate the relationship.

Multiple regression

Often, a response variable is affected by more than one explanatory variable. To study such multivariable linear relationships we expand the model for simple linear regression, $\hat{y} = \beta_0 + \beta_1 x + \varepsilon$, to

$$\hat{y} = \beta_0 + \beta_1 x_1 + \beta_2 x_2 + \cdots + \beta_i x_i + \varepsilon,$$

where subscripts 1 through i denote different independent explanatory variables. Multiple regression analysis generalizes simple linear regression and rests on similar assumptions. Multiple regression analysis allows us to estimate the independent effect of a particular explanatory variable on an outcome while accounting for the effects of other explanatory variables. This accounting is called adjusting for, or controlling for, the effects of the variables in the model. If we can add to the model explanatory variables that are also strongly associated with the response variable, we reduce the component of variation unexplained by the model. This decreases the SE of the other regression coefficients, which improves the estimate of the coefficients and thereby increases the power of the analysis to detect an effect for the model.[113] However, be aware that there is a maximum number of variables for any model and that is related to the number of observations. As a rule of thumb, you need about 10 observations per variable in the model.[115]

Let's expand the simple linear regression analysis started earlier.

The `hctonadm` **variable measures hematocrit of an infant on admission to the NICU. This was stored as a string and must be reformatted.**

```
. gen hct_adm = real( hctonadm)
(6 missing values generated)

. codebook hct_adm
```

```
--------------------------------------------------------------------------------
--------------------------------------------------------------------
hct_adm
(unlabeled)
--------------------------------------------------------------------------------
--------------------------------------------------------------------

                    type:  numeric (float)

                   range:  [0,94.2]                    units:  .001
           unique values:  400                       missing .:  6/3048

                    mean:  38.3635
                std. dev:   20.545
```

```
         percentiles:        10%       25%       50%       75%       90%
                              0        36.2      45.8      51.7      56.5
```

```
. sum hct_adm,det

                                 hct_adm
-------------------------------------------------------------
        Percentiles      Smallest
 1%          0                0
 5%          0                0
10%          0                0        Obs                  3042
25%         36.2              0        Sum of Wgt.          3042

50%         45.8                       Mean             38.36351
                           Largest     Std. Dev.        20.54503
75%         51.7            72.2
90%         56.5            75.4       Variance         422.0982
95%         59.9            81.3       Skewness        -1.056525
99%         66.7            94.2       Kurtosis         2.700627
```

**Mean and median don't coincide, and there are several 0 values, which I
suspect someone entered to represent "missing." I don't want to change the
original data set, so I won't drop any observations. I'll execute analytical
commands with conditions that exclude 0 and missing values. As an exercise,
think of how you would create a new variable that satisfies the same conditions.**

```
. sum hct_adm if hct_adm ~=0 & hct_adm <100,det

                                 hct_adm
-------------------------------------------------------------
        Percentiles      Smallest
 1%         18             7.131
 5%         34.7           7.249
10%         38.4           7.28        Obs                  2440
25%         43.1           7.28        Sum of Wgt.          2440

50%         48.1                       Mean             47.82861
                           Largest     Std. Dev.        8.567006
75%         52.9            72.2
90%         57.75           75.4       Variance         73.3936
95%         60.75           81.3       Skewness        -.6650217
99%         67.6            94.2       Kurtosis         6.210209
```

```
. histogram hct_adm if hct_adm ~=0 & hct_adm <100 & gestage<=38,normal
(bin=32, start=7.131, width=2.7209062)        Output appears in Fig. 33.7.
```

A good approximation to the normal distribution.

```
. pwcorr lowestsystolicbp hct_adm if gestage<=38 & hct_adm~=0 & hct_adm<100,sig

             | lowest~p  hct_adm
-------------+------------------
lowestsyst~p |  1.0000
             |
             |
    hct_adm  |  0.2671    1.0000
             |  0.0000
             |
```

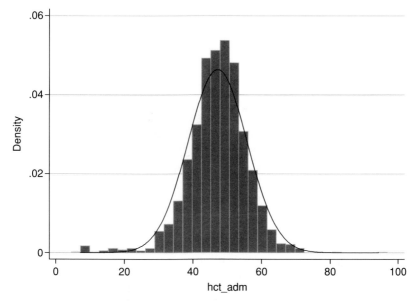

Figure 33.7 histogram hct_adm if hct_adm ~=0 & hct_adm <100 &
gestage<=38, normal.

Modest positive correlation, highly significant.

. twoway scatter lowestsystolicbp hct_adm if gestage<=38 & hct_adm~=0 &
hct_adm<100 **Output appears in Fig. 33.8.**
**Lots of outliers, but I can detect a positive correlation. Let's now explore
the multivariate linear regression analysis.**

. regress lowestsystolicbp BWsqrt hct_adm if gestage<=38 & hct_adm~=0 &
hct_adm<100

```
      Source |       SS       df       MS              Number of obs =    1593
-------------+------------------------------           F(  2,  1590) =  425.50
       Model |  51895.465      2  25947.7325           Prob > F      =  0.0000
    Residual |  96960.8376   1590  60.9816589           R-squared     =  0.3486
-------------+------------------------------           Adj R-squared =  0.3478
       Total |  148856.303   1592  93.5027026           Root MSE      =  7.8091
```

```
-------------------------------------------------------------------------------
lowestsyst~p |     Coef.   Std. Err.      t    P>|t|     [95% Conf. Interval]
-------------+-----------------------------------------------------------------
      BWsqrt |   .577594   .0222017    26.02   0.000     .5340465    .6211416
     hct_adm |  .1491521    .024255     6.15   0.000     .1015769    .1967272
       _cons |    15.293   1.282713    11.92   0.000     12.77702    17.80899
-------------------------------------------------------------------------------
```

**Compared with the simple regression that explained about 30% of the variation,
our model now explains 35%. Unlike R^2, which cannot decrease as additional
variables are added to the model, the adjusted R^2 can decrease when an
additional variable does not contribute to the model's predictive ability.[109]
Next, we examine the plot of residuals against fitted values.**

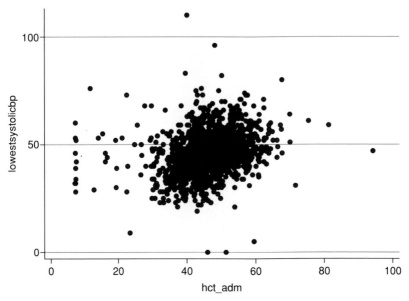

Figure 33.8 `twoway scatter lowestsystolicbp hct_adm if gestage<=38 &`
`hct_adm~=0 & hct_adm<100.`

```
. rvfplot, yline(0)   Output appears in Fig. 33.9.
```

Random scatter with no discernable pattern.

Explanatory variables need not be only continuous. Nominal variables work
fine. The following Stata output illustrates the model including five categories
of gestational age.

```
. regress  lowestsystolicbp BWsqrt hct_adm  gestcat if gestage<=38 & hct_adm~=0
& hct_adm<100
```

Source	SS	df	MS		
Model	56244.0602	3	18748.0201		
Residual	92612.2424	1589	58.2833495		
Total	148856.303	1592	93.5027026		

	Number of obs =	1593
	F(3, 1589) =	321.67
	Prob > F =	0.0000
	R-squared =	0.3778
	Adj R-squared =	0.3767
	Root MSE =	7.6344

lowestsyst~p	Coef.	Std. Err.	t	P>|t|	[95% Conf. Interval]
BWsqrt	.291171	.0396314	7.35	0.000	.2134357 .3689062
hct_adm	.1102264	.0241367	4.57	0.000	.0628832 .1575696
gestcat	3.065869	.354937	8.64	0.000	2.369674 3.762063
_cons	18.89692	1.321601	14.30	0.000	16.30466 21.48919

The model now explains about 38% of the variation in the response variable.

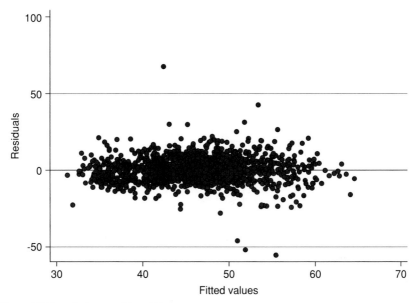

Figure 33.9 `rvfplot, yline(0)`.

Conditional probability

Have you noticed that the explanatory variable coefficients change as additional variables are added to the model? To understand this, consider that each regression model represents a conditional probability equation. The coefficients of each variable in a model are computed based on the other variables as a given condition. Some variables may share the same information, so as we add such variables to the model we remove some of the relative influence that the model first attributed to the variables originally specified. Thus, the coefficients and even their P values may change as their explanatory contribution is diluted by the added variable.

Interaction term

We next integrate the notion of effect modification (Chapter 28), or interaction. We must explore whether the exposure has the same effect across the various subgroups represented by other model covariates. For example, if the effect of the exposure on the outcome differs between males and females, then there is an interaction between gender and the exposure. To explore this possibility, we add an interaction term to the model. We generate a new variable that represents the product of the two variables we suspect may interact. In the following, we generate an interaction term for hct_adm (exposure) and gestcat (subgroups) and then add it to our model.

```
. gen hctgest=hct_adm*gestcat
(6 missing values generated)
```

```
. regress  lowestsystolicbp  BWsqrt hct_adm  gestcat   hctgest if gestage<=38 &
hct_adm~=0 & hct_adm<100
```

Source	SS	df	MS		
				Number of obs =	1593
Model	56850.6832	4	14212.6708	F(4, 1588) =	245.31
Residual	92005.6193	1588	57.9380474	Prob > F =	0.0000
				R-squared =	0.3819
				Adj R-squared =	0.3804
Total	148856.303	1592	93.5027026	Root MSE =	7.6117

lowestsyst~p	Coef.	Std. Err.	t	P>|t|	[95% Conf. Interval]	
BWsqrt	.293142	.0395185	7.42	0.000	.2156281	.3706558
hct_adm	.3323534	.0727433	4.57	0.000	.1896704	.4750364
gestcat	6.02461	.9804772	6.14	0.000	4.101445	7.947776
hctgest	-.0667317	.0206231	-3.24	0.001	-.1071831	-.0262803
_cons	9.142888	3.289854	2.78	0.006	2.689974	15.5958

```
The amount of variation explained by the model doesn't substantially improve,
but note the P value for the interaction term coefficient: 0.001. We may
reject the null hypothesis that hematocrit on admission has the same effect
on y regardless of gestational age category.
```

Indicator variables

Having identified this interaction, we should evaluate a model that accounts
for each gestational age category. The point is to determine the individual
relationships between lowestsystolicbp and each category of gestational age. To
facilitate doing this we use an indicator or a so-called dummy variable: another
derived variable. For each gestational age category, we create an indicator
variable that for every observation has the value of 0 or 1. This is why they're
called indicators or dummies: the numerical values for the variable don't have
any quantitative meaning. Indicators indicate the condition represented by
the variable that applies to a particular observation. Here's an easy way to
evaluate such a model using Stata.

```
. tab gestcat, gen(Igestcat)
```

1 <=25wks				
2 >25 & <=28wks				
3 >28 & <=32wks				
4 >32 & <=36wks				
5 >36wks		Freq.	Percent	Cum.
1		143	4.69	4.69
2		224	7.35	12.04
3		582	19.09	31.14
4		876	28.74	59.88
5		1,223	40.12	100.00
Total		3,048	100.00	

The command created five indicator variables, one corresponding to each value of gestcat. Stata automatically appended the digits 1 through 5 to the end of the variable name I supplied in the command line. To clarify how to use an indicator value to denote the appropriate categorization for a particular observation, Table 33.1 illustrates how to code Igestcat1 through Igestcat5 for an infant with gestational age 29 weeks. For such an infant, gestcat = 3.

Table 33.1 How to code the indicators for an infant with gestational age 29 weeks

Indicator variable	Value
Igestcat1	0
Igestcat2	0
Igestcat3	1
Igestcat4	0
Igestcat5	0

Now, we add these indicator variables to our regression model.

```
. regress  lowestsystolicbp BWsqrt hct_adm Igestcat1 Igestcat2 Igestcat3
Igestcat4 Igestcat5 if gestage<=38 & hct_adm~=0 & hct_adm<100

      Source |       SS       df       MS              Number of obs =    1593
-------------+------------------------------           F(  6,  1586) =  166.53
       Model |  57533.0799     6  9588.84665           Prob > F      =  0.0000
    Residual |  91323.2227  1586  57.5808466           R-squared     =  0.3865
-------------+------------------------------           Adj R-squared =  0.3842
       Total |  148856.303  1592  93.5027026           Root MSE      =  7.5882


------------------------------------------------------------------------------
lowestsyst~p |     Coef.   Std. Err.      t    P>|t|     [95% Conf. Interval]
-------------+----------------------------------------------------------------
      BWsqrt |   .2848064    .039587     7.19   0.000     .2071581    .3624547
     hct_adm |   .1076037   .0241094     4.46   0.000     .0603142    .1548933
   Igestcat1 |  -13.37068    1.52395    -8.77   0.000    -16.35985   -10.38151
   Igestcat2 |  -11.15825    1.24612    -8.95   0.000    -13.60246   -8.714034
   Igestcat3 |  -5.990593   .9307426    -6.44   0.000    -7.816209   -4.164978
   Igestcat4 |  -4.740939   .7540191    -6.29   0.000    -6.219918    -3.26196
   Igestcat5 |  (dropped)
       _cons |   35.50859   2.570644    13.81   0.000     30.46638    40.55081
------------------------------------------------------------------------------
```

The coefficients for Igestcat1, Igestcat2, Igestcat3, and Igestcat4 have P values that support rejecting H_0: the coefficient is equal to 0. Stata dropped Igestcat5 from the computation because when all the other categories take on a value of 0, Igestcat5 is assumed to take the value of 1 and therefore is built into the model without an explicit variable. Note that the interaction variable has now been removed from the model because it is redundant.

Modeling approach

We conclude with a brief overview of the process to determine which variables to try in a model and which to keep. If the P value for a coefficient supports H_0, it makes sense to work with a simpler model and drop that variable. When the data set includes many candidate explanatory variables, examining all possible combinations can be impractical. In these cases, one of two stepwise approaches may be used. Forward selection adds variables one at a time on the basis of a statistical criterion, such as the rank ordering of each variable's contribution to R^2. The process ends, for example, when adding more variables doesn't change R^2. Backward elimination begins with a saturated model (all variables) and determines the effect on R^2 of a dropped variable.

CHAPTER 34

Predicting dichotomous outcomes: logistic regression, and receiver operating characteristic

The aim of logistic regression

Logistic regression is a general approach to predict a dichotomous outcome such as lived/died, or disease/no disease. Logistic regression estimates the *probability* of the outcome occurring on the basis of one or more explanatory variables. The modeling method differs from that for linear regression because we apply the logit transform to the outcome variable. In this and the following chapter, we work with increasingly complex mathematical notation, but the emphasis remains on narrative explanation.

Suppose we wish to explore the outcome of death while in the NICU for infants $\leq$ 36-weeks gestation. In Chapter 28 we created the survived variable; survived $= 0$, if an infant died, and survived $= 1$, if an infant survived. We may estimate the probability that an infant dies while in the NICU as follows:

```
. tab survived if gestage<=36

   0 if died, |
   1 if lived |      Freq.       Percent         Cum.
  ------------+-----------------------------------------
           0 |        123          6.78          6.78
           1 |      1,692         93.22        100.00
  ------------+-----------------------------------------
       Total |      1,815        100.00
```

$123/1815 = 0.068 = 6.8\%$.

By restricting the analysis to gestational age $\leq$36 weeks, I tried to exclude deaths due to lethal congenital malformations in relatively mature infants. However, we know that risk of dying also relates to birth weight. How might we account for this effect? We could create a few sensible categories of BW and stratify the analysis.

```
. sum BW,det

                              BW
  -------------------------------------------------------------
         Percentiles       Smallest
  1%          515             400
```

```
  5%           755            400
 10%          1025            420        Obs                    3048
 25%          1610            425        Sum of Wgt.            3048

 50%          2330                       Mean               2409.226
                            Largest      Std. Dev.           1038.61
 75%        3247.5          5380
 90%          3805          5422         Variance           1078711
 95%          4090          5500         Skewness           .151844
 99%          4593          5557         Kurtosis          2.212458
```

```
. gen BWcat=1 if BW <750
(2900 missing values generated)

. replace BWcat=2 if BW>=750 & BW <1000
(136 real changes made)

. replace BWcat=3 if BW>=1000 & BW <1500
(358 real changes made)

. replace BWcat=4 if BW>=1500 & BW <2500
(1042 real changes made)

. replace BWcat=5 if BW>=2500
(1364 real changes made)

. tab BWcat

    BWcat |      Freq.     Percent        Cum.
----------+-----------------------------------
        1 |        148        4.86        4.86
        2 |        136        4.46        9.32
        3 |        358       11.75       21.06
        4 |      1,042       34.19       55.25
        5 |      1,364       44.75      100.00
----------+-----------------------------------
    Total |      3,048      100.00
```

```
. tab survived BWcat if gestage<=36

0 if died, |                       BWcat
1 if lived |     1       2       3       4       5 |     Total
-----------+-----------------------------------------+----------
         0 |    68      18      10      20       7 |       123
         1 |    76     116     342     903     255 |     1,692
-----------+-----------------------------------------+----------
     Total |   144     134     352     923     262 |     1,815
```

The probability of dying when BWcat = 1 is 68/144, or .47; when BWcat = 2 is 18/134, or .13; when BWcat = 3 is 10/352, or .028; when BWcat = 4 is

20/923, or .022; and when BWcat $= 5$ is 7/262, or .027. Risk is rather high in the two lowest weight categories and then levels off at much lower values.

We also know that less mature infants have an increased risk of dying. If we also want to account for gestational age as well as BWcat, the foregoing analytical approach becomes much more complicated.

Why not, then, account for explanatory variables by creating a model similar to what we used for multiple linear regression $\hat{y} = P = \beta_0 + \beta_1 x_1 + \beta_2 x_2 + \cdots + \beta_i x_i$? Such a model is unsatisfactory because the value of P must range between 0 and 1, and we have no way to assure that the terms on the right side of the equation will always add up to something between these limits. To assure the model operates within these limits, we make use of the logistic function: $f(z) = \frac{1}{1+e^{-z}}$, where z is called an index, representing all the coefficients and explanatory variables on the right side of the above regression equation, $z = \beta_0 + \beta_1 x_1 + \beta_2 x_2 + \cdots + \beta_i x_i$. Each variable x may be continuous, categorical, or may be an interaction term.

The logistic model

Here's how the logistic function works. For all values of z between $-\infty$ and $+\infty$, $f(z)$ will range between 0 and 1. How convenient – exactly the range we need for probability estimates! By means of the logistic function, the logistic model provides a conditional probability estimate: the probability of the outcome occurring. Let's call it D for disease, given a particular observation's profile of explanatory variables. Symbolically, $P(D = 1|x_1, x_2, \ldots, x_i)$. We may therefore represent the logistic model this way: $P(D = 1|x_1, x_2, \ldots, x_i) = \frac{1}{1+e^{-(\beta_0 + \sum \beta_i x_i)}}$. The equation may look different in some references, only because some terms may be algebraically rearranged. The left side of the equation, the conditional probability statement, is sometimes represented as $p(\mathbf{X})$, so $p(\mathbf{X}) = \frac{1}{1+e^{-(\beta_0 + \sum \beta_i x_i)}}$.

Applying the logit transform to $p(\mathbf{X})$, logit $p(\mathbf{X}) = \ln_e [\frac{p(\mathbf{X})}{1-p(\mathbf{X})}]$. Now, $[\frac{p(\mathbf{X})}{1-p(\mathbf{X})}]$ happens to represent the odds for an individual satisfying the particular conditional probability statement, $\mathbf{X}$, of developing the disease, D. Recall from Chapter 27, odds $= \frac{p}{1-p}$, when we compute P from a crude, unadjusted proportion. When we have specific knowledge of the values of particular risk factors, we express the same notion this way: $[\frac{p(\mathbf{X})}{1-p(\mathbf{X})}]$. Thus, to apply the logit transform is to take the natural logarithm of the odds for D to occur given an individual with the profile $\mathbf{X}$. After rearranging terms, we can represent the odds for an individual to satisfy the conditional probability statement, $\mathbf{X}$, of developing the disease, D, this way:[124] $[\frac{p(\mathbf{X})}{1-p(\mathbf{X})}] = e^{(\beta_0 + \sum \beta_i x_i)}$. Taking the natural logarithm of both sides of the equation, we get $\ln_e [\frac{p(\mathbf{X})}{1-p(\mathbf{X})}] = \beta_0 + \sum \beta_i x_i$. The right side of the equation now resembles the array of variables and coefficients used for multiple linear regression.

We don't use the least squares method to fit the best model, as we did for linear regression. Instead, we use the maximum-likelihood method. For the methodological details, see Refs. 113 and 124.

Using Stata for logistic regression analysis

Stata offers two commands: `logit` and `logistic`. Both do the same basic computations, but `logit` presents the estimates in terms of coefficients and `logistic` presents the estimates in terms of odds ratios for a one-unit change in the explanatory variable.

Very important: when running a logistic regression, Stata interprets a dichotomous outcome value of 0 as a "failure" and a 1, or missing, as a "success." Stata may decode 0 and 1 *oppositely* when performing survival analysis (see Chapter 35).

Let's explore the logit command.

```
. logit survived BW if gestage<=36

Iteration 0:   log likelihood = -449.80849
Iteration 1:   log likelihood = -378.65977
Iteration 2:   log likelihood = -359.08496
Iteration 3:   log likelihood = -357.31006
Iteration 4:   log likelihood = -357.27425
Iteration 5:   log likelihood = -357.27423
```

```
Logit estimates                           Number of obs   =        1815
                                          LR chi2(1)      =      185.07
                                          Prob > chi2     =      0.0000
Log likelihood = -357.27423               Pseudo R2       =      0.2057
```

survived	Coef.	Std. Err.	z	P>|z|	[95% Conf. Interval]
BW	.0023279	.0002079	11.20	0.000	.0019204 .0027355
_cons	-.5769464	.2455864	-2.35	0.019	-1.058287 -.0956059

The sequentially numbered iterations at the top of the output concern maximum likelihood estimation. The survived **variable is coded 0 = died ("failure) and 1 = survived ("success"). The model includes 1815 observations (the same number we obtained in earlier tabulations). The model is highly statistically significant and explains about 21% of the variance in the outcome. The BW coefficient =** .0023279; **heavier infants are more likely to have their value of survived = 1(the coefficient may be a small number, but it's a positive number). BW is a highly statistically significant predictor of** survived.

Following model creation, running the command predict **computes the predicted probability of** surviving.

```
. predict survhat
(option p assumed; Pr(survived))
```

```
. label var survhat "predicted probability of surviving"
```

Let's display the values of survhat **graphically:**

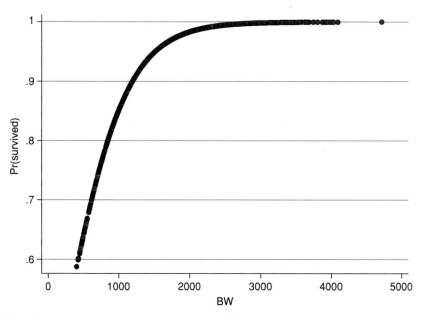

Figure 34.1 `twoway scatter survhat BW if gestage<=36`.

. `twoway scatter survhat BW if gestage<=36`   **Output appears in Fig. 34.1.**

Next, we create the same model using the logistic command.

. `logistic survived BW if gestage<=36`

```
Logistic regression                          Number of obs   =        1815
                                             LR chi2(1)      =      185.07
                                             Prob > chi2     =      0.0000
Log likelihood = -357.27423                  Pseudo R2       =      0.2057

-----------------------------------------------------------------------------
    survived | Odds Ratio   Std. Err.      z    P>|z|     [95% Conf. Interval]
-------------+---------------------------------------------------------------
          BW |   1.002331    .0002084    11.20   0.000     1.001922    1.002739
-----------------------------------------------------------------------------
```

The results are displayed in terms of odds ratio: increasing slightly for each unit increment in BW (gram increase in birth weight).

Now let's explore the effect of another possible explanatory variable. For brevity, I don't include here the univariate analyses that should precede your adding a variable to a model.

. `logit survived BW gestage if gestage<=36`

(maximum likelihood estimation output omitted for brevity)

```
Logit estimates                              Number of obs   =        1815
                                             LR chi2(2)      =      236.50
                                             Prob > chi2     =      0.0000
```

```
Log likelihood = -331.56018                    Pseudo R2       =      0.2629


------------------------------------------------------------------------------
   survived |      Coef.    Std. Err.      z     P>|z|     [95% Conf. Interval]
------------+-----------------------------------------------------------------
         BW |   -.000328    .0004057    -0.81    0.419     -.0011231    .0004672
    gestage |    .4501115   .0674913     6.67    0.000       .317831    .5823921
      _cons |   -10.10507   1.456753    -6.94    0.000     -12.96025   -7.249886
------------------------------------------------------------------------------
```

Adding gestage to the model increases the proportion of variance it explains
to about 26%. At first glance, in a model that also adjusts for gestational
age, heavier infants seem a little less likely to have their value of the
survived variable = 1 (coefficient has changed to a very small, but negative
number). However, the P value = 0.4, so we have little basis to reject the null
hypothesis that the BW coefficient = 0. When adjusted for BW and gestage,
only gestage predicts survived. Here's the logistic version:

```
. logistic survived BW gestage if gestage<=36

Logistic regression                            Number of obs   =       1815
                                               LR chi2(2)      =     236.50
                                               Prob > chi2     =     0.0000
Log likelihood = -331.56018                    Pseudo R2       =     0.2629


------------------------------------------------------------------------------
   survived | Odds Ratio   Std. Err.      z     P>|z|     [95% Conf. Interval]
------------+-----------------------------------------------------------------
         BW |   .9996721   .0004056    -0.81    0.419      .9988775    1.000467
    gestage |   1.568487   .1058593     6.67    0.000      1.374144    1.790316
------------------------------------------------------------------------------
```

The receiver operating characteristic curve

To assess a model's ability to discriminate individuals that do and do not experience the outcome, we may measure the area under the receiver operating
characteristic (ROC) curve.[125] The name of this curve derives from its original
purpose of discriminating signal from noise in radar signals. Recall the general formulation of a test statistic in terms of signal and noise, in Chapter 25.
To produce such a curve, we calculate the sensitivity and specificity of every
observation and plot sensitivity against 1 − specificity. Sensitivity measures
the proportion of true positives identified by the model and specificity, the
proportion of true negatives. To brush up on these concepts, see Refs. 125 and
126. A model that perfectly discriminates has an area of 1 under the curve. No
discriminatory ability yields an area of 0.5 under the curve. This makes sense
because an uninformative model performs no better than tossing a coin.

After creating a logistic model using Stata, run the `lroc` command:

```
. lroc          Output appears in Fig. 34.2.

Logistic model for survived

number of observations =      1815
area under ROC curve   =    0.8225
```

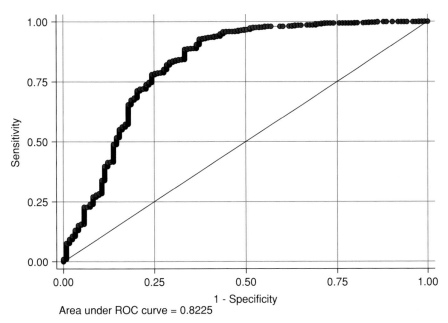

Figure 34.2 `lroc, to produce an ROC curve.`

To evaluate competing models, determine which yields the largest area under
the curve.

Now that we know BW is not a significant explanatory variable after adjusting
for gestational age, let's remove it from the model we just evaluated.

`. logistic survived gestage if gestage<=36`

```
Logistic regression                          Number of obs   =       1815
                                             LR chi2(1)      =     235.86
                                             Prob > chi2     =     0.0000
Log likelihood = -331.88026                  Pseudo R2       =     0.2622
```

```
------------------------------------------------------------------------------
    survived | Odds Ratio   Std. Err.      z    P>|z|     [95% Conf. Interval]
-------------+----------------------------------------------------------------
     gestage |   1.495096   .0451295    13.32   0.000     1.409209    1.586217
------------------------------------------------------------------------------
```

Of course, R^2 remains essentially the same. Next, let's evaluate the ROC curve
for this model.

`. lroc`   **Output appears in Fig. 34.3.**

```
Logistic model for survived

number of observations =      1815
area under ROC curve   =    0.8247
```

Not surprisingly, the model's discriminatory ability also remains essentially
the same.

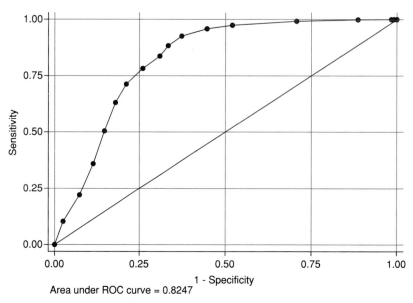

Area under ROC curve = 0.8247

Figure 34.3 `lroc`, with BW removed from the model.

Indicator variables in logistic regression

Some readers may have difficulty reconciling the analytical findings about BW
with their clinical experience. Indeed, sometimes the influence on outcome
of a continuous variable varies within its range. Let's reconsider the previous
model, now using the categorical BWcat, created in Chapter 20, instead of the
continuous BW. Indicator variables are very helpful in this regard. If we type
xi: in front of the logistic command and enter i.BWcat as an explanatory
variable, Stata creates and evaluates indicator variables for BWcat:

```
. xi: logistic survived i.BWcat gestage if gestage<=36
i.BWcat            _IBWcat_1-5       (naturally coded; _IBWcat_1 omitted)

Logistic regression                          Number of obs   =       1815
                                             LR chi2(5)      =     270.87
                                             Prob > chi2     =     0.0000
Log likelihood = -314.37123                  Pseudo R2       =     0.3011

-----------------------------------------------------------------------------
    survived |  Odds Ratio   Std. Err.      z    P>|z|     [95% Conf. Interval]
-------------+---------------------------------------------------------------
   _IBWcat_2 |   2.901105   .9790459     3.16   0.002     1.497289    5.621101
   _IBWcat_3 |   7.171224   3.319132     4.26   0.000     2.894828    17.76494
   _IBWcat_4 |   3.130834   1.872087     1.91   0.056     .9698013    10.10735
   _IBWcat_5 |   1.282729   1.03029      0.31   0.757     .2657345    6.191867
     gestage |   1.363681   .0902994     4.68   0.000     1.197701    1.552663
-----------------------------------------------------------------------------
```

**Interestingly, this model explains a greater proportion of the variation (30%)
than did the models with or without BW (26%). Notice that Stata dropped
IBWcat_1, using it as the reference. After adjusting for gestage, compared to**

an infant in IBWcat_1 the odds of surviving are 2.9 times greater for an infant
in IBWcat_2 and 7.2 times greater for an infant in IBWcat_3. The P values for
the other indicators (although coming close to significance for _IBWcat_4) do
not support rejecting the null hypothesis: OR = 1. Thus, some ranges of BW,
when adjusted for gestational age, seem to matter for survival; some don't.

Testing the linear trend

We may explicitly test the hypothesis that a linear trend exists among ordered
categories of an explanatory variable in a logistic model. When Stata runs the
model that includes the categorical variable BWcat, it treats this variable as a
continuous variable, and the test statistic addresses the linear component of
trend. The following Stata output should clarify the point.

```
. logistic survived BWcat gestage if gestage<=36

Logistic regression                         Number of obs    =       1815
                                            LR chi2(2)       =     243.37
                                            Prob > chi2      =     0.0000
Log likelihood = -328.12153                 Pseudo R2        =     0.2705

-------------------------------------------------------------------------------
    survived | Odds Ratio   Std. Err.      z    P>|z|     [95% Conf. Interval]
-------------+-----------------------------------------------------------------
       BWcat |   1.653084   .2993445     2.78   0.006     1.159197    2.357396
     gestage |   1.287825   .0775254     4.20   0.000       1.1445    1.449099
-------------------------------------------------------------------------------
```

With each step in value of BWcat from 1 to 5, an infant has 65% higher odds of
surviving, *assuming* a linear trend. The P value of 0.006 supports rejecting the
null hypothesis. *Beware*: we know from the preceding analysis (using indicator
variables) that the trend in fact is not completely linear. (It's also a good
idea to explore cross-tabulations (for example: tab survived BWcat) and
associated graphical displays.) The fact that this model explains 27% of the
variance compared to 30% for the previous model further emphasizes the need to
consider carefully our analytical interpretation.

Evaluating how well the logistic model fits the data

Recall that the linear regression model predicts some value of a continuous
outcome variable given one or more explanatory variables. To assess how well
the model fits the data, we examine the plot of residuals against predicted
values. This makes good sense because it amounts to comparing observed
with expected values.

Although logistic regression predicts some probability value that is continuous between 0 and 1, the value of the outcome variable for a given observation is not continuous; it's either 0 or 1. For example, although a model might
predict an 80% probability of survival for a particular profile of explanatory
variables, the outcome for an actual individual fitting that profile is not 80%
survived. Any actual individual either "succeeds" (survives; outcome = 1) or

"fails" (dies; outcome = 0). We therefore need a different approach to evaluating observed and expected values than what we use for linear regression.

The Hosmer–Lemeshow goodness-of-fit test groups the data according to predicted probabilities. The test compares observed (O) and expected (E) values among deciles of outcome values for the entire sample. To illustrate this test, create the following model: `xi: logistic survived i.BWcat gestage if gestage<=36`; then run the following Stata command:

```
. lfit, group(10) table

Logistic model for survived, goodness-of-fit test

  (Table collapsed on quantiles of estimated probabilities)
  +--------------------------------------------------------+
  | Group |   Prob | Obs_1 | Exp_1 | Obs_0 | Exp_0 | Total |
  |-------+--------+-------+-------+-------+-------+-------|
  |     1 | 0.8430 |   130 | 129.3 |    79 |  79.7 |   209 |
  |     2 | 0.9525 |   176 | 176.0 |    13 |  13.0 |   189 |
  |     3 | 0.9647 |   177 | 174.1 |     4 |   6.9 |   181 |
  |     4 | 0.9739 |   294 | 289.7 |     4 |   8.3 |   298 |
  |     5 | 0.9748 |    76 |  76.0 |     2 |   2.0 |    78 |
  |-------+--------+-------+-------+-------+-------+-------|
  |     6 | 0.9807 |   259 | 260.7 |     7 |   5.3 |   266 |
  |     7 | 0.9814 |   108 | 108.0 |     2 |   2.0 |   110 |
  |     8 | 0.9858 |   230 | 231.6 |     5 |   3.4 |   235 |
  |     9 | 0.9895 |   145 | 149.4 |     6 |   1.6 |   151 |
  |    10 | 0.9966 |    97 |  97.3 |     1 |   0.7 |    98 |
  +--------------------------------------------------------+

          number of observations =     1815
                number of groups =       10
       Hosmer-Lemeshow chi2(8) =      17.07
                    Prob > chi2 =     0.0294
```

Obs_1, Exp_1, Obs_0, and **Exp_0** columns describe the number of observed and expected values of 1 or 0. The Hosmer–Lemeshow null hypothesis maintains that O − E = 0. A model that fits the data well is consistent with the null hypothesis. The *P* value for our model is 0.0294, supporting our rejecting the null hypothesis and suggesting an unacceptable model fit.

Perhaps we have data in our data set that can help us better understand survival. Let's explore the Apgar score at 1 minute of life, coded as `apgar`.

```
. codebook apgar

-------------------------------------------------------------------------------
-------------------------------------------------------------------
apgar
(unlabeled)
-------------------------------------------------------------------------------
-------------------------------------------------------------------

                type:  numeric (byte)

               range:  [0,99]                   units:  1
       unique values:  12                    missing .:  20/3048

                mean:  6.98646
            std. dev:  8.08851
```

```
          percentiles:        10%      25%      50%      75%      90%
                                2        5        7        8        9

. sum apgar,det
```

```
                                    apgar
-----------------------------------------------------------------
      Percentiles        Smallest
  1%           1                 0
  5%           1                 0
 10%           2                 0      Obs                  3028
 25%           5                 0      Sum of Wgt.          3028

 50%           7                        Mean              6.98646
                          Largest       Std. Dev.         8.08851
 75%           8                99
 90%           9                99      Variance           65.424
 95%           9                99      Skewness         10.16569
 99%          10                99      Kurtosis         116.2561
```

**Some observations are coded as 99, but are unlabeled. We might guess that 99
means "missing." Let's include** apgar **as an explanatory variable, omitting
observations where** apgar = 99.

```
. xi: logistic survived i.BWcat gestage apgar if gestage<=36 & apgar ~=99
i.BWcat            _IBWcat_1-5          (naturally coded; _IBWcat_1 omitted)
Logistic regression                          Number of obs    =       1796
                                             LR chi2(6)       =     322.51
                                             Prob > chi2      =     0.0000
Log likelihood = -281.9747                   Pseudo R2        =     0.3638
-----------------------------------------------------------------------------
    survived | Odds Ratio  Std. Err.      z    P>|z|     [95% Conf. Interval]
-------------+---------------------------------------------------------------
   _IBWcat_2 |    3.11802   1.138851     3.11   0.002     1.52398    6.379383
   _IBWcat_3 |   6.887066   3.368261     3.95   0.000     2.640807    17.96105
   _IBWcat_4 |   3.457298   2.180212     1.97   0.049     1.004522    11.8991
   _IBWcat_5 |   1.678545   1.400152     0.62   0.535     .3272701    8.609138
     gestage |    1.21597    .084709     2.81   0.005     1.060779    1.393865
       apgar |   1.422465   .0688832     7.28   0.000     1.293665    1.564088
-----------------------------------------------------------------------------
```

The model now explains 36% of the variation, and apgar **is a highly significant
predictor of survival among these infants. Does this model fit the data better
than the last one?**

```
. lfit, group(10) table
```

Logistic model for survived, goodness-of-fit test

```
(Table collapsed on quantiles of estimated probabilities)
+--------------------------------------------------------+
| Group |   Prob | Obs_1 | Exp_1 | Obs_0 | Exp_0 | Total |
|-------+--------+-------+-------+-------+-------+-------|
|     1 | 0.8413 |    99 | 100.9 |    81 |  79.1 |   180 |
|     2 | 0.9377 |   169 | 165.4 |    14 |  17.6 |   183 |
|     3 | 0.9670 |   168 | 169.9 |    10 |   8.1 |   178 |
|     4 | 0.9787 |   178 | 176.3 |     3 |   4.7 |   181 |
|     5 | 0.9843 |   179 | 180.7 |     5 |   3.3 |   184 |
|-------+--------+-------+-------+-------+-------+-------|
|     6 | 0.9876 |   177 | 175.5 |     1 |   2.5 |   178 |
|     7 | 0.9898 |   180 | 181.0 |     3 |   2.0 |   183 |
```

```
|    8 | 0.9920 |    179 | 178.4 |    1 |    1.6 |    180 |
|    9 | 0.9936 |    170 | 168.8 |    0 |    1.2 |    170 |
|   10 | 0.9978 |    176 | 178.1 |    3 |    0.9 |    179 |
+-----------------------------------------------------------+

         number of observations =      1796
                number of groups =        10
        Hosmer-Lemeshow chi2(8) =      10.69
                  Prob > chi2 =       0.2196
```

P is now 0.2196, the fit is acceptable. As you might expect, the area under
the ROC curve is increased, too.

```
. lroc          Output appears in Fig. 34.4.
```

Logistic model for survived

```
number of observations =      1796
area under ROC curve   =    0.8859
```

Using Stata to compute sensitivity and specificity

Stata makes it simple to compute the underlying test characteristics of the ROC
curve: sensitivity and specificity, and their related measures. After running the
analysis presented immediately above:

```
. lstat
```

Logistic model for survived

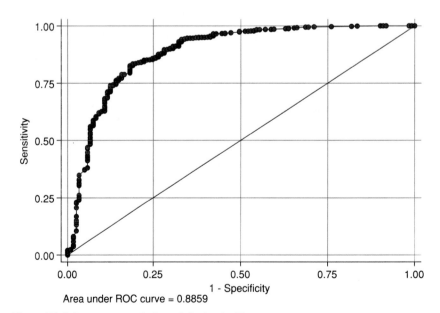

Area under ROC curve = 0.8859

Figure 34.4 lroc; expanded model including apgar.

```
                -------- True --------
Classified |        D              ~D |      Total
-----------+-------------------------+----------
     +     |      1650             71 |       1721
     -     |        25             50 |         75
-----------+-------------------------+----------
   Total   |      1675            121 |       1796

Classified + if predicted Pr(D) >= .5
True D defined as survived != 0
------------------------------------------------------
Sensitivity                      Pr( + | D)     98.51%
Specificity                      Pr( - | ~D)    41.32%
Positive predictive value        Pr( D | +)     95.87%
Negative predictive value        Pr(~D | -)     66.67%
------------------------------------------------------
False + rate for true ~D         Pr( + | ~D)    58.68%
False - rate for true D          Pr( - | D)      1.49%
False + rate for classified +    Pr(~D | +)      4.13%
False - rate for classified -    Pr( D | -)     33.33%
------------------------------------------------------
Correctly classified                            94.65%
------------------------------------------------------
```

This model has 98.5% sensitivity, but only 41% specificity, based on a cutpoint of 50% probability of surviving. You can vary the cutpoint using the option cutoff(), **placing an alternate decimal value than 0.5 within the parentheses. The next command displays what happens to sensitivity and specificity as the diagnostic cutpoint varies.**

. lsens   **Output appears in Fig. 34.5.**

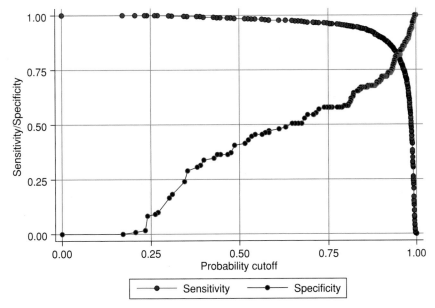

Figure 34.5 lsens.

Key points in evaluating a logistic model

- Check the overall χ^2 statistic and P value for the model. These are indicated in bold font (for emphasis) in the upper half of the logistic regression output given below. If the model does not support rejecting the null hypothesis, you need not go further down this list.

```
. xi: logistic survived i.BWcat gestage apgar if gestage<=36 & apgar~=99
i.BWcat           _IBWcat_1-5          (naturally coded; _IBWcat_1 omitted)


Logistic regression                          Number of obs   =       1796
                                             LR chi2(6)      =     322.51
                                             Prob > chi2     =     0.0000
Log likelihood =   -281.9747                 Pseudo R2       =     0.3638
```

- lfit: Does the model acceptably fit the data?
- lroc: How well does the model discriminate between the individuals who do and do not experience the outcome event?

CHAPTER 35
Predicting outcomes over time: survival analysis

Analyzing the time to an event

Some outcome variables are defined by the time between the start point of some process and the occurrence of an event. The event might be an infection or death. Whatever the event might be, what we measure and analyze is the *time to that event*. Doing so enables us to account for more information than we could with a model predicting a dichotomous outcome. The terminology for this analytical method is framed in terms of survival, so we call the time to the event survival time. With this perspective, we consider events "failures," even though some events may represent positive outcomes, for example, return to normal activity level. Survival analysis estimates the probability of an individual "surviving" – not having an event – for a specified interval of time and compares the "survival" – actually, event occurrence – patterns for individuals in different groups.

Time to event is a continuous variable but the outcome values usually are not normally distributed. Thus, it is inappropriate to use least square methods to fit the model, as we do for multiple regression analysis. Survival analysis encompasses a variety of other modeling techniques.

Survival data

The random variable describing survival time is denoted by T. The value of a particular observation within T is denoted by t. The random variable indicating whether the event of interest occurred during the period of observation is denoted by $\_d$ in Stata, and δ in many texts. If a failure, that is, event, occurred, $\_d$ or $\delta = 1$. If $\_d$ or $\delta = 0$, it means the event did not occur during the period of observation.

- *Analytical caution*
  - **(a)** In logistic regression, what you consider a failure may be coded either as a $\underline{0}$ or a $\underline{1}$. It depends on how you frame the outcome variable.

    The "survived" variable in Chapter 34 is coded as 0 = died and 1 = survived. If the variable was called "died" and you considered that outcome as a failure, you would code "failure" as a 1. But in the analytical framework of logistic regression analysis by Stata, a 1 is considered a "success." The point is logistic regression predicts the probability of an individual with a given covariate profile becoming a 1. So be mindful of how you have framed your outcome variable, particularly when you analyze the data using both logistic regression and survival analysis methods.

(b) In survival analysis, by default Stata codes failure as a $\underline{1}$, unless you establish another *explicit* coding scheme.

Censoring

If the event does not occur, we call that situation censoring. Censoring can mean we have data for

- the entire study interval, but the failure did not occur during that interval; we know that failure time, the time to event, exceeds the study interval.
- some of the study interval, but at some point during that interval we could not collect data for one or more individuals; some of these individuals are considered lost to follow-up; in other cases, information gaps exist for a variety of reasons.

See Refs. 20 and 21 for a discussion of the different ways for data to be unavailable.[127,128]

The key point for us is that survival analysis can use data from censored observations and data from failures (events). Also important is that the method assumes that censoring is *uninformative*: the probability of being censored is not related to the probability of failure.

Survivor and hazard functions

The distribution of survival times is called the survivor function, and is denoted by $S(t)$. This function gives the probability that an individual survives beyond time t. Another way to think about this function is that it gives the proportion of individuals who have not experienced failure at time t. Survivor functions start at maximum value when $t = 0$. Therefore, $S(0) = 1$ means at the instant the observation period begins, no individual has yet failed, so the probability that an individual survives beyond time $t = 0$ is 1. All survivor functions decrease in value over time, toward a theoretical value of 0. A survivor curve drawn from an observed data set looks like an irregular staircase seen end-on (Fig. 35.1); it goes to 0 only if there is no censoring.

The survivor function is framed in terms of *absence* of failure. If instead, we focus on the *occurrence* of failure, we have the hazard function, or hazard rate: *h(t)*. Other names for the hazard function further illuminate the concept: the conditional failure rate, the age-specific failure rate, and the force of mortality.[127] The hazard function gives the instantaneous rate of failure during some small time interval, given that the individual has survived up to the beginning of that interval. The cumulative hazard is the integral of the hazard function from $t = 0$ to some specific value of t.

The hazard rate gives a probability of failure per unit of time, so the value of the rate will depend on the chosen unit of time. For example, if the numerator, that is, probability, has a value of 0.25 and the denominator is in units of 1 day, then the hazard rate will be expressed as 0.25/day. However, if the numerator remains the same but the same time interval for the denominator is expressed in units of 1 week, then we have 0.25/(1/7 week) = 0.25/.14 = 1.75/week. And if the unit of time is 1 year, then the hazard rate is 0.25/(1/365 year) = 0.25/.0027 = 91.25/year. Knowing the hazard function for a data set helps you choose the optimal parametric survival analysis method (generally beyond our scope). $S(t)$ and $h(t)$ may be derived from each other; a point soon illustrated.

Setting up a survival data set in Stata

The data set we use to illustrate concepts in this chapter is set up differently from the other practice data set accompanying the book. To facilitate flexible analysis, a survival analysis data set includes variables describing when the observation period begins and ends, and a categorical outcome variable (failure/success). In practice_nosocomial.dta [again, I removed identifying variables to protect patient confidentiality], t0 gives start time and te, end time. The outcome variable is status. Sometimes, as with our data set, outcome can take on values other than 0 or 1. Success is still indicated by a 0, but some outcome events can occur more than one time. Our data set describes occurrences of nosocomial infections in infants [positive blood culture result beyond 3 days of life] in an NICU. Most infants who experience this complication experience it only one time but some have repeated events. Therefore, status = 1, 2, or 3 refers to the sequential infection number. We shall consider only the method to analyze a single event, so in what follows Stata considers any value of status other than 0 as a failure.

The stset command configures a data set for survival analysis. At a minimum, you must identify the variables that describe observation time and event occurrence. Stata automatically creates the observation time variable if you identify which variable records start time and which records end time. This permits greater analytical flexibility.

```
.stset te, failure(status) origin(t0)

failure event:  status != 0 & status < .  != 0 means not equal to 0
obs. time interval:  (origin, te]
 exit on or before:  failure
    t for analysis:  (time-origin)
           origin:  time t0

-----------------------------------------------------------------
       657  total obs.
         2  obs. end on or before enter()
-----------------------------------------------------------------
       655  obs. remaining, representing
```

```
    49  failures in single record/single failure data
 11558  total analysis time at risk, at risk from t =          0
                         earliest observed entry t =          0
                            last observed exit t =          162
```

**Stata performs a one-time structuring of the data, which applies
for all subsequent survival analytical procedures while the loaded
data set remains in your computer's RAM memory. Stata also checks
the data, as you see above. In addition, running** stset **creates some
new variables:**

- **_t0: Note the underscore, distinguishing it from the original t0
  variable. Stata considers analysis time to start at the value of
  _t0 for each record.**
- **_t: This describes the value for the time at which
  observation ended for each record. Thus,** t **for analysis:**
  (time-origin), **means t for analysis = (_t - _t0).**
- **_d: Stata's failure variable; 1 if failure, 0 if not.**
- **_st: Records the results of Stata's evaluating which records to
  include in the analysis. This variable has a value of 1 if the
  record can be used and 0 if not. Running the command** list if
  _st == 0 **reveals that the 2 observations not included had a value
  of 0 for observation time. Thus, Stata found a flaw in the way
  this data set was set up. If we want to include the dropped
  observations, we need to change the time unit so that t for
  analysis >0 (e.g. set values <1 to be 0.5).**

**If Stata found serious problems with the data set, the output would
have included the alert: PROBABLE ERROR. Stata tells us that it's
using 655 of the initial 657 observations. Among those records 49
failures occurred during the total exposure time of 11558 days.**

**Explore the data set to assure yourself that the values Stata
assigned to these variables make sense within particular records.
Then run**

```
. stdes
```

```
       failure _d:  status
  analysis time _t:  (te-origin)
           origin:  time t0
```

Category	total	mean	min	median	max
		|------------ per subject ------------|		
no. of subjects	655				
no. of records	655	1	1	1	1
(first) entry time		0	0	0	0
(final) exit time		17.6458	1	10	162
subjects with gap	0				
time on gap if gap	0				
time at risk	11558	17.6458	1	10	162
failures	49	.0748092	0	0	1

The category Subjects with gap **flags censoring issues that are**
beyond our scope. Nonetheless, we may ignore this because the
value = 0. In many ways, stdes **produces something similar to what**
you get when you type the summarize *varname,* detail **command for an**
ordinary variable. Note where the table indicates that the
median time for occurrence of a nosocomial infection is 10 days.

Kaplan–Meier nonparametric method

Let's sort our records in order of increasing observation time, _t, to examine
them in so-called life table format.

```
. sort _t
. sts list

          failure _d:  status
   analysis time _t:  (te-origin)
            origin:  time t0
```

Time	Beg. Total	Fail	Net Lost	Survivor Function	Std. Error	[95% Conf. Int.]	
1	655	0	50	1.0000	.	.	.
2	605	0	57	1.0000	.	.	.
3	548	2	49	0.9964	0.0026	0.9855	0.9991
4	497	1	37	0.9943	0.0033	0.9826	0.9982
5	459	3	22	0.9878	0.0049	0.9731	0.9945
6	434	3	29	0.9810	0.0063	0.9638	0.9901
7	402	2	31	0.9761	0.0071	0.9572	0.9868
8	369	2	12	0.9708	0.0080	0.9501	0.9830
9	355	1	22	0.9681	0.0085	0.9465	0.9811
10	332	4	16	0.9564	0.0102	0.9314	0.9725

(Remainder of output omitted to save space.)

The survivor function provided in the Stata output above is computed by
the Kaplan–Meier method; also known as product–limit method. This is a
nonparametric technique based on the observed survival times. The method
computes the value of the survivor function during each of a series of time
intervals.

Let us denote by the letter A the outcome that an individual remains in
the group that we are observing, up to and not including Time=3 in the above
tabular output. We denote by the letter B the outcome that an individual does
not develop a nosocomial infection, that is, the individual survives, at Time=3.
The probability of the outcome that the individual survives beyond Time=3,
that is, does not get a nosocomial infection until any time *after* that point
in time, is *P(A)* * *P(B | A)*; in words: the probability of remaining infection-
free through Time=2 multiplied by the probability of not becoming infected at
Time=3, given that the individual remained infection-free through Time=2.

Continuing with this formulation, we denote the value of the Survivor Function (fourth column from left) at Time=3 as $S(3)$. Therefore, $S(3) = S(2)$ * [the probability of not developing a nosocomial infection at Time=3]. To estimate the probability of "failing," that is, developing a nosocomial infection, during a given time interval, we compute the following proportion:

$$\frac{\text{\#individuals that fail during that interval}}{\text{\#individuals that could have failed during that interval}}$$

To compute the probability estimate of *not* developing a nosocomial infection during that interval, we subtract from 1 the estimated probability of failing during the interval (the time particular interval we consider is Time=2 to Time=3):

$$S(3) = 1.0000^* \, (1 - 2/548) = 1.000^* \, (1 - .00364964) = 0.9964.$$

This is exactly the result in the Survivor Function column on the line for Time=3. Incidentally, censored observations do not contribute to the probability estimate for the subsequent interval.

Generalizing our illustration yields the formula for the Kaplan–Meier or the product–limit estimate S(t): $\hat{S}(t) = \prod_{j|t_j \leq t} \left(\frac{n_j - d_j}{n_j} \right)$, where n_j denotes the number of at-risk individuals at time t_j (in the above Stata output, look down the column Beg.Total) and d_j denotes the number of failures at t_j (look down the column Fail). See Refs. 127 and 128 for more discussion.

The survival curve shown in Fig. 35.1 corresponds to the complete output of the sts list command. The vertical axis of the Kaplan–Meier (KM) plot shows the proportion surviving, the estimate of survival probability. The horizontal axis shows the value of the time variable. It is evident why the plot is also described as a step function. Vertical lines indicate each failure – infection, in our data set. Horizontal lines indicate time intervals with no failures.

```
. sts graph            Output appears in Fig. 35.1.

        failure _d:  status
  analysis time _t:  (te-origin)
         origin:  time t0

. stsum

        failure _d:  status
  analysis time _t:  (te-origin)
         origin:  time t0
```

| | time at risk | incidence rate | no. of subjects | |----- Survival time ----| |
				25%	50%	75%
total		11558	.0042395	655	61	.	.

This summary output tells us that there were 655 subjects followed for a total of 11558 days (we know this much from previous output).

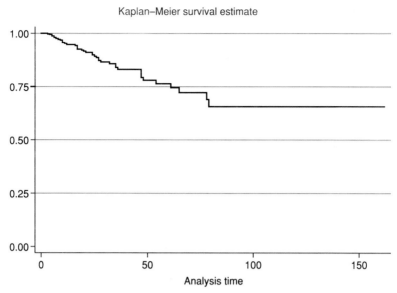

Kaplan–Meier survival estimate

Figure 35.1 sts graph.

**The median survival time can't be computed from this data because
not enough failures occurred during the observation interval for
50% of the group to remain (the first quartile is reported,
however). The incidence rate describes the daily incidence rate of
about 4.2 infections per 1000 patient days.**

We can calculate the confidence intervals for the KM plot. Figure 35.2 illustrates the commonly used method by Greenwood. At least 20–30 uncensored survival times are commonly recommended.

```
. sts graph, gwood                      Output appears in Fig. 35.2.

        failure _d:  status
  analysis time _t:  (te-origin)
           origin:  time t0
```

I mentioned that the hazard function can be derived directly from the survivor function. sts list with the option na produces the cumulative (Nelson–Aalen) hazard function for the same data set.

```
. sts list, na

        failure _d:  status
  analysis time _t:  (te-origin)
           origin:  time t0
```

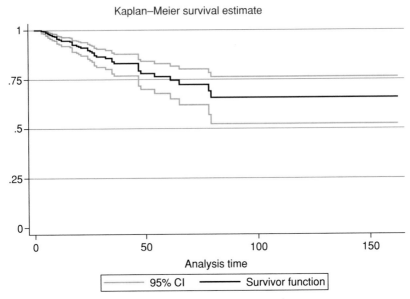

Figure 35.2 sts graph, gwood.

Time	Beg. Total	Fail	Net Lost	Nelson-Aalen Cum. Haz.	Std. Error	[95% Conf. Int.]	
1	655	0	50	0.0000	0.0000	.	.
2	605	0	57	0.0000	0.0000	.	.
3	548	2	49	0.0036	0.0026	0.0009	0.0146
4	497	1	37	0.0057	0.0033	0.0018	0.0176
5	459	3	22	0.0122	0.0050	0.0055	0.0272
6	434	3	29	0.0191	0.0064	0.0099	0.0368
7	402	2	31	0.0241	0.0073	0.0133	0.0436
8	369	2	12	0.0295	0.0082	0.0171	0.0510
9	355	1	22	0.0323	0.0087	0.0191	0.0548
10	332	4	16	0.0444	0.0106	0.0278	0.0708

(Remainder of output omitted to save space.)

Comparing survival outcomes: Kaplan–Meier method

Suppose we think that an infant with an umbilical arterial catheter in place for ≥ 3 days is at increased risk to develop a nosocomial infection. Here's how we could compare the outcomes of those who did and did not have this exposure.

```
. sum ua,det

                              ua
-----------------------------------------------------------------
        Percentiles       Smallest
 1%            0               0
 5%            0               0
10%            0               0       Obs                  649
```

```
25%              0               0      Sum of Wgt.        649

50%              0                      Mean           .7041602
                              Largest   Std. Dev.      2.034122
75%              0              12
90%              2              12      Variance       4.137652
95%              5              12      Skewness       3.834062
99%             10              17      Kurtosis       19.77098
```

. gen UAcat = 1 if ua <=3
(58 missing values generated)

. replace UAcat = 2 if ua >3
(58 real changes made)

. tab UAcat

```
    UAcat |      Freq.     Percent        Cum.
------------+-----------------------------------
        1 |        599       91.17       91.17
        2 |         58        8.83      100.00
------------+-----------------------------------
    Total |        657      100.00
```

Did you notice the discrepancy in numbers of observations: 649 vs. 657? Running codebook reveals 8 missing values for ua (output omitted). We shall drop those observations, drop UAcat, and then repeat the process of generating UAcat.

. drop if ua==.
(8 observations deleted)

. drop UAcat

. gen UAcat = 1 if ua <=3
(50 missing values generated)

. replace UAcat = 2 if ua >3
(50 real changes made)

. tab UAcat

```
    UAcat |      Freq.     Percent        Cum.
------------+-----------------------------------
        1 |        599       92.30       92.30
        2 |         50        7.70      100.00
------------+-----------------------------------
    Total |        649      100.00
```

. sts graph, by(UAcat)   **Output appears in Fig. 35.3.**

```
        failure _d:  status
   analysis time _t:  (te-origin)
           origin:  time t0
```

To compare the cumulative hazard functions simply add the option na.
. sts graph, by(UAcat) na   **Output appears in Fig. 35.4.**

```
        failure _d:  status
   analysis time _t:  (te-origin)
           origin:  time t0
```

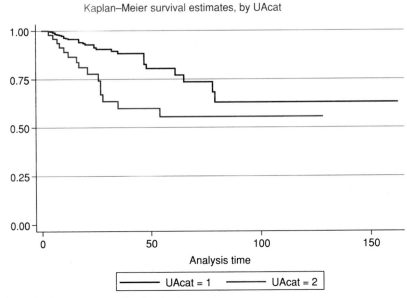

Figure 35.3 sts graph, by(UAcat).

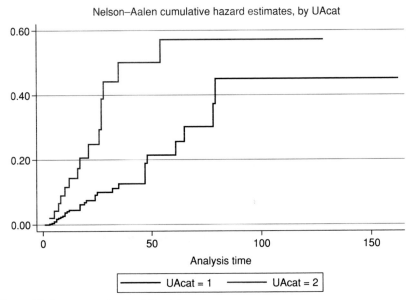

Figure 35.4 sts graph, by(UAcat) na.

```
. stsum, by(UAcat)
          failure _d:  status
    analysis time _t:  (te-origin)
             origin:   time t0
```

		incidence	no. of	|----- Survival time -----|		
UAcat	time at risk	rate	subjects	25%	50%	75%
1	9358	.0035264	598	65	.	.
2	1710	.0087719	49	26	.	.
total	11068	.0043368	647	61	.	.

The incidence rate of nosocomial infection among infants with umbilical arterial catheters in place for more than 3 days is more than twice that of those with umbilical arterial catheters in for ≤ 3 days.

Again, did you notice the discrepancy in numbers of observations: 647 vs. 649? One subject was dropped from each group. I suspect that these dropped subjects were the missing data necessary for analysis. Here are the commands and output confirming my hunch:

```
. list  _t if  UAcat==1 in -5/-1

       +-----+
       | _t  |
       |-----|
646.   | 141 |
647.   | 162 |
648.   |  .  |
       +-----+

. list  _t if  UAcat==2 in -5/-1

       +-----+
       | _t  |
       |-----|
645.   | 128 |
649.   |  .  |
       +-----+
```

Survivor functions and the incidence rates in the preceding analysis *appear* to be different. We can evaluate the observed and expected numbers of failures using the log-rank test. It evaluates the null hypothesis that the distributions – survivor functions – are the same:[109] $H_0 = S_1(t) = S_2(t)$.

```
. sts test UAcat

          failure _d:  status
    analysis time _t:  (te-origin)
             origin:   time t0

Log-rank test for equality of survivor functions
```

	Events	Events
UAcat	observed	expected

```
1      |       33              40.30
2      |       15               7.70
------+-------------------------
Total |       48              48.00

           chi2(1) =        8.57
           Pr>chi2 =      0.0034
```

The P value of 0.003 supports rejecting H_0. The test statistic reflects a comparison of observed and expected events at all times.

Running the following command yields incidence rates and tests the null hypothesis that those rates are the same.

```
. stir UAcat

         failure _d:  status
   analysis time _t:  (te-origin)
             origin:  time t0

note:  Exposed <-> UAcat==2 and Unexposed <-> UAcat==1

                     | UAcat                    |
                     | Exposed    Unexposed     |     Total
       --------------+--------------------------+----------
           Failure   |    15            33      |      48
              Time   |  1710          9358      |   11068
       --------------+--------------------------+----------
                     |                          |
    Incidence Rate   | .0087719     .0035264    |  .0043368
                     |                          |
                     |    Point estimate        | [95% Conf. Interval]
                     |--------------------------+---------------------
Inc. rate diff.  |         .0052455         | .0006462    .0098448
Inc. rate ratio  |        2.487507          | 1.255405    4.709165  (exact)
Attr. frac. ex.  |         .597991          | .2034441    .7876481  (exact)
Attr. frac. pop  |        .1868722          |
                 +----------------------------------------------------
                      (midp)    Pr(k>=15) =                 0.0031  (exact)
                      (midp)  2*Pr(k>=15) =                 0.0062  (exact)
```

The two-tailed P value of 0.006 supports rejecting the null hypothesis that the rates are the same.

Nonparametric survival analysis limits adjusting for covariates, but a little is possible. Suppose our data set included a variable for gender and we want to explore whether the survivor functions for each UAcat group differ by gender. This would be particularly important if we thought gender was unequally distributed among the UAcat groups. We could stratify the analysis to see the gender specific KM plots:

```
sts graph if gender==0, by(UAcat)
sts graph if gender==0, by(UAcat)
```

Next, to obtain a stratified log-rank test:

```
sts test UAcat, logrank strata(gender) detail
```

This command will produce a separate log-rank test for each stratum of gender (male;female) and for all strata combined.

Cox semiparametric method, and a brief mention of parametric methods

An infant's requiring an umbilical artery catheter and the outcome of a nosocomial infection each may be associated with gestational age. Stata offers an option for displaying a KM plot that adjusts for a covariate; to illustrate, let's adjust for gestational age. Note that we could alternatively stratify the analysis by gestational age category, but this approach collapses the values of the stratifying variable (we must convert a continuous to a categorical variable) and becomes increasingly complicated as the number of adjustment variables increases.

```
. sum ga

    Variable |        Obs        Mean    Std. Dev.        Min        Max
-------------+----------------------------------------------------------
          ga |        649    34.20031    4.822139         20         42

. gen cent_ga = ga-34.20031

. label var cent_ga "ga-mean (ga-34.20031)"
. sts graph, by(UAcat) adjustfor(cent_ga) Output appears in Fig. 35.5.

        failure _d:  status
   analysis time _t:  (te-origin)
            origin:  time t0
```

Compare Fig. 35.5 with Fig. 35.3: after adjusting for centered gestational age (I'll explain this notion soon) the survivor functions appear similar. Centered gestational age does not appear to matter. Although the results in Fig. 35.5 are displayed on a KM plot, the adjustment is based on a semiparametric technique called the Cox proportional hazards (PH) method. In a Cox model, continuous covariates may require special treatment, as we did in generating `cent_ga`, the centered gestational age variable, from `ga`. Covariate adjustment and predictive modeling for survival data requires more assumptions about the data than do nonparametric techniques.

The Cox proportional hazards method is a regression model to predict the hazard rate for the jth individual in a data set. Central to the Cox method is the *cumulative* hazard function: $H(t) = \int_0^t h(u)du$, where $h(u)$ describes the hazard function. Earlier, I mentioned that the hazard and survival functions may be

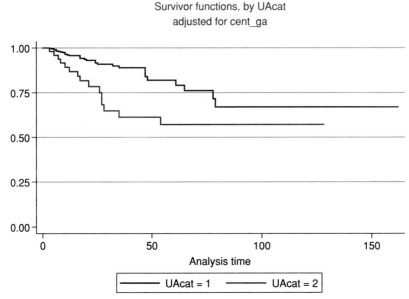

Figure 35.5 `sts graph, by(UAcat) adjustfor(cent_ga).`

derived from each other. The relationship is $H(t) = -\ln\{S(t)\}$, where $S(t)$ can represent the Kaplan–Meier estimator. We could alternatively represent the same relationship this way: $S(t) = e^{-H(t)}$. These relationships are fundamental to adjusting a survival analysis for covariates.

The model may be represented this way: $h(t|X_j) = h_0(t)e^{(X_j\beta_x)}$. Now, recall the logistic regression model in Chapter 34: $\ln_e\left[\frac{p(x)}{1-p(x)}\right] = \beta_0 + \sum \beta_i x_i$. Let's consider differences and similarities between the logistic regression and Cox models.

- Of course, the dependent variables differ:
  (a) In the logistic model, the dependent variable is the natural logarithm of the odds of success.
  (b) In the Cox model, the dependent variable is the hazard rate for the jth individual.
- The logistic model contains the intercept term, β_0. No intercept term appears on the right side of the Cox equation.
  (a) Instead, $h_0(t)$ appears: *the baseline hazard.*
- The logistic model entails a conditional probability estimate: $p(\mathbf{X}) = p(D = 1|x_1, x_2, \ldots, x_i,)$; the probability of disease, given a particular observation's profile of explanatory variables.
- In the Cox equation, $\mathbf{x}_j$ denotes the covariate vector: the array of one or more explanatory variables, including interaction terms.

Returning to the equation describing the Cox model, $h(t|\mathbf{x}_j) = h_0(t)e^{(X_j\beta_x)}$, an individual's hazard of failure at time t is the product of the baseline hazard at time t and the exponential expression involving the covariate vector. Notice, the baseline hazard, $h_0(t)$, is a function of time but not of the covariate vector; the exponential expression is related to the covariate vector and not to time. Sometimes the covariate vector *may* vary with time; when it does, we use something called the extended Cox model. If all covariates are equal to zero, the expression reduces to the baseline hazard ($e^0 = 1$).

I can now explain the earlier statement about continuous covariates in a Cox model sometimes requiring special treatment. I created the centered gestational age variable, cent_ga, to facilitate interpreting the model against a baseline hazard: $h_0(t)$. Essentially, a value of cent_ga that equals the mean value for ga causes the cent_ga term to drop out of the model. If the cent_ga variable and its coefficient drop out of the regression equation, then we have the baseline hazard that exists before accounting for that variable. See Ref. 129 for a more complete discussion of situations where continuous covariates require special treatment.

The distribution of the values for the baseline hazard is not specified in the Cox model. For this reason, Kleinbaum[128] calls the Cox model nonparametric. Most authors refer to the Cox model as semiparametric.

Parametric models specify particular distributional characteristics for the baseline hazard. Terms such as Weibull, gamma, and log-normal specify the distributional characteristics assumed of the baseline hazard. Each varies with the values of their distributional parameters. They are used to model health care outcomes because they may closely approximate the hazard functions of certain groups of patients. For example, one such function might approximate the survival experience of patients in remission from cancer.

Cox PH assumptions

You may be wondering why didn't we just go straight to a Cox model to analyze the nosocomial data set, why did we spend time on KM analysis? Readers familiar with neonatal patients can think of several plausible adjustment covariates. Moreover, the Cox model usually does a good job estimating the regression coefficients for the correct parametric model. Well, we can't charge directly ahead because although the Cox model makes no assumptions about the shape of the distribution of the hazard function, it does make some assumptions about the data. And that's why many authors refer to it as a *semi*parametric method.

The Cox model assumes
- the baseline hazard is the same for all individuals.
- the hazard ratio predicted by the covariate matrices stays the same over time.
  - **(a)** If we plotted the hazard ratio comparing any two individuals over time, regardless of which group the individuals are in, the plot would be a horizontal straight line at $y =$ the constant value of the hazard ratio.

- the explanatory variables are independent: the multiplicative assumption.[129]

  (a) The model equation entails adding up the exponentiated covariate terms. Adding logarithmic terms is the same as multiplying arithmetic terms. And to compute the probability of two independent events both occurring, we take the product of their individual probabilities.

    Thus, we assume the effects of two covariates that each are associated with the outcome will be the product of their individual effects on the outcome.

  (b) In reality, some explanatory variables are not independent of each other. To identify this circumstance and incorporate it into the model, you must explore the effects of adding interaction terms (see Chapter 33).

Cox PH analysis using Stata

Let's analyze the nosocomial data using the Cox PH method.

```
. stcox UAcat cent_ga

        failure _d:  status
  analysis time _t:  (te-origin)
           origin:  time t0

Iteration 0:    log likelihood = -248.03245
Iteration 1:    log likelihood = -244.61408
Iteration 2:    log likelihood = -244.24584
Iteration 3:    log likelihood = -244.24535
Refining estimates:
Iteration 0:    log likelihood = -244.24535

Cox regression -- Breslow method for ties

No. of subjects =          647          Number of obs   =        647
No. of failures =           48
Time at risk    =        11068
                                        LR chi2(2)      =       7.57
Log likelihood  =    -244.24535         Prob > chi2     =     0.0227

------------------------------------------------------------------------------
        _t | Haz. Ratio   Std. Err.      z    P>|z|     [95% Conf. Interval]
-----------+------------------------------------------------------------------
     UAcat |   2.245879   .7726312     2.35   0.019     1.144339    4.407763
   cent_ga |    .974125   .0363148    -0.70   0.482     .9054874    1.047966
------------------------------------------------------------------------------
```

This model is significant at the 0.05 level. The χ^2 statistic evaluates the null hypothesis that all the coefficients are equal to 0. In other words, the covariates together are unrelated to the outcome. The coefficients estimate the ratio of the hazards for a one-unit change in the covariate. We would speak of, for example, a 2.2-fold relative hazard of nosocomial infection associated with an umbilical artery catheter in place for longer than 3 days. The interval estimate of this effect is 1.144339, 4.407763.

```
. stcurve, survival        Output appears in Fig. 35.6.
```

Figure 35.6 displays the predicted survival at the mean values of all the explanatory variables. You could specify particular values, for example,

```
. stcurve, survival at1(UAcat=1) at2(UAcat=2) Output appears in Fig. 35.7.
```

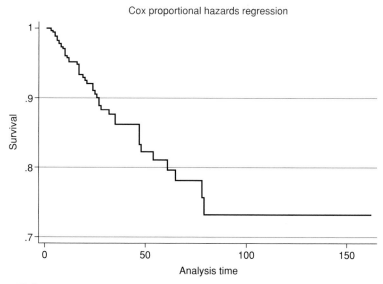

Figure 35.6 `stcurve, survival.`

Or,

`. stcurve, survival at1(cent_ga=-10) at2(cent_ga=6)` **Output appears in Fig. 35.8.**

Here's how to obtain a hazard plot:

`. stcurve, hazard at1(UAcat=1) at2(UAcat=2) yscale(log)` **Output appears in Fig. 35.9.**

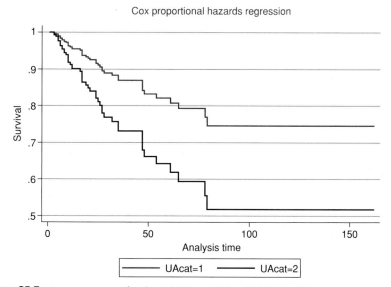

Figure 35.7 `stcurve, survival at1(UAcat=1) at2(UAcat=2).`

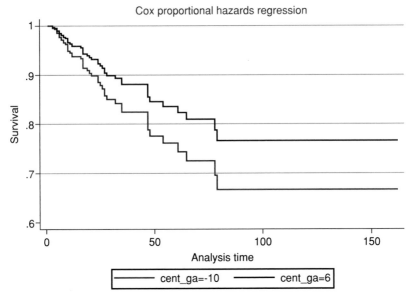

Figure 35.8 `stcurve, survival at1(cent_ga=-10) at2(cent_ga=6).`

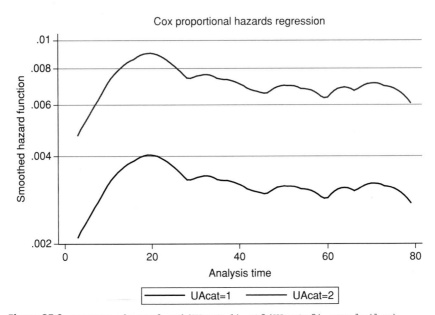

Figure 35.9 `stcurve, hazard at1(UAcat=1) at2(UAcat=2) yscale(log).`

I plotted Fig. 35.9 on a log scale to demonstrate the proportionality of the hazards. Stata offers some more rigorous ways to evaluate the PH assumption. The overall topic is beyond our scope and I don't want to give you the impression that a model may be comprehensively evaluated along the lines of the following graphical illustrations. Passing one test does not assure that other tests will give similar results.[127] Keeping these caveats in mind, let's compare the Cox and KM survivor functions by plotting them simultaneously. If you use this method, note that you should not first run the `stcox` command. Start out by testing the PH assumption before you work on the Cox model.

```
. stcoxkm, by(UAcat)          Output appears in Fig. 35.10.

            failure _d:  status
    analysis time _t:  (te-origin)
              origin:  time t0
```

The closer the observed (KM) and predicted (Cox) plots, the more likely the PH assumptions apply. Figure 35.10 shows an area where observed and predicted deviate substantially for infants in UAcat = 2.

Another way to evaluate the PH assumption is a "log–log" plot ($-\ln(-\ln$ (survival)) against $\ln$(analysis time)). The curves are expected to be parallel. In Fig. 35.11, this appears to be the case over most, but not all, of the observation period (note that the time scale is different from Fig. 35.9).

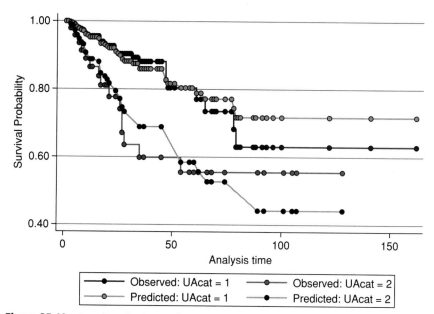

Figure 35.10 `stcoxkm, by(UAcat)`.

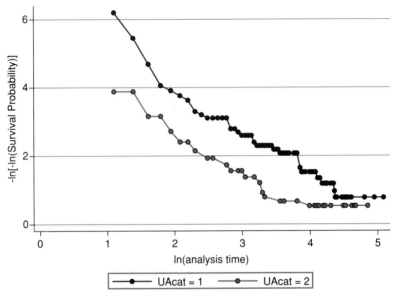

Figure 35.11 stphplot, by(UAcat).

```
. stphplot, by(UAcat)          Output appears in Fig. 35.11.

         failure _d:  status
   analysis time _t:  (te-origin)
            origin:  time t0
```

So exactly how close is "close" for these graphical tests? Kleinbaum says the log–log plot should be "approximately parallel," and for the Cox/KM plot no categories should appear to be "quite discrepant."[128] There are other methods discussed in Refs. 127 and 128 and the Stata survival analysis reference manual[130].

Survival analysis: summary and comparison to logistic regression

We use survival analysis methods to answer the following types of questions from observed data:

- What are the estimated exposure-specific distributions of time to event?
  - **(a)** Do the exposure-specific distributions differ?
  - **(b)** Does exposure status vary according to the value of some baseline characteristic?
- Is it possible to control for possible baseline differences among the exposure groups?
  - **(a)** Were the PH assumptions tested?
  - **(b)** Was the multiplicative assumption tested?

Both logistic regression and survival analysis can assess the independent contribution of multiple covariates to a binary outcome. However, particularly for outcomes where the goal of intervention is to delay *when* the outcome ultimately occurs, survival analysis can teach us things that logistic regression cannot. Additionally, logistic regression cannot use data for a patient who was lost to follow-up; we must know the outcome of each observation. Survival analysis can incorporate censored observations – nonoccurrence information – even though the patient was lost to follow-up. Katz and Hauck recommend logistic regression over Cox PH when few subjects were lost to follow-up and the outcome occurs in a small proportion of the subjects.[129] Further, for commonly occurring outcomes, the relative hazards from a Cox PH model and the odds ratios from a logistic model will differ substantially.[129]

CHAPTER 36

Choosing variables and hypotheses: practical considerations

Ideal vs. operational variables

Let's return to the problem of how to decide on the variables you need. I omitted an important issue from my discussion of conceptual frameworks in Chapter 18. Usually, what we would ideally *like* to measure and what we realistically *can* measure are not the same. We now explore some implications of this inequality and considerations for selecting exactly what we *shall* measure.

In Chapter 18, we pondered which question(s) the MaternalEtOH field actually allows a database user to answer.

1 Did this mother ingest any ethanol during this pregnancy?
2 Was this infant exposed to any ethanol during this gestation?
3 What is the association between a mother's admitting to using ethanol during pregnancy and phenotypic features of fetal alcohol syndrome in her infant?
4 Did this mother admit to any ethanol ingestion during this pregnancy?

Of the choices, only the last on the list is answered by the data in MaternalEtOH. We require different data to answer questions 1–3.

Consider what drives our collecting data about prenatal ethanol exposure. It might be that we want to identify a patient who has had some "high risk" exposure, or we may want to investigate a *particular* exposure–outcome relationship. In any case, the basis to collect the data ought to be explicit and sound. To collect data for vague reasons, unconnected to an explicit conceptual framework, often amounts to wasted effort. To further ensure that the data we collect will be the data we require, we must explicitly articulate the *precise* factor or relationship about which we wish to be better informed. Essentially, useful data collection is predicated on having a clear idea of what might be different once we have the data we seek.

The data we seek may be provided via several alternative variables. For example, if we seek data about adequacy of perfusion we might consider measuring blood pressure or capillary refill time. Note that we seek to know about adequacy of perfusion, that is, our ideal measurement variable, but we measure something else, that is, our operational measurement variable. However, operational measures of exposure may differ from ideal measures of exposure in important ways. As Savitz[103] lucidly explains (I summarize his Chapter 8 in this section), we identify the strongest association between exposure and outcome for the exposure variable with the greatest causal effect on the outcome. This may seem obvious, but it's analytically profound. Exposure has several dimensions, including when it occurred (timing), its intensity, and how long it lasted (duration). Often we don't know these specifications, and even when we do, it may be difficult to measure them exactly. We are confined to measuring what we think is in the causal chain and what we *can* measure.

Operational measures of exposure bundle along with the element we want, a component of variability unconnected to the outcome. This variability that is not relevant to the outcome will diminish the strength of the exposure–outcome association. Thus, the extent to which our proxy or operational exposure variable departs from the ideal measure of exposure interferes with our ability to identify an exposure–outcome relationship. This concept is central to selecting a variable from a list of candidates.

Returning to our MaternalEtOH variable, we do not fully know the timing, intensity, and duration of exposure that produce the strongest association with fetal alcohol syndrome or with some particular expression of the exposure. We nonetheless can advance our understanding of disease related to ethanol exposure, provided

- our operational exposure measure (MaternalEtOH) correlates strongly with the ideal exposure marker and
- the strength of the association between ideal exposure marker and outcome is so great that the operational exposure measure's irrelevant variability does not dilute the association such that $P > \alpha$ – the chosen cutpoint for statistical significance.

Thus, if the association between ideal exposure marker and outcome, though real, is weak, we may not identify the association by means of an operational exposure marker. Therefore, ensure that your conceptual framework reflects the foregoing discussion.

At times, it may be hard to distinguish exposure from outcome. For example, we may treat a genetic marker as an exposure variable when it actually represents an early stage of the outcome.[103] In such cases, our analysis would essentially put the same information on either side of the = sign in a regression equation. We might be fooled into thinking we've discovered an association.

Collinearity

In discussing regression methods, I said that we assume the predictor variables are independent of each other. When this is not so, when we include two or more closely correlated explanatory variables in a regression analysis, we introduce collinearity. An extreme example: suppose that in the multiple regression model in Chapter 33 we included not only the variable BWsqrt but also a variable BWsqrt^3, the cube of BWsqrt. The derived variable would not contain any information not also contained in BWsqrt. Although I did not make this point earlier, it's a good idea to check for very strong correlation among variables that are plausible candidates for this problem.

```
. gen BWsqrt3=BWsqrt^3

. pwcorr BWsqrt BWsqrt3,sig

             |  BWsqrt  BWsqrt3
-------------+------------------
      BWsqrt |  1.0000
             |
             |
     BWsqrt3 |  0.9681   1.0000
             |  0.0000
             |
```

```
. regress  lowestsystolicbp BWsqrt BWsqrt3 hct_adm Igestcat1 Igestcat2
Igestcat3 Igestcat4 Igestcat5 if gestage<=38 & hct_adm~=0 & hct_adm<100
```

Source	SS	df	MS		Number of obs =	1593
					F(7, 1585) =	142.83
Model	57577.4526	7	8225.35037		Prob > F =	0.0000
Residual	91278.85	1585	57.5891798		R-squared =	0.3868
					Adj R-squared =	0.3841
Total	148856.303	1592	93.5027026		Root MSE =	7.5888

lowestsyst~p	Coef.	Std. Err.	t	P>|t|	[95% Conf. Interval]	
BWsqrt	.3839676	.1197041	3.21	0.001	.1491726	.6187627
BWsqrt3	-.0000161	.0000183	-0.88	0.380	-.000052	.0000198
hct_adm	.1080888	.0241174	4.48	0.000	.0607834	.1553943
Igestcat1	(dropped)					
Igestcat2	1.877299	1.01489	1.85	0.065	-.1133697	3.867967
Igestcat3	6.761867	1.210705	5.59	0.000	4.387116	9.136619
Igestcat4	7.952664	1.405065	5.66	0.000	5.196684	10.70864
Igestcat5	12.98133	1.587295	8.18	0.000	9.867912	16.09475
_cons	19.85299	3.048841	6.51	0.000	13.8728	25.83317

Let's include an interaction term in the regression analysis.

```
. gen BW2_BW3=BWsqrt*BWsqrt3

. regress  lowestsystolicbp BWsqrt BWsqrt3 BW2_BW3 hct_adm Igestcat1 Igestcat2
Igestcat3 Igestcat4 Igestcat5 if gestage<=38 & hct_adm~=0 & hct_adm<100
```

Source	SS	df	MS		Number of obs =	1593
					F(8, 1584) =	124.96
Model	57594.6777	8	7199.33472		Prob > F =	0.0000
Residual	91261.6248	1584	57.6146621		R-squared =	0.3869
					Adj R-squared =	0.3838
Total	148856.303	1592	93.5027026		Root MSE =	7.5904

lowestsyst~p	Coef.	Std. Err.	t	P>|t|	[95% Conf. Interval]	
BWsqrt	.2065702	.3458261	0.60	0.550	-.4717548	.8848953
BWsqrt3	.0000782	.0001734	0.45	0.652	-.0002619	.0004184
BW2_BW3	-1.03e-06	1.88e-06	-0.55	0.585	-4.70e-06	2.65e-06
hct_adm	.1090841	.0241913	4.51	0.000	.0616336	.1565345
Igestcat1	(dropped)					

```
Igestcat2 |    2.107348    1.098851    1.92   0.055    -.0480075    4.262704
Igestcat3 |    7.032796    1.308423    5.38   0.000     4.466373    9.599219
Igestcat4 |    8.131857    1.443081    5.64   0.000     5.301308    10.96241
Igestcat5 |    13.17985     1.62863    8.09   0.000     9.985351    16.37435
    _cons |    23.19565    6.831705    3.40   0.001     9.795513    36.59578
```

Collinearity leads to unstable estimates of regression coefficients, increases their standard errors, and affects their computed P values.[131] Look at BWsqrt and BWsqrt^3 in the two analyses above and at the interaction term (BW2_BW3) in the second analysis. In the analysis with the interaction term, the coefficient for BWsqrt is smaller by almost a factor of 2, its standard error is larger by almost a factor of 3, and its P value changes from 0.001 to 0.550. This instability reflects the difficulty in distinguishing the influence of one or the other of the highly correlated variables on the outcome, so the estimated effect becomes unreliable.[131] Not surprisingly, R^2 will not improve and the adjusted R^2 may decrease. The take-away message: predictive models don't tolerate strongly redundant information, nor, as you may recall, do normalized data models.

Misclassification

Even after you've worked hard to clean a data set, consider the possibility that a subject's exposure or disease classification may be incorrect. Whether misclassification of exposure or disease is independent of the other – random – determines the implications of such errors. Random misclassification is termed nondifferential; and nonrandom, differential.

What a study subject tells you about exposure may depend on whether the associated outcome occurred. For example, a mother whose infant has been diagnosed with fetal alcohol syndrome may feel inhibited about providing an accurate history of her ethanol consumption during pregnancy. This kind of bias leads to differential misclassification of exposure. Nondifferential misclassification of exposure may be more likely when exposure data is obtained before the related outcome occurs.

On average, nondifferential misclassification puts a similar proportion of misclassified subjects in each category. This tends to produce underestimates of the actual relative risk: bias toward the null. So an association of borderline statistical significance may in fact be stronger than the data suggest. Of course, the risk of type II error is increased.

Differential misclassification does not have a predictable effect on an exposure–outcome association. The specifics of the relationship determine the extent to which exposure and nonexposure proportions are erroneously altered. The effect may be biased toward or away from null.

If we erroneously assign a value of a categorical variable, it's simply called misclassification. Doing so for a continuous variable is called measurement error. Disease outcomes are commonly considered to be categorical, but often this is so simply because we dichotomized a continuous outcome.[132] For example, what happens when we change the cutpoint for the critical value of blood glucose to establish a diagnosis of diabetes mellitus? We can create millions of diabetics overnight.

Take time to reflect on your variable choices and your analysis

How do you know that you are collecting the data you need? Before reading this book, you may have considered this question trivial and the answer self-evident. As you collect and analyze your data, reflect often on *how* you know the "important" questions are the *right* questions. And are these questions the ones the data indeed *enable* you to answer? Be mindful of misclassification – the gap between, for example, a 0/1 and actual or no alcohol intake.

Be sure you understand the difference between a hypothesis test and a measure of association. Interpreting a hypothesis test addresses only random error, that is, sampling variation, or chance effects. Interpreting a measure of association entails thinking about clinical significance, chance, bias, and confounding.

If you collect data because you think the chosen variables predict or adjust for risk of some outcome, to what extent has the association been validated in the literature? If you collect important patient outcome variables, do you also collect validated or candidate predictor variables? Just think: a study of 94,110 infants that included a wide array of patient- and hospital-level variables could ultimately explain very little of the variation in mortality across hospitals. Systematic but *unexplained* differences in mortality across participating hospitals accounted for 84% of variation in mortality.[133] When models prove uninformative, we ought to reconsider how we determine the factors to which we think we need to pay attention.

Conclusion – The challenge of transforming data and information to shared knowledge: tools that make us smart

When IBM discovered that it was not in the business of making office equipment or business machines, but that it was in the business of processing information, then it began to navigate with clear vision.
MARSHALL MCLUHAN, 1964 (von Baeyer,[36] p. 5)

Every day, we clinicians collect vast amounts of data to fuel our prodigious information processing industry. But processing information is only a part of our mission. Ultimately, we *use* information: as defined in Chapter 5, we are knowledge workers. We implement the results of data management and analysis.

Although this book may be unique in surveying both data management and analysis, you now appreciate why the two go hand in hand. Only by understanding the relationships between antecedents and outcomes can we determine the data and information elements to which we should attend. You now also appreciate how particular methods of managing, analyzing, and interpreting data and information can bolster our efforts to use information – to *transform* data and information into knowledge. How to maximize our knowledge and transfer it to others is another story.

Early in the book I pointed to attitudes of technological laggards among us, those reluctant to give up the traditional ways by which they manage and learn from patient information. To be fair, health care workers tend to be rather intelligent and reasonable people. So we should ask why would intelligent and reasonable people obstinately prefer technology that imposes the shortcomings we examined in Chapters 1–4?

At every opportunity, I ask these workers to talk about their concerns with new technology. One common strain reverberates in their replies. They, indeed all of us, are accustomed to engaging with a patient problem on the basis of a narrative – a *story* about what happened. Similarly, we are accustomed to transferring our knowledge of a patient via a story. Telling stories can tie together into a coherent whole items of information that individually may seem disparate. When they are about unsolved problems, stories, creating a coherent account of events, may clarify the nature of the true problem and inspire new candidate solutions. If we did not tell the story we might not coherently organize the components. Thus, stories are a means to discover new knowledge.[38] Further, by their retelling, stories can establish a common interpretive framework.[38] If this is so, then the widespread variation in health care[10,11] suggests we have yet much to learn about telling good stories.

In any event, our predisposition for story formats conflicts with computer outputs. These don't tell a story in the traditional way: typically, they simply provide information. Although graphs may tell stories,[47] not all stories lend themselves to graphical display. Do not be deceived by software applications that offer narrative report formats. Such formats entail inserting field values into spaces in a fixed template. I know of no software that consistently creates accurate, apropos, clear, coherent, and complete stories from our data. Superficially, the computational product may look like a traditional story, but rarely will it gratify our human need for one. It lacks the richly nuanced functionality of the real thing. Storytellers calibrate details to the story aims. At times, stories are telling by what we leave out. Storytellers arrange story elements to reflect their importance and chronology for the thesis. Generic rank- or time-ordering may be pointless, or worse, distracting. Storytellers may select one word only subtly different from an alternate, or may use especially vivid vocabulary, because word choice may be crucial to accurately communicating a particular idea. No, computers are not real storytellers.

The stories we are accustomed to using in our work may seem compelling, but they are not always accurate, apropos, clear, coherent, and complete. We cannot reliably identify the details that matter, or interpret them. If we could, I would not have written, and you would not have read, this book. Nonetheless, stories are a communication modality – and often, a cognitive tool – rooted in our cultural evolution, a deep and essential part of how we engage with others' experience and with our own. To show we understand, we tell our story. Indeed, it is by *telling* the story that we may first understand (see Ref. 134, especially Ch. 5). Our challenge is to use our new technology to facilitate accurate, apropos, clear, coherent, and complete stories; stories that reflect our accrual of fresh experience and knowledge, connect it to what has gone before, and communicate what we know to others.

The problem with our stories about patients is we've tended to consider these stories within the long tradition of oral storytelling. This tradition permits enormous variation in details among iterations of the same tale (see p. 150 in Ref. 134). From the same situation, people can tell different stories. From the same story, people can draw different conclusions. The cognitive tools we've considered in this book are designed to help with this problem. To the extent that the tools help us determine to what we should attend and enable us to attend to them accurately and reliably, our tools can make us smarter. But the problem is broader still. When you buy a book, you expect not the author's first draft but the final product of reiterative composition and revision. For at that stage of refinement are the ideas likely to be clear and coherent, the reading easy as possible. From this perspective, both traditional pen- and paper-based patient notes and related oral communication with colleagues – the stories we tell about our patients – are commonly "first-drafts." New cognitive tools for patient information may automate composition and revision, but beware: we know little about how to do this well.

The goal is to develop tools that quickly help us turn data and information into knowledge articulated as final drafts; tools that provide the correct answers and only the correct answers to our important questions; tools that even point us to the questions we should be asking.[134]

Science is built of facts the way a house is built of bricks; but an accumulation of facts is no more science than a pile of bricks is a house

HENRI POINCARÉ

References

1. Gawande A. The Bell Curve. *The New Yorker* 2004:82–91.
2. Brookfield SD. *Becoming a Critically Reflective Teacher.* San Francisco: Jossey-Bass, 1995.
3. Choudhry NK, Fletcher RH, Soumerai SB. The Relationship between Clinical Experience and Quality of Health Care. *Annals of Internal Medicine* 2005;142(4):260–273.
4. Schoen DA. *Educating the Reflective Practitioner.* San Francisco: Jossey-Bass, 1987.
5. Weinberger SE, Duffy FD, Cassel CK. "Practice Makes Perfect". Or Does It? *Annals of Internal Medicine* 2005;142(4):302–303.
6. Eddy DM. *Clinical Decision Making.* Sudbury, MA: Jones and Bartlett, 1996.
7. Weick KE. *Sensemaking in Organizations.* Thousand Oaks, CA: Sage Publications, 1995.
8. Eddy DM. Evidence-Based Medicine: A Unified Approach. *Health Affairs* 2005;24(1):9–17.
9. Weinstein MC, Fineberg HV, Elstein AS, *et al. Clinical Decision Analysis.* Philadelphia: W.B. Saunders, 1980.
10. Blumenthal D. The Variation Phenomenon in 1994. *The New England Journal of Medicine* 1994;331(15):1017–1018.
11. The Center for the Evaluative Clinical Sciences DMS. *The Dartmouth Atlas of Health Care 1998.* Chicago: American Hospital Publishing, 1998.
12. Committe on Quality of Health Care in America IoM. *Crossing the Quality Chasm: A New Health System for the 21st Century.* Washington, DC: National Academy Press, 2001.
13. Dick RS, Steen EB, Detmer DE, Eds. *The Computer-Based Patient Record: An Essential Technology for Health Care,* revised ed. Washington: National Academy Press, 1997.
14. Smith R. Doctors Are Not Scientists. *British Medical Journal* 2004;328:7454.
15. Thompson TG, Brailer DJ. The Decade of Health Information Technology: Delivering Consumer-Centric and Information-Rich Health Care. United States Department of Health and Human Services, Office for the National Coordinator for Health Information Technology (ONCHIT), Washington, DC, 2004. Available at: http://www.hhs.gov/onchit/framework/hitframework.pdf (accessed Aug 2, 2005).
16. Stata 8 [program]. 8.0 Version. College Station, TX: Stata Press, 2003.
17. Wyatt JC, Wright P. Design Should Help Use of Patients' Data. *Lancet* 1998;352:1375–1378.
18. Sellen AJ, Harper RHR. *The Myth of the Paperless Office.* Cambridge, MA: MIT Press, 2002.
19. Department of Health, UK. Delivering 21st Century IT Support for the NHS: National Specification for Integrated Care Records Service, Version 1.22, 2002. Available at: http://www.dh.gov.uk/assetRoot/04/07/16/76/04071676.pdf (accessed Aug 2, 2005).

20. Nemeth CP, Cook RI, Woods DD. The Messy Details: Insights from the Study of Technical Work in Healthcare. *IEEE Transactions on Systems, Man, and Cybernetics,* 2004;34:689–692.

21. Wears RL, Berg M. Computer Technology and Clinical Work. *Journal of American Medical Association* 2005;293(10):1261–1263.

22. Woods DD. Designs Are Hypotheses About How Artifacts Shape Cognition and Collaboration. *Ergonomics* 1998;41(2):168–173.

23. Sprague L. Electronic Health Records: How Close? How Far to go? In: *National Health Policy Forum Issue Brief.* Washington, DC: National Health Policy Forum, 2004.

24. Stead WW, Kelly BJ, Kolodner RM. Achievable Steps Toward Builing a National Health Information Infrastructure in the United States. *Journal of the American Medical Informatics Association* 2005;12(2):113–120.

25. Waegemann CP, Tessier C, Barbash A, *et al.* Healthcare Documentation: A Report on Information Capture and Report Generation. Consensus Workgroup on Health Information Capture and Report Generation, 2002. Available at: http://www.medrecinst.com/resources/infoCap/FinalReport.pdf (accessed Aug 2, 2005).

26. Fuller S. Designing a Data Collection Process. Chicago, IL: American Health Information Management Association, 1998.

27. Tessier C. The Essentials of Healthcare Documentation. *Healthcare Informatics* 2003:87–90.

28. Committee on Data Standards for Patient Safety IoM. Key Capabilities of an Electronic Health Record System. Washington, DC: National Academy Press, 2003.

29. Javitt JC. How to Succeed in Health Information Technology. *Health Affairs* 2004;W4:321–324.

30. Powsner SM, Wyatt JC, Wright P. Opportunities for and Challenges of Computerisation. *Lancet* 1998;352:1617–1622.

31. Zimmerman B, Lindberg C, Plsek P. *Edgeware: Insights from Complexity Science for Health Care Leaders.* Dallas, TX: VHA, 1998.

32. Schulman J. NICU Notes: A Palm OS® and Windows® Database Software Product and Process to Facilitate Patient Care in the Newborn Intensive Care Unit. *Proceedings of AMIA Symposium* 2003:999.

33. Schulman J. *Evaluating the Processes of Neonatal Intensive Care.* London: BMJ Books, 2004.

34. Floridi L. Information. In: Florida L, Eds. *The Blackwell Guide to the Philosophy of Computing and Information.* Oxford, UK: Blackwell, 2004:40–61.

35. Devlin K. *InfoSense.* New York: W.H. Freeman, 2001.

36. von Baeyer HC. *Information: The New Language of Science.* Cambridge, MA: Harvard University Press, 2004.

37. Lucent T. Introduction to Information Theory. Available at: http://www-lmmb.ncifcrf.gov/~toms/paper/primer/index.html. Lucent Technologies Bell Labs Innovation, 2004.

38. Brown JS, Duguid P. *The Social Life of Information.* Boston: Harvard Business School Press, 2002.

39. Wurman RS. *InformationAnxiety2.* Indianapolis, IN: Que, 2000.

40. Surowiecki J. Net Worth. *The New Yorker* 2005:62.

41. Smith B. Ontology. In: Florida L, Ed. *The Blackwell Guide to the Philosophy of Computing and Information.* Oxford, UK: Blackwell, 2004:155–166.

42. Brailer DJ. Translating Ideals for Health Information Technology into Practice. *Health Affairs* 2004;W4:318–320.

43. Connolly TM, Begg CE. *Database Systems: A Practical Approach to Design, Implementation, and Management,* 2nd ed. Harlow, England: Addison Wesley, 1999.

44. Roman S. *Access Database Design and Programming,* 3rd ed. Sebastopol, CA: O'Reilly & Associates, 2002.

45. Simsion GC. *Data Modeling Essentials,* 2nd ed. Scottsdale, AZ: The Coriolis Group, 2001.

46. Whitehorn M, Marklyn B. *Inside Relational Databases,* 2nd ed. London: Springer-Verlag London, 2001.

47. Lidwell W, Holden K, Butler J. *Universal Principles of Design.* Gloucester, MA: Rockport Publishers, 2003.

48. Litwin P, Getz K, Gunderloy M. *Access 2002 Desktop Developer's Handbook.* San Francisco: Sybex, 2001.

49. Hernandez MJ. *Database Design for Mere Mortals,* 2nd ed. Boston: Addison Wesley, 2003.

50. Bagui S, Earp R. *Learning SQL: A Step by Step Guide Using Access®.* Boston: Pearson Education, 2004.

51. Pendragon Forms Software Corporation. Pendragon Forms 4.0. Libertyville, IL: Pendragon Forms Software Corporation, 2003.

52. Balter A. *Mastering Microsoft Office Access 2003.* Indianapolis, IN: Sams, 2004.

53. Phillips I. Personal communication (Libertyville, IL), March 23, 2005.

54. Pierce J, Pardi P. *Mircrosoft® Office Access 2003 Inside Track.* Redmond, WA: Microsoft Press, 2004.

55. Leszynski S, Reddick G. Naming Conventions for Microsoft Access. Microsoft Corporation, 2004.

56. Pierce J, Pardi P. *Microsoft Office Access 2003 Inside Track.* Redmond, WA: Microsoft Press, 2004.

57. Whitehorn M, Marklyn B. *Accessible Access 2000.* London: Springer-Verlag London, 2000.

58. Saksena D, Berkowitz N. *Access 97-2000 Database Development Outside VBA.* Plano, TX: Wordware Publishing, 2001.

59. Jones E. *Microsoft Access 2000 Developer's Guide.* Foster City, CA: M & T Books, 1999.

60. Microsoft Office Online. Microsoft, 2004 (http://office.microsoft.com/en-us/default.aspx).

61. Riordan RM. Relational Algebra. *Designing Relational Database Systems.* Redmond, WA: Microsoft Press, 1999.

62. Callahan E. *Microsoft® Access 2002 Visual Basic® for Applications Step by Step.* Redmond, WA: Microsoft Press, 2001.

63. Smith R, Sussman D, Blackburn I, *et al. Beginning Access 2002 VBA.* Birmingham, UK: Peer Information, 2003.

64. Barker FS. *Access 2003: Your Visual Blueprint™ for Creating and Maintaining Real-World Databases.* Hoboken, NJ: Wiley, 2004.

65. Fehily C. *SQL.* Berkeley, CA: Peachpit Press, 2002.

66. Forta B. *Sams Teach Yourself SQL in 10 Minutes,* 2nd ed. Inidanapolis, IN: Sams Publishing, 2001.

67. Getz K, Litwin P, Baron A. *Access Cookbook.* Sebastopol, CA: O'Reilly & Associates, 2002.

68. Intellisync MobileApp Designer [program]. Intellisync Corporation, 2003. Available at: http://www.sync.com/index.html (accessed Aug 2, 2005).

69. Bunch AJ. *Fundamental Microsoft Jet SQL for Access 2000.* Redmond, WA: Microsoft Corporation, 2000.

70. Norman DA. *The Design of Everyday Things.* New York: Currency Doubleday, 1988.

71. Cooper A. *About Face: The Essentials of User Interface Design,* 1st ed. New York: Hungry Minds, 1995.

72. The International Neonatal Network. The CRIB (clinical risk index for babies) Score: A Tool for Assessing Initial Neonatal Risk and Comparing Performance of Neonatal Intensive Care Units. *The Lancet* 1993;342(8865):193–198.

73. Petersen LA, Orav EJ, Teich JM, *et al.* Using a Computerized Sign-Out Program to Improve Continuity of Inpatient Care and Prevent Adverse Events. *The Joint Commission Journal on Quality Improvement* 1998;24(2):77–87.

74. PalmSource Inc. Zen of Palm. Sunnyvale, CA: PalmSource, Inc., 2003.

75. Cougias DJ, Heiberger EL, Koop K. *The Backup Book: Disaster Recovery from Desktop to Data Center,* 3rd ed. Lecanto, FL: Schaser-Vartan Books, 2003.

76. Robinson G. *Real World Microsoft Access Database Protection and Security.* New York: Apress/Springer-Verlag, 2004.

77. Mel HX, Baker D. *Cryptography Decrypted.* Boston: Addison-Wesley, 2001.

78. Singh S. *The Code Book.* New York: Anchor, 2000.

79. Pancoast PE, Patrick TB, Mitchell JA. Physician PDA Use and the HIPAA Privacy Rule. *Journal of the American Medical Informatics Association* 2003;10(6):611–612.

80. Barman S. *Writing Information Security Policies.* Indianapolis, IN: New Riders, 2001.

81. United States Government, Department of Health and Human Services, Office of Civil Rights. Standards for Privacy of Individually Identifiable Health Information. Section 45, CFR Parts 160 and 164, 2003:29–30. Available at: http://www.hhs.gov/ocr/combinedregtext.pdf (accessed Aug 2, 2005).

82. Van Der Meijden MJ, Tange HJ, Troost J, *et al.* Determinants of Success of Inpatient Clinical Information Systems: A Literature Review. *Journal of the American Medical Informatics Association* 2003;10(3):235–243.

83. Littlejohns P, Wyatt JC, Garvician L. Evaluating Computerised Health Information Systems: Hard Lessons Still to be Learnt. *British Medical Journal* 2003;326:860–863.

84. Rogers EM. *Diffusion of Innovations,* 4th ed. New York: Free Press, 1995.

85. Lorenzi NM, Riley RT. Managing Change: An Overview. *Journal of the American Medical Informatics Association* 2000;7(2):116–124.

86. Goodman DC, Fisher ES, Little GA, *et al.* The Uneven Landscape of Newborn Intensive Care Services: Variation in the Neonatology Workforce. *Effective Clinical Practice* 2001;4(4):143–149.

87. Goodman DC, Fisher ES, Little GA, *et al.* Are Neonatal Intensive Care Resources Located According to Need? Regional Variation in neonatologists, Beds, and Low Birth Weight Newborns. *Pediatrics* 2001;108(2):426–431.

88. Wennberg J, Gittelsohn. Small Area Variations in Health Care Delivery. *Science* 1973;182:1102–1108.

89. Coiera E. Designing Interactions. In: Berg M, Ed. *Health Information Management: Integrating Information Technology in Health Care Work.* London: Routledge, 2004:101–123.

90. Koppel R, Metlay JP, Cohen A, *et al.* Role of Computerized Physician Order Entry Systems in Facilitating Medication Errors. *Journal of American Medical Association* 2005;293(10):1197–1203.

91. Kemper DW, Mettler M. *Information Therapy: Prescribed Information as a Reimbursable Medical Service*. Boise, ID: Healthwise, 2002.

92. Garg AX, Adhikari NKJ, McDonald H, *et al*. Effects of Computerized Clinical Decision Support Systems on Practitioner Performance and Patient Outcomes. *Journal of American Medical Association* 2005;293(10):1223–1238.

93. Berg M. *Health Information Management: Integrating Information Technology in Health Care Work*. London: Routledge, 2004.

94. Ash JS, Berg M, Coiera E. Some Unintended Consequences of Information Technology in Health Care: The Nature of Patient Care Information System-related Errors. *Journal of the American Medical Informatics Association* 2004;11(2):104–112.

95. Dowell J, Long J. Conception of the Cognitive Engineering Design Problem. *Ergonomics* 1998;41(2):126–139.

96. Von Hippel E. *Democratizing Innovation*. Cambridge, MA: MIT Press, 2005.

97. Fineberg HV. The Quest for Causality in Health Services Research. In: Sechrest L, Perrin E, Bunker J, Eds. *Research Methodology: Strengthening Causal Interpretation of Nonexperimental Data*. Rockville, MD: Agency for Health Care Policy and Research, 1990:215–220.

98. Lyell DJ. Hypertensive Disorders of Pregnancy: Relevance for the Neonatologist. *NeoReviews* 2004;5(6):e240–e245.

99. Taeusch HW, Ballard RA. *Avery's Diseases of the Newborn*, 7th ed. Philadelphia: W.B. Saunders, 1998.

100. Elwood JM. *Critical Appraisal of Epidemiological Studies and Clinical Trials*, 2nd ed. Oxford: Oxford University Press, 1998.

101. Hennekens CH, Buring JE. *Epidemiology in Medicine*. Boston: Little, Brown and Company, 1987.

102. Rothman KJ, Greenland S. *Modern Epidemiology*, 2nd ed. Philadelphia: Lippincott Williams & Wilkins, 1998.

103. Savitz DA. *Interpreting Epidemiologic Evidence: Strategies for Study Design and Analysis*. New York: Oxford University Press, 2003.

104. Kiely JL. Some Conceptual Problems in Multivariable Analyses of Perinatal Mortality. *Paediatric and Perinatal Epidemiology* 1991;5:243–257.

105. Crombie IK. The Foundations of Research. In: Crombie IK, Ed. *Research in Health Care*. New York: Wiley, 1996.

106. Hills M, De Stavola BL. *A Short Introduction to Stata 8 for Biostatistics*. London: Timberlake Consultants Press, 2003.

107. Hamilton LC. *Statistics with Stata*. Belmont, CA: Duxbury, 2003.

108. UCLA Academic Technology Services. Resources to Help You Learn Stata (http://www.ats.ucla.edu/stat/stata/).

109. Pagano M, Gauvreau K. *Principles of Biostatistics*. Belmont, CA: Duxbury Press, 1993.

110. Rowntree D. *Statistics Without Tears*, Classic edition. Boston, MA: Pearson Education, 2004.

111. Isaac R. *The Pleasures of Probability*. New York: Springer-Verlag, 1995.

112. Maor E. *e: The Story of a Number*. Princeton, NJ: Princeton University Press, 1994.

113. Kirkwood BR, Sterne JAC. *Essential Medical Statistics*, 2nd ed. Oxford, UK: Blackwell, 2003.

114. United States Government Department of Health and Human Services, Office of the Secretary. Standards for Privacy of Individually Identifiable Health Information; Final Rule. Federal Register, National Archives and Records Administration,

Washington, DC, Aug 14, 2002. Available at: http://www.hipaadvisory.com/regs/regs_in_PDF/finalprivmod.pdf (accessed Aug 8, 2005).

115. van Belle G. *Statistical Rules of Thumb*. New York: Wiley-Interscience, 2002.

116. Hulley SB, Cummings SR, Browner WS, *et al. Designing Clinical Research: An Epidemiological Approach,* 2nd ed. Philadelphia: Lippincott Williams & Wilkins, 2001.

117. Upton G, Cook I. *A Dictionary of Statistics*. Oxford: Oxford University Press, 2004.

118. Senn S. *Dicing with Death: Chance, Risk, and Health*. Cambridge, UK: Cambridge University Press, 2003.

119. Abelson RP. *Statistics as Principled Argument*. Hillsdale, NJ: Lawrence Erlbaum Associates, 1995.

120. *The American Heritage College Dictionary*. Boston: Houghton Mifflin Company, 1997.

121. Browner WS. *Publishing and Presenting Clinical Research*. Baltimore, MD: Williams and Wilkins, 1999.

122. Godfrey K. Comparing the Means of Several Groups. *New England Journal of Medicine* 1985;313(23):1450–1456.

123. Godfrey K. Simple Linear Regression in Medical Research. *New England Journal of Medicine* 1985;313(26):1629–1636.

124. Kleinbaum DG. *Logistic Regression*. New York: Springer, 1994.

125. Altman DG, Bland JM. Statistics Notes: Diagnostic tests 3: Receiver Operating Characteristic Plots. *British Medical Journal* 1994;309:188.

126. Sox HCJ, Blatt MA, Higgins MC, et al. *Medical Decision Making*. Boston: Butterworth-Heinemann, 1988.

127. Cleves MA, Gould WW, Gutierrez RG. *An Introduction to Survival Analysis Using Stata*. College Station, TX: Stata Press, 2002.

128. Kleinbaum DG. *Survival Analysis*. New York: Springer, 1996.

129. Katz MH, Hauck WW. Proportional Hazards (Cox) Regression. *Journal of General Internal Medicine* 1993;8:702–711.

130. Stata Corporation. *Stata Survival Analysis and Epidemiological Tables Reference Manual*. Release 8 ed. College Station, TX: Stata Press, 2003.

131. Dallal GE. Collinearity, 2001. Available at: http://www.tufts.edu/~gdallal/collin.htm (accessed Aug 2, 2005).

132. Schulman J. Sorting Out the Ways to Sort Out Fetal Growth. *Journal of Perinatology* 2002;22:339–340.

133. Rogowski JA, Horbar JD, Staiger DO, *et al.* Indirect vs Direct Hospital Quality Indicators for Very Low-Birth-Weight Infants. *Journal of American Medical Association* 2004;291(2):202–209.

134. Norman DA. *Things That Make Us Smart*. Cambridge, MA: Perseus Books, 1993.

Index

Pages numbers in *italic* represent figures, those in **bold** represent tables.